Physiotherapy and Occupational Therapy for People with Cerebral Palsy

Dedication

This book is dedicated to the people with cerebral palsy and their families that we have worked with over the many years who have inspired us and contributed to our learning.

Physiotherapy and Occupational Therapy for People with Cerebral Palsy: A Problem-Based Approach to Assessment and Management

Edited by Karen J Dodd, Christine Imms and Nicholas F Taylor

2010

Mac Keith Press

© 2010 Karen J Dodd, Christine Imms and Nicholas F Taylor

Editor: Hilary M. Hart
Managing Director, Mac Keith Press: Caroline Black
Production Manager: Udoka Ohuonu
Project Manager: Annalisa Welch
Indexer: Dr Laurence Errington

The Editors and publisher would like to thank Oliver Hunter and his family
(Anthony, Frances, Spencer, Harrison, and Felix) for allowing us to use their
photographs on our cover.

First published in this edition 2010 by
Mac Keith Press, 6 Market Road, London N7 9PW, UK

British Library Cataloguing-in-Publication data
A catalogue record of this book is available from the British Library

ISBN: 978-1-898683-68-1

Typeset by Keystroke Typesetting and Graphic Design Ltd,
Tettenhall, Wolverhampton
Printed by Latimer Trend & Company Ltd, Plymouth
Mac Keith Press is supported by Scope

Contents

Contents

Contributors

Helen Bourke-Taylor, Lecturer, School of Occupational Therapy, La Trobe University, Melbourne, Victoria, Australia

Karen Dodd, Associate Dean, Division of Allied Health, School of Physiotherapy, La Trobe University, Melbourne, Victoria, Australia

Josie Duncan, Senior Occupational Therapist, Occupational Therapy Department, The Royal Children's Hospital, Melbourne, Victoria, Australia

Sarah Foley, Senior Clinician, Physiotherapy, Kids Plus Foundation, Geelong, Victoria, Australia

Kerr Graham, Professor of Orthopaedic Surgery, Hugh Williamson Gait Analysis Laboratory, The Royal Children's Hospital, Melbourne, Victoria, Australia

Susan Greaves, Senior Occupational Therapist, Occupational Therapy Department, The Royal Children's Hospital, Melbourne, Victoria, Australia

Adrienne Harvey, Post-Doctoral Fellow, CanChild Centre for Childhood Disability Research, McMaster Child Health Research Institute, Hamilton, Ontario, Canada and the Murdoch Children's Research Institute, Melbourne, Victoria, Australia

Brian Hoare, Senior Occupational Therapist, Victorian Paediatric Rehabilitation Service, Monash Medical Centre, Clayton, Victoria, Australia

Christine Imms, Senior Lecturer, School of Occupational Therapy, La Trobe University, and Senior Occupational Therapist (Research), The Royal Children's Hosptial Research Affiliate, Murdoch Children's Research Institute, Royal Children's Hospital, Melbourne, Victoria, Australia

Contributors

Mary Law, Professor and Associate Dean (Health Sciences) Rehabilitation Science, Co-Founder, CanChild Centre for Childhood Disability Research, McMaster University, Institute of Applied Health Sciences, Hamilton, Ontario, Canada

Margaret Mayston, Senior Teaching Fellow, Department of Neuroscience, Physiology and Pharmacology, Division of Biosciences, University College London, London, UK

Dinah Reddihough, Associate Professor, Developmental Medicine, The Royal Children's Hospital, Melbourne, Victoria, Australia

Barbara Scoullar, Senior Clinician, Occupational Therapy, Young Adult Complex Disability Service, St Vincent's Hospital, Melbourne, Victoria, Australia

Debra Stewart, Assistant Dean, Occupational Therapy Program, School of Rehabilitation Science, McMaster University, Institute of Applied Health Sciences, Hamilton, Ontario, Canada

Nicholas Taylor, Professor of Physiotherapy, School of Physiotherapy, La Trobe University, Melbourne, Victoria, Australia

Pam Thomason, Senior Physiotherapist and Service Manager, Hugh Williamson Gait Analysis Laboratory, The Royal Children's Hospital, Melbourne, Victoria, Australia

Margaret Wallen, Senior Occupational Therapist (Research), Occupational Therapy Department, The Children's Hospital at Westmead, Westmead, New South Wales, Australia

Foreword

This book is a practical guide for physiotherapists and occupational therapists who provide therapy for children and adults with cerebral palsy. As well as being a useful resource for these developmental therapists, the book is also targeted at physiotherapy and occupational therapy students and at people with cerebral palsy and their families and carers. It is also likely to be of interest to other health professionals who support the needs of people with cerebral palsy, such as medical practitioners, nurses, speech therapists, orthotists and dieticians.

Over the past four decades there have been a number of very important developments in the field of neurodisability, many of which inform this book. Furthermore, there is an emerging sense that we are moving beyond the confining notions of 'normal' and 'abnormal' and are ready to think about individual capacity, capability, performance and the factors that promote or inhibit the realization of people's best capacity. This approach is both challenging – each child and family must be considered and engaged as a unique constellation – and liberating, insofar as it allows us to seek and work with the particular characteristics of that specific constellation in a strengths-based approach, and not simply apply formulaic approaches to a 'typical case' of this or that condition, or focus on the deficits.

The editors have drawn on several current ways of thinking about our field to inform their text. These include the application of the Occupational Performance Process Model; a strong emphasis on the concepts and language of the World Health Organization's International Classification of Functioning, Disability and Health; and consistent reference to the application of the principles of a family-centred approach to the provision of services to children and their families. They have encouraged their contributing authors to use a common template to present and discuss the case illustrations that constitute the main body of the book. This structural and conceptual consistency provides the book with a sound architecture, such that after a few chapters the reader can anticipate what is coming, recognize easily the ideas that are being promoted, and begin to think like the authors!

The book is divided into four sections. The first four chapters provide background information about the approach to clinical reasoning that informs the whole text. Their discussion of cerebral palsy includes a focus on family and an overview of therapy. These chapters effectively set up the rest of the text. The five chapters that comprise Part 2 address the preschool years, cross-linking a number of themes about this phase of development and the challenges faced by parents. Each chapter is thoughtfully built around a case illustration to bring to life the concepts that have been introduced, and to provide an approach that it is hoped will prove useful to others. Chapters 10–13 in Part 3 explore issues of importance to children and young people through the school years, including the increasingly recognized complexity associated with transition to adulthood. Importantly for a book about cerebral palsy (often thought of as a 'children's condition') the final three chapters in Part 4 address adult issues.

This book is not meant as a definitive account of all the therapies or schools of thought about 'management' of cerebral palsy. Rather, it has been cleverly structured to present a problem-based approach to address issues across the full range of motor impairments (i.e. all Gross Motor Function Classification System [GMFCS] levels). The ages of the people in the case illustrations range from 6 months to 45 years, and the kinds of challenges they face also vary to cover the broad scope of what professionals might encounter in our practices with people of virtually any age with motor impairments found in the cerebral palsy spectrum. As a result, readers should come away with a sound understanding of approaches to problem-solving with, and on behalf of the children, youth and families with whom we work. In this respect the book is an excellent example of a practical approach to a wide range of complex problems that never have been straightforward, and never will lend themselves to formulaic answers.

When I began my training in developmental disability as a raw paediatric recruit I was very naïve about the nature of the roles, responsibilities and capabilities of my colleagues. I simply had no idea what people like therapists, psychologists and others contributed to the assessment and management of children with disabilities. The truth was, and sadly still is, that as physicians many of us are poorly informed about what therapies colleagues in related disciplines can offer the children and young people with whom we work. In my early training I clearly would have benefited from the content and the approaches that are so well presented in the pages of this excellent book.

Readers are encouraged to share and discuss this book with colleagues and to consider the ways that the ideas herein can be applied to their own settings. If that happens then the authors will have succeeded in their goal of moving the field forward just a bit more.

Peter Rosenbaum
Hamilton, Canada

Chapter 1

Introduction to the clinical reasoning approach of the book

Christine Imms, Karen J Dodd and Nicholas F Taylor

How to use this book

Cerebral palsy is the most common physical disability in childhood (Rosenbaum, 2003). The disturbances that occur in the developing fetal or infant brain with cerebral palsy result in a wide variety of movement disorders that persist from childhood into the adult years. Physiotherapists and occupational therapists play a key role in helping people with cerebral palsy to solve problems with movement and the range of other impairments that so often accompany cerebral palsy, so that they can be more active and better able to participate in roles such as study, work, recreation and relationships. The aim of this book is to provide a practical guide for physiotherapists and occupational therapists who support the needs of people with cerebral palsy but it will also be a useful resource for those with cerebral palsy, their families, carers and teachers. It may also be of interest to physiotherapy and occupational therapy students, and other allied health professionals.

The book includes an introductory background section (Part 1) where key issues in defining and classifying cerebral palsy (Chapter 2), understanding the family's perspective (Chapter 3) and an overview of therapy interventions (Chapter 4) are described and discussed. Parts 2, 3 and 4 (Chapters 5–16) take a case-based approach to managing cerebral palsy across the lifespan and include chapters on the preschool years, the school years, and, finally, the adult years. Each chapter describes a case, and how the physiotherapist or occupational therapist managed that individual's problems. These chapters include the reasoning behind assessment and treatment choices, and describe the interventions and outcomes. This book will not and does not aim to describe the management of every possible problem area associated with cerebral palsy. Rather, it provides in-depth descriptions of common clinical situations that many physiotherapists and occupational therapists who are working with people with cerebral palsy may encounter.

The intervention process model

A key feature of the book is the intervention process model described below and used throughout the case-based chapters in Parts 2, 3 and 4. The model describes the clinical reasoning process that informs assessment, intervention and evaluation. It was adapted from the Occupational Performance Process Model (Canadian Association of Occupational Therapists [CAOT], 2002) to accommodate generic language with which both physiotherapists and occupational therapists are familiar. The eight steps of the intervention process model explicitly describe the clinical reasoning process underlying the interventions described in Parts 2, 3 and 4 of the book (Figure 1.1). The eight steps are as follows.

(1) Initial data collection. The process begins with the referral and includes the early information gathered from the client, family and other sources that begins to contextualize the person and their potential therapy needs.

(2) Identify and prioritize the concerns. This is a client-centred process that identifies, acknowledges and prioritizes the concerns of the client, family and other key individuals.

(3) Identify relevant theory. With initial information gathered and the concerns of the client and others identified, relevant theory is considered to inform and guide the remaining steps in the process.

(4) Assess body function and structure, activity and participation. The therapist identifies the components that facilitate performance as well as those that may contribute to the concerns through appropriate assessment or observation.

(5) Identify contextual factors: environmental and personal. Factors relating to the individual (for example age, sex, temperament) and the environment (for example social, physical, institution supports and barriers) are identified so that they can be considered in relation to implementing a management plan.

(6) Negotiate a management plan. Using the information gained initially, as well as from appropriate assessment, a management plan is negotiated with the client, family and others as required, including, for example, other health professionals, teachers, classroom aides, sports coaches, or recreational leaders or organizations.

(7) Implement the plan. The negotiated treatment plan is implemented. This includes ongoing evaluation of progress and need for adjustment or modification of the plan as required.

(8) Evaluate the outcomes. The final step is a review of the outcomes for the client. This includes whether the concerns were addressed in a manner that suited the individual, and whether the issues were resolved or further intervention is required. In most cases, this step includes some formal re-evaluation to identify how much and what sort of change occurred following intervention. The client is discharged if the issues are resolved to the satisfaction of the client, his/her family and key others. If the issues are not resolved a further round of intervention, beginning at Step 2, may be initiated.

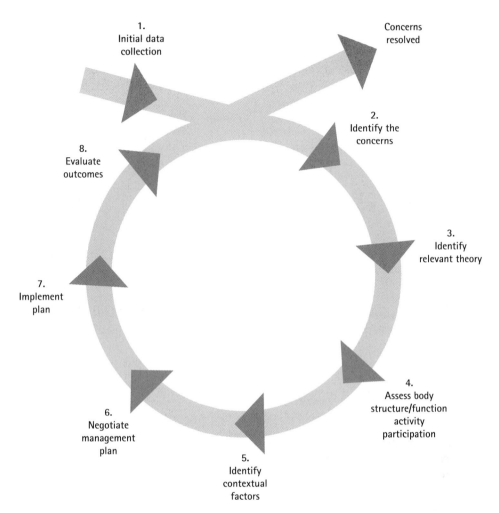

Figure. 1.1 The intervention process: model adapted with permission from the Canadian Occupational Performance Process Model (CAOT, 2002).

International Classification of Functioning, Disability and Health

Another feature of the book is the use of International Classification of Functioning, Disability and Health (ICF, World Health Organization, 2001) as a framework to assist in the clinical reasoning process. Recent international acceptance of the ICF has resulted in a more overt appreciation of the complex interactions between a person, their environment and activities in the presence of a health condition (Figure 1.2).

The ICF defines functioning and disability as umbrella terms that encompass the body functions and structures of people, the activities people do and the life areas in which they participate, taking account of the interactions of these factors with contextual factors (World Health Organization, 2001). In the management of people with cerebral

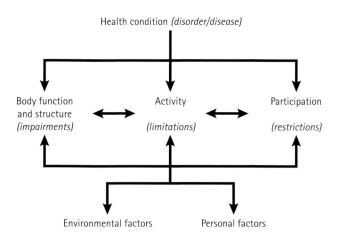

Figure 1.2 The International Classification of Functioning, Disability and Health. Figure used with permission from WHO (2001) International Classification of Functioning, Disability and Health: Short version. Geneva: World Health Organization: 26. Copyright 2001 by the World Health Organization.

palsy, the ICF helps to expand thinking beyond fixing primary impairments of body structure and function, by acknowledging that the relationships between the components that affect functioning are complex and non-linear. The ICF therefore highlights the importance of promoting the person's full participation in all aspects of functioning and life (Rosenbaum and Stewart, 2004). The recognition of the role of contextual factors is also very applicable in the management of people with cerebral palsy, particularly in acknowledging the important contribution of the family environment to the person's health and well-being (Rosenbaum and Stewart 2004).

As well as providing a broad conceptual framework to understand the health condition of cerebral palsy, the ICF can also be a useful practical guide for parents and therapists when determining priorities for assessment and treatment. Throughout the clinical cases described in Parts 2, 3 and 4 of the book, assessments are organized according to the ICF components (step 4 of the intervention process model), and include sections where contextual factors are considered (step 5 in the model). Descriptions of the more commonly used assessments in this book can be found in the Appendix.

The ICF is also considered when devising and implementing the management plans in Parts 2, 3 and 4 of the book (steps 6 and 7 of the intervention process model), as the parents and therapist decide where intervention is best targeted to improve functioning: that is, if the intervention should be primarily directed at reducing impairments, improving activity or increasing life participation.

A family-centred approach to therapy
Throughout this book an emphasis has also been placed on implementing a family-centred approach to therapy. Gaining the confidence and trust of the child's family and other key support people is critical to the success of therapy for children and young people with cerebral palsy. It is important for therapists to understand the fundamental need to be sensitive to and respectful of the family culture and to work closely as a team

with the family and significant support people (e.g. daycare staff, teachers, support workers) to successfully support the individual. Therapy directed at technical and short-term rehabilitation interventions that focus only on the individual with cerebral palsy is rarely successful. Rather, success comes from using a family-centred approach that includes families in decision-making, and recognizes the importance of acknowledging the family environment and making all reasonable accommodations to suit the family when providing services. Chapter 3 summarizes some of the important things that therapists can do when working with young people with cerebral palsy.

Multidisciplinary practice models

Another underlying principle in this book is that of multidisciplinary team work. The problems and issues faced by people with cerebral palsy are not confined to physical impairments that impact on the individual alone. Rather a diagnosis of cerebral palsy can bring with it a range of physical, sensory, psychological, as well as social-emotional issues that cannot effectively be managed in isolation from each other. No one discipline can individually manage all of the concerns, but working together the multidisciplinary team can provide better outcomes.

The multidisciplinary health care team is a group of professionals with diverse training and backgrounds who can work together in a coordinated and collaborative way. Team members collaborate to solve client problems that are too complex to be solved by one discipline. To provide care as efficiently as possible, the team creates 'formal' and 'informal' structures that encourage collaborative problem-solving. Team members work interdependently to define and help clients solve problems, and learn to accept and capitalize on disciplinary differences and overlapping roles (Drinka and Clark, 2000). For these reasons, practice models that include a range of individuals from different health disciplines can more effectively and efficiently support the needs of people with cerebral palsy and their families.

Concluding remarks

The key themes emphasized throughout the book are the use of the clinical reasoning approach of the intervention process model, the use of the ICF as a framework to help therapists inform child and parent decision-making about priorities of assessment and treatment, the use of family-centred approaches in developing and implementing therapeutic strategies and the use of multidisciplinary team work. We do not expect that therapists will read the book from cover to cover. Instead we expect that the reader will start by looking at one of the case-based chapters that is most pertinent to them in terms of the areas of their particular clinical roles and responsibilities. If an element of the background or theory in the case-based chapter needs further explanation, the therapist can refer back to the relevant section or chapter in Part 1, or for more detail about a particular assessment to the Appendix. We hope that this book will provide a clinically relevant resource for therapists.

References

Canadian Association of Occupational Therapists (CAOT) (2002) *Enabling Occupation: An Occupational Therapy Perspective.* Ottawa: Canadian Association of Occupational Therapists.

Drinka TJK & Clark PG (2000) *Health Care Teamwork: Interdisciplinary Practice & Teaching.* Westport, CT: Greenwood Publishing Group.

Rosenbaum P (2003) Cerebral palsy: what parents and doctors want to know. *BMJ,* 326, 970–4.

Rosenbaum P & Stewart D (2004) The World Health Organization International Classification of Functioning, Disability, and Health: a model to guide clinical thinking, practice and research in cerebral palsy. *Seminars in Pediatric Neurology,* 11, 5–10.

World Health Organization (2001) *International Classification of Functioning, Disability and Health. Short Version.* Geneva: WHO.

Chapter 2

What is cerebral palsy?

Christine Imms and Karen J Dodd

Cerebral palsy has been defined as

> *a group of permanent disorders of the development of movement and posture, causing activity limitation[s] that are attributed to non-progressive disturbances that occurred in the developing fetal or infant brain. The motor disorders of cerebral palsy are often accompanied by disturbances of sensation, perception, cognition, communication and behaviour, by epilepsy and by secondary musculoskeletal problems.*
>
> *(Rosenbaum et al, 2007a: p. 9)*

As this definition suggests, cerebral palsy is a potentially complex condition. The impact of cerebral palsy on individuals varies widely, from someone who cannot mobilize independently, has little communication and has associated impairments such as epilepsy and severe intellectual impairment, to someone who has a very mild impairment of motor control that might lead to one foot dragging when the individual is tired or unwell but who has no other impairments. As a result of this variability in presentation, the focus and role of physiotherapy and occupational therapy vary widely for different individuals.

In this chapter, we describe the impact that cerebral palsy can have on the body, and on the activities and participation of individuals. In addition, we present briefly what is known about how environmental and personal factors affect outcomes for people with cerebral palsy, along with a description of procedures used to identify individuals at particular risk for associated impairments or conditions that have an impact on the long-term health and well-being of people with cerebral palsy. This information provides background to each of the subsequent chapters.

Cerebral palsy as a health condition

Cerebral palsy affects about 1 in every 400 children born or 2–2.5 children per 1000 live births (Blair and Stanley, 1997; Odding et al, 2006; Westbom et al, 2007). More males than females are affected in a ratio of 1.3:1 (Blair and Stanley, 1997). However, the prevalence of cerebral palsy varies according to birthweight, with approximately 50% of all children with cerebral palsy being of low birthweight (<2500 grams) (Pharoah et al, 1996).

As children can present with different forms of cerebral palsy we require descriptive classifications that include several components. By consensus (Rosenbaum et al, 2007a) these components have been identified as (1) motor abnormalities, (2) anatomical and neuroimaging findings, (3) associated impairments, and (4) causation and timing of the neural injury.

Motor abnormalities

The primary motor disorder of cerebral palsy is described in terms of the nature of the movement disorder and the resultant level of motor function. This includes identifying the presence of abnormal muscle tone and specific movement disorders. Muscle tone, whether it be high, low or normal, is 'the sensation of resistance that is encountered as a joint is passively moved through a range of motion' (Lance and McLeod, 1981: p. 128). When a joint is moved passively through range the muscles are usually electrically silent, but resistance is felt because of the inertia of the limb and the compliance of the soft tissues (Katz and Rymer, 1989).

Spasticity

Spasticity is present in 75 to 88% of people with cerebral palsy (Blair and Stanley, 1997; Odding et al, 2006; Westbom et al, 2007; Krägeloh-Mann and Cans, 2009). Spasticity is one component of the upper motor neurone syndrome, and it is this damage to the central nervous system corticospinal (pyramidal) tract function, rather than spasticity per se, that is the cause of motor problems in people with cerebral palsy. Spasticity is 'characterised by a velocity-dependent increase in tonic stretch reflexes (muscle tone) with exaggerated tendon jerks (phasic stretch reflex), resulting from hyper-excitability of the stretch reflex' (Lance, 1980: p. 485). Spasticity therefore is present when the resistance to movement increases with increasing speed and when the resistance to movement differs with varying direction of joint movement (e.g. differs with flexion versus extension of a joint) (Sanger et al, 2003). In addition, spasticity is present when the resistance increases rapidly after a threshold of movement is reached – that is after the 'catch' is felt (Sanger et al, 2003).

Chronic spasticity can lead to changes in the properties of soft tissues. Muscle stiffness, contracture, atrophy and fibrosis may interact with spasticity to produce 'hypertonia', which is the term often used to refer to the excessive resistance felt when the joints of people with neurological disorders such as cerebral palsy are moved passively. In clinical practice, it is important to distinguish between resistance due to spasticity and that due to changes to soft tissues, because the distinction has therapeutic implications in terms of the effectiveness of different therapeutic interventions. For example, anti-spasticity agents such as botulinum toxin A are only useful for true spasticity and not muscle contracture, whereas muscle lengthening procedures such as surgery are more effective if the person has muscle contractures or stiffness.

Dyskinesia
Dyskinetic (dystonia or choreo-athetosis) cerebral palsy occurs in around 15% of people with cerebral palsy (Odding et al, 2006; Himmelmann et al, 2007; Westbom et al, 2007). Dystonia is characterized by 'involuntary sustained or intermittent muscle contractions causing twisting and repetitive movements, abnormal postures or both' (Sanger et al, 2003: p. e92). Dystonia is distinguished from spasticity by the fact that it can be triggered by voluntary activity, tasks or emotional states but it is not influenced by the velocity at which the limb is moved (Sanger et al, 2003). Choreo-athetosis is characterized by hyperkinesia (i.e. increased activity) and hypotonia (Surveillance of Cerebral Palsy in Europe [SCPE], 2000). The involuntary, slow, writhing, muscle tone fluctuations seen in dyskinetic cerebral palsy generally affect the hands, arms, feet or legs, but can affect the entire body, resulting in difficulties with maintaining an upright posture, or with sitting or walking. Dyskinesia can cause a person to appear restless, only being still when fully relaxed or asleep.

These involuntary fluctuations of muscle tone can also make it difficult for people with dyskinesia to hold and manipulate objects in their hands and to use their hands to carry out otherwise simple acts like rubbing their face or feeding themselves. Uncontrolled movement is also common in the face. This can severely affect speech, a condition called dysarthia. Some degree of dysarthria is common because of the individual's difficulty coordinating the actions of the tongue and pharynx during breathing and speaking. Oral dyskinesia can also result in difficulties with eating and drooling.

Ataxia
Ataxia is a feature of central nervous system (CNS) extrapyramidal motor dysfunction, particularly cerebellar abnormality, and is present in around 4% of people with cerebral palsy (Bax et al, 2006; Odding et al, 2006; Westbom et al, 2007). Ataxia is defined as an 'inability to activate the correct pattern of muscles during movement' (Sanger et al, 2006: p. 2160) resulting in an abnormal trajectory of movement and inaccurate limb placement.

Children with ataxia often present as infants with hypotonia. Their voluntary movements can be affected by gross intentional tremors and most commonly a lack of postural stability. Ataxia can be present in the trunk or limbs and affect the individual's gait. Difficulties with judging speed, distance and power of hand movements affect precise upper limb activities such as holding a pen or pencil for writing, or tying a shoe lace (Bax and Brown, 2004; Sanger et al, 2006).

Hypotonia

Hypotonia (low muscle tone) is more common in young children, and particularly in children with quadriplegic cerebral palsy who often begin life with a significant amount of hypotonia in their trunk and their limbs. Population prevalence overall is reported as relatively low at around 1% (Blair and Stanley, 1997) although more recent reports indicate that 'pure hypotonia is not a feature of cerebral palsy' (Krägeloh-Mann and Cans, 2009: p. 2). Like those with hypertonia, people with hypotonia have a reduced ability to respond to movement demands.

Mixed presentation

More than one type of motor disorder can be present in an individual, with spasticity most often occurring in combination with other types of motor disorders. A useful classification tree for identifying subtypes of cerebral palsy has been developed by the Surveillance of Cerebral Palsy in Europe register (Surveillance of Cerebral Palsy in Europe [SCPE], 2000: p. 821). This simple decision tree provides clinicians with a hierarchical pathway of questions that enables them to classify the subtype of cerebral palsy (i.e. spastic bilateral cerebral palsy, spastic unilateral cerebral palsy, ataxic cerebral palsy, dyskinetic cerebral palsy) present in individuals with cerebral palsy.

Classification of dysfunction

By definition, all people with cerebral palsy have impaired motor function of CNS origin. The severity of this dysfunction can be classified using the Gross Motor Function Classification System (GMFCS, Palisano et al, 1997, 2008) and the Manual Ability Classification System (MACS, Eliasson et al, 2006). In addition, a five-level Communication Function Classification System is currently being developed (Hidecker et al, 2008; Rosenbaum et al, 2008). This tool classifies the individual's ability to send and receive communications. At present the reported prevalence of communication disorders in cerebral palsy varies greatly because there is no established method for classifying communication function (Hidecker et al, 2008).

The Gross Motor Function Classification System

The GMFCS classifies a person's ability to self-initiate movements related to sitting and walking. Typical performance rather than maximal performance is rated using a five-level scale. Specific criteria vary for each of the following five age groups: before the second birthday; between the second and fourth birthday; between the fourth and sixth birthday; between the sixth and twelfth birthday; and between the twelfth and eighteenth birthday. Figure 2.1 summarizes the five levels for children aged 6 to 12 years, and Figure 2.2 summarizes the levels for youth aged 12–18 years. The GMFCS has undergone continued psychometric development since its publication in 1997, and the revised version (Palisano et al, 2008) is available at http://motorgrowth.can child.ca/en/GMFCS/resources/GMFCS-ER.pdf.

A growing body of literature supports the soundness of the psychometric properties and the utility of the GMFCS in describing levels of severity of gross motor limitations in

GMFCS E & R between 6th and 12th birthday: Descriptors and illustrations

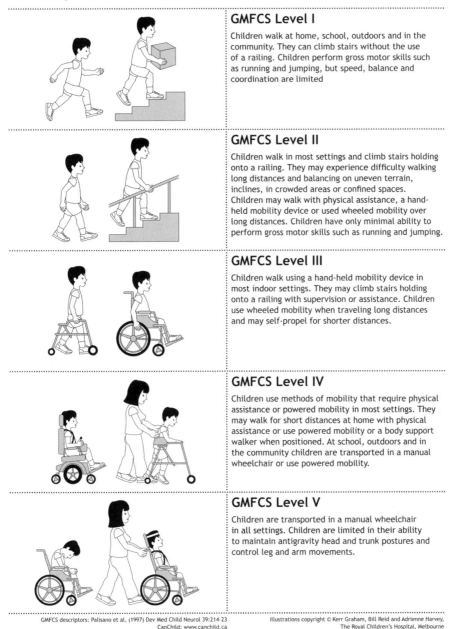

GMFCS Level I

Children walk at home, school, outdoors and in the community. They can climb stairs without the use of a railing. Children perform gross motor skills such as running and jumping, but speed, balance and coordination are limited

GMFCS Level II

Children walk in most settings and climb stairs holding onto a railing. They may experience difficulty walking long distances and balancing on uneven terrain, inclines, in crowded areas or confined spaces. Children may walk with physical assistance, a hand-held mobility device or used wheeled mobility over long distances. Children have only minimal ability to perform gross motor skills such as running and jumping.

GMFCS Level III

Children walk using a hand-held mobility device in most indoor settings. They may climb stairs holding onto a railing with supervision or assistance. Children use wheeled mobility when traveling long distances and may self-propel for shorter distances.

GMFCS Level IV

Children use methods of mobility that require physical assistance or powered mobility in most settings. They may walk for short distances at home with physical assistance or use powered mobility or a body support walker when positioned. At school, outdoors and in the community children are transported in a manual wheelchair or use powered mobility.

GMFCS Level V

Children are transported in a manual wheelchair in all settings. Children are limited in their ability to maintain antigravity head and trunk postures and control leg and arm movements.

GMFCS descriptors: Palisano et al. (1997) Dev Med Child Neurol 39:214-23
CanChild: www.canchild.ca

Illustrations copyright © Kerr Graham, Bill Reid and Adrienne Harvey,
The Royal Children's Hospital, Melbourne

Figure 2.1 The five levels of the Gross Motor Function Classification System for children aged 6 to 12 years of age. Figure used with permission from Peter Rosenbaum, CanChild and Kerr Graham, Bill Reid & Adrienne Harvey, Royal Children's Hospital, Melbourne.

GMFCS E & R between 12th and 18th birthday: Descriptors and illustrations

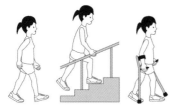

GMFCS Level I

Youth walk at home, school, outdoors and in the community. Youth are able to climb curbs and stairs without physical assistance or a railing. They perform gross motor skills such as running and jumping but speed, balance and coordination are limited.

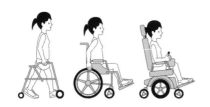

GMFCS Level II

Youth walk in most settings but environmental factors and personal choice influence mobility choices. At school or work they may require a hand held mobility device for safety and climb stairs holding onto a railing. Outdoors and in the community youth may use wheeled mobility when traveling long distances.

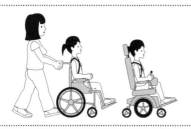

GMFCS Level III

Youth are capable of walking using a hand-held mobility device. Youth may climb stairs holding onto a railing with supervision or assistance. At school they may self-propel a manual wheelchair or use powered mobility. Outdoors and in the community youth are transported in a wheelchair or use powered mobility.

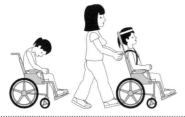

GMFCS Level IV

Youth use wheeled mobility in most settings. Physical assistance of 1-2 people is required for transfers. Indoors, youth may walk short distances with physical assistance, use wheeled mobility or a body support walker when positioned. They may operate a powered chair, otherwise are transported in a manual wheelchair.

GMFCS Level V

Youth are transported in a manual wheelchair in all settings. Youth are limited in their ability to maintain antigravity head and trunk postures and control leg and arm movements. Self-mobility is severely limited, even with the use of assistive technology.

GMFCS descriptors: Palisano et al. (1997) Dev Med Child Neurol 39:214-23
CanChild: www.canchild.ca

Illustrations copyright © Kerr Graham, Bill Reid and Adrienne Harvey,
The Royal Children's Hospital, Melbourne

Figure 2.2 Gross Motor Function Classification System (GMFCS) levels for young people aged 12–18 years. Figure used with permission from Peter Rosenbaum, CanChild and Kerr Graham, Bill Reid & Adrienne Harvey, Royal Children's Hospital, Melbourne.

children with cerebral palsy (for example, Rosenbaum et al, 1996; Palisano et al, 1997; Görter et al, 2004). The tool has

- high inter-rater reliability between parent and clinician scorings (intraclass correlation coefficients [ICCs]: 0.92–0.97) (Morris et al, 2004);
- high inter-rater reliability between adults with cerebral palsy who rate their own level and a therapist rating (ICC: 0.93, 95% confidence interval [CI]: 0.89–0.96) (Jahnsen et al, 2006).

The GMFCS promotes communication between clinicians about a child's gross motor function, and this facilitates referrals and reciprocal information sharing between professionals within health, education and community settings.

THE MANUAL ABILITY CLASSIFICATION SYSTEM

The Manual Ability Classification System (MACS) classifies the child's ability to handle objects in important daily activities, for example during play and leisure, eating and dressing (Eliasson et al, 2006). Classification can be determined by asking the parents or someone else familiar with the child. The child's ability is classified into one of five levels reflecting the child's typical manual performance, not maximal capacity (see Figure 2.3). Manual Ability Classification System rating forms are available in 16 languages at www.macs.nu.

As with the GMFCS the MACS does not attempt to classify the reason why a person has a certain level of manual ability. The ability to use the hands to achieve the tasks of everyday life is influenced by many factors including motor, sensory, cognitive and affective (Eliasson, 2005). If each factor is measured, knowledge is gained about the components themselves, but not about how they inter-relate; for example, how one child can compensate for poor sensation by using their vision and another, despite good motor function, cannot achieve this because of poor cognition. The MACS pulls all aspects of hand function together into a unified, holistic descriptive of ability, making it a useful classification tool.

- The MACS has demonstrated evidence of validity for children with cerebral palsy aged 4–18 years (Eliasson et al, 2006).
- Inter-rater reliability between two therapist raters was 0.97 (ICC, 95% CI: 0.96–0.98) in 74 children aged 5–18 years (Eliasson et al, 2006).
- Inter-rater reliability between therapists and parents was 0.96 (ICC, 95% CI: 0.89–0.98) in 25 children aged 8 to 12 years (Eliasson et al, 2006).
- Stability of caregiver ratings over 12 months was high with an ICC of 0.92 (95% CI 0.87–0.95) and it is recommended that caregivers be given the MACS rating scale in their native language (Imms et al, 2009).

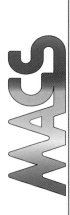

MACS

What do you need to know to use MACS?

The child's ability to handle objects in important daily activities, for example during play and leisure, eating and dressing.

In which situation is the child independent and to what extent do they need support and adaptation?

I. **Handles objects easily and successfully.** At most, limitations in the ease of performing manual tasks requiring speed and accuracy. However, any limitations in manual abilities do not restrict independence in daily activities.

II. **Handles most objects but with somewhat reduced quality and/or speed of achievement.** Certain activities may be avoided or be achieved with some difficulty; alternative ways of performance might be used but manual abilities do not usually restrict independence in daily activities.

III. **Handles objects with difficulty; needs help to prepare and/or modify activities.** The performance is slow and achieved with limited success regarding quality and quantity. Activities are performed independently if they have been set up or adapted.

IV. **Handles a limited selection of easily managed objects in adapted situations.** Performs parts of activities with effort and with limited success. Requires continuous support and assistance and/or adapted equipment, for even partial achievement of the activity.

V. **Does not handle objects and has severely limited ability to perform even simple actions.** Requires total assistance.

Distinctions between Levels I and II

Children in Level I may have limitations in handling very small, heavy or fragile objects which demand detailed fine motor control, or efficient coordination between hands. Limitations may also involve performance in new and unfamiliar situations. Children in Level II perform almost the same activities as children in Level I but the quality of performance is decreased, or the performance is slower. Functional differences between hands can limit effectiveness of performance. Children in Level II commonly try to simplify handling of objects, for example by using a surface for support instead of handling objects with both hands.

Distinctions between Levels II and III

Children in Level II handle most objects, although slowly or with reduced quality of performance. Children in Level III commonly need help to prepare the activity and/or require adjustments to be made to the environment since their ability to reach or handle objects is limited. They cannot perform certain activities and their degree of independence is related to the supportiveness of the environmental context.

Distinctions between Levels III and IV

Children in Level III can perform selected activities if the situation is prearranged and if they get supervision and plenty of time. Children in Level IV need continuous help during the activity and can at best participate meaningfully in only parts of an activity.

Distinctions between Levels IV and V

Children in Level IV perform part of an activity, however, they need help continuously. Children in Level V might at best participate with a simple movement in special situations, e.g. by pushing a simple button.

Figure 2.3 The Manual Ability Classification System (MACS) validated for children and youth aged 4–18 years. Figure used with permission from Ann–Christin Eliasson, copyright Marianne Arner, Eva Beckung, Ann–Christin Eliasson, Lena Krumlinde-Sundholm, Peter Rosenbaum & Birgit Roseblad, 2005.

Anatomical and neuroimaging findings

Anatomical (or topographical) distribution identifies the body parts affected by the motor disorder including limb distribution (unilateral or bilateral involvement), trunk and oropharynx. People with dystonia and ataxia tend to have whole body involvement (Bax and Brown, 2004). For people with predominantly spastic cerebral palsy:

- 35% have hemiplegia;
- 28% have diplegia;
- 37% have quadriplegia (Howard et al, 2005).

These proportions vary according to birthweight; more children with extremely low birthweight (<1000 g) experience hemiplegia or quadriplegia, and those of low birthweight (1500–2499 g) are more likely to have diplegia (Jessen et al, 1999).

The terms *hemiplegia* (one side of the body), *diplegia* (only the lower limbs are affected or, as more usually seen, the whole body is involved but the lower limbs are more affected than upper limbs) and *quadriplegia* (all four limbs are affected) are commonly used clinical descriptors of the topographical distribution. Although these terms appear clinically meaningful, there has not been international consensus on the definition of terms (Rosenbaum et al, 2007a). More recently it has been recommended that rather than using the terms hemiplegia, diplegia and quadriplegia, the descriptions unilateral or bilateral distribution be used (Rosenbaum et al, 2007a). The Surveillance of Cerebral Palsy in Europe (SCPE) group report a prevalence of 58% bilateral spastic cerebral palsy and 30% unilateral cerebral palsy (Krägeloh-Mann and Cans, 2009). Because of variations in definitions, it is important to articulate clearly what is meant by terms used in communications.

Neuroimaging findings

Although cerebral palsy is usually diagnosed by excluding all other likely causes for the clinical presentation of individuals, magnetic resonance imaging (MRI) and computed tomography (CT) are being used to identify the site and extent of neural lesions and to further our understanding of the aetiology of the condition (Korzeniewski et al, 2008). Approximately 85% of children will have abnormal MRI or CT findings, with over half of these children having periventricular white matter injuries (Krägeloh-Mann et al, 2007). Variations in brain lesions are associated with the timing of the insult and related to the clinical presentation in terms of severity and associated impairments (Krägeloh-Mann and Cans, 2009). Neuroimaging techniques are advancing and it is recommended that all children with cerebral palsy be investigated where possible (Rosenbaum et al, 2007a).

Associated impairments

Associated impairments are common and therapists therefore must consider how they might affect performance and ensure that children are referred to appropriate professionals for thorough assessment and management.

- Epilepsy occurs in up to a third of children with cerebral palsy. The incidence is highest in those with spastic quadriplegia (Carlsson et al, 2003; Venkateswaran and Shevell, 2008), in those with dyskinetic cerebral palsy (Himmelmann et al, 2007) and with severe intellectual impairment (Carlsson et al, 2003). Seizure types vary and include generalized tonic–clonic, simple or complex partial seizures and many individuals will have more than one type (Carlsson et al, 2003).

- Cognitive impairments are common although reported incidence varies between studies because of differing definitions. Carlsson et al (2003) report the incidence of intellectual impairment as around 45%, with 25% classified as severe (IQ <50 assessed on the Griffiths scale at 4 years of age). The SCPE group report frequencies ranging from 23 to 44% with any learning disability (IQ <70), and with severe disability (IQ <50) of 30 to 41% (SCPE, 2000).

- Behavioural and psychosocial problems are more common in children with cerebral palsy (25%) than children with other chronic conditions (12%) and those in the general population (5%) (McDermott et al, 1996).

- Although severe visual impairments are reported in 10–12% of children, up to 70% have visual acuity problems (Reid et al, 2005; Odding et al, 2006; Krägeloh-Mann and Cans, 2009).

- Hearing impairment is much less common, occurring in less than 8% (Reid et al, 2005; Odding et al, 2006; Surman et al, 2006).

- Tactile sensation, proprioception, two-point discrimination and haptic perception are impaired in up to 50% of children with cerebral palsy (Odding et al, 2006).

- A range of problems with motor control can occur including muscle incoordination, which can lead to muscle weakness, stereotyped and restricted patterns of movement, slow initiation of voluntary movement, as well as sudden and involuntary muscle activity

- There is a high risk of secondary musculoskeletal impairments related to muscle and tendon shortening that may result in soft tissue or bony contractures and/or joint subluxation or dislocation, which in turn can lead to abnormal alignment of body parts.

  - A study of 212 children with cerebral palsy followed from 9 to 16 years of age reported that 0% of children with pure ataxia experience hip displacement, whereas almost 80% of children with bilateral symmetrical spasticity (quadriplegia) have some degree of hip displacement (Hägglund et al, 2007).

  - Children with the spastic motor type are at particular risk of contractures of the muscles of the spine and the lower extremities, including equinus deformity of the foot, knee and hip flexion contractures, or in severe cases 'windswept hips' with abduction, semi-flexion and external rotation of one hip and adduction, semi-flexion and internal rotation of the other. In the upper extremity, thumb-in-palm, swan-neck deformities of the fingers, wrist flexion, ulna deviation, forearm pronation, elbow flexion and internal rotation and adduction of the shoulder are common (Johnstone et al, 2003).

Throughout the case-based chapters in Parts 2, 3 and 4 of this book, we have added a snapshot of associated impairments reported for individuals within each of the five GMFCS levels. The data reported in these snapshots are from a variety of sources (Liptak et al, 2001; Nordmark et al, 2001; Palisano et al, 2003, Vargus-Adams, 2005; Himmelmann et al, 2006; Soo et al, 2006; Hägglund et al, 2007; Westbom et al, 2007 Knox, 2008). The snapshots are intended to provide some indication of the likelihood that an individual seen in clinical practice who is similar to those described in the cases will present with associated impairments.

Causation and timing
The exact cause and timing of the neural injury that results in cerebral palsy can be difficult to ascertain (Koman et al, 2004) and remains unknown for most individuals. The multitude of potential pathways to cerebral palsy (Stanley et al, 2000) goes some way to explaining the variability of neural insult and presentation of motor type and distribution as well as associated comorbidities in the condition. Events on the causal pathway to cerebral palsy include congenital brain malformations, vascular events such as arterial blockage, maternal infections, hypoxia during delivery, neonatal encephalopathy, acquired brain injury early in life and infection (Reddihough and Collins, 2003). In addition, there are factors that increase the risk of cerebral palsy, the most important of which have been identified as intrauterine infection, preterm birth and multiple births (Odding et al, 2006). Recent reviews have also highlighted the growing evidence of genetic pathways that may predispose to events that cause cerebral palsy (Keogh and Badawi, 2006; Schaefer, 2008). Proportions of cases attributed to prenatal, labour and delivery or postnatal events have been reported as approximately 75% (Reddihough and Collins, 2003), 6–9% (Reddihough and Collins, 2003; Odding et al, 2006) and 8–10% (Brown, 2003; Reid et al, 2006; Surman et al, 2006), respectively.

Outcomes of cerebral palsy
Once a diagnosis of cerebral palsy has been established and discussed with the parents, the parents want information about likely long-term outcomes (Rosenbaum, 2003). In terms of overall survival, the children born with cerebral palsy between 1956 and 1994 in Western Australia had an overall mortality rate of 6% before 5 years of age, and 11% between 5 and 40 years (Blair et al, 2001: p. 511). Respiratory illness was the most common cause of death, and those who had severe cerebral palsy plus an intellectual disability were the most likely to die in childhood. Overall longevity for today's children is unknown, but one UK study reported 85% survival to 50 years of age, compared with 96% in the general population in a cohort born between 1940 and 1950 (Hemming et al, 2006). Children with cerebral palsy in GMFCS levels III–V have reduced growth in comparison to peers without impairment, and smaller children with cerebral palsy had poorer outcomes in terms of school days missed and limitations in participation in usual activities (Samson-Fang et al, 2002; Stevenson et al, 2006).

The GMFCS has been shown to predict outcomes related to sitting and walking (Rosenbaum, 2003). Data suggest that by 3 years of age, children in level V will have achieved 90% of their gross motor skills and will on average achieve a score on the Gross Motor Function Measure of around 20. Children in level I take longer to achieve 90% of their gross motor skills (by age 5) and achieve many more skills, with an average Gross Motor Function Measure–66 score of just under 90 (out of 100). Less is known about the development of manual ability in children with cerebral palsy. One preliminary study using the MACS and data from the Assisting Hand Assessment (AHA – see Appendix, p. 291 for brief description) demonstrated distinctions between the MACS levels in the development of use of the assisting hand in children with hemiplegia in performance of bimanual skills (Holmefur et al, 2009). This study was limited by the selection of children for whom the AHA is appropriate, and thus exluded children with bilateral impairments and those in MACS levels IV and V. In this study rapid development is seen in the first 3 years of life for most children followed by a slowing trajectory of change. Children with greater impairments (i.e. MACS level III) achieve less and have a longer, slower rate of achievement in comparison to those with less impairment (i.e. MACS levels I and II) (Holmefur et al, 2009).

Outcomes in terms of well-being and quality of life are also critical. Studies have consistently found strong relationships between severity of functional impairment as measured by the GMFCS and health-related quality of life components, such as mobility and physical function (Kennes et al, 2002; Vargus-Adams, 2005; Rosenbaum et al, 2007b). However, there appeared to be little relationship between severity of impairments and physical functioning and many psychosocial domains of health-related quality of life (Kennes et al, 2002; Livingston et al, 2007; Majnemer et al, 2007; Rosenbaum et al, 2007b). In comparison with normative data, however, children with cerebral palsy have reduced health-related quality of life (Wake et al, 2003; Vargus-Adams, 2005).

It is important to make a distinction between measures of health-related quality of life and the individual's personal valuation of their life quality. Measures of health-related quality of life focus on functional attributes. A personal valuation of life quality may not. Two recent studies that used instruments that defined and measured the subjective aspects of quality of life found that children with cerebral palsy report their life quality to be similar to that of non-disabled peers (Dickinson et al, 2007) and that quality of life defined in this way is a separate dimension to that of health-related quality of life (Rosenbaum et al, 2007b). These recent findings support those of previous studies that found high levels of well-being in children and adolescents with disability (Kennes et al, 2002; Jemtå et al, 2005) although, as children become older, their perceived well-being is reduced (Jemtå et al, 2005). Capturing subjective well-being as distinct from health and function is important because older adolescents define success in life in terms of being happy, which includes being believed in by others, believing in oneself and being accepted (King et al, 2000).

Transition to adulthood is a critical phase of development. Although most individuals with cerebral palsy live to adulthood, outcomes for adults with cerebral palsy have been reported in terms of decreasing social interaction and activity, increasing isolation (Stevenson et al, 1997; Ng et al, 2003), reductions in access to health care despite no reduction in need (Stevenson et al, 1997; Stewart et al, 2001; Ng et al, 2003; Hilberink et al, 2007) and limited access to employment and leisure opportunities (Morris, 1999; Hilberink et al, 2007). Jahnsen and colleagues' (2002) study of the coping potential of adults with cerebral palsy found that they 'experience life as less manageable and meaningful and . . . more unpredictable and incomprehensible than the general population' (p. 517). Supporting and advocating for families as they negotiate transitions to and from health, education and community services provides an opportunity for youth to learn strategies and skills they can use as they transition into adulthood.

Effect of environmental and personal factors
The effect that cerebral palsy has on people is explained not only by the severity of their impairments. In addition, environmental factors extrinsic to the individual such as the physical and material features of the environment, formal and informal social structures as well as services and systems in the community may influence an individual's experience of cerebral palsy. The individual's personal characteristics such as their personality, age, sex, ethnic group, fitness, habits, education and social background also interact with the health condition and environment to affect the level and extent of functioning for an individual. For example, different environments may differentially affect the ability of the same individual to perform successfully or participate in an activity. Similarly, two people might have severe impairment and yet one person's level of fitness may be better than the other's, which may positively affect their ability to perform a physical activity. For these reasons, it is important for therapists to consider environmental and personal factors when working with people with cerebral palsy.

Identification of individuals at risk
This section highlights specific areas in which early identification of difficulties or ongoing monitoring of those at particular risk for poor outcomes is recommended. Earlier in this chapter we highlighted the numerous impairments that may be associated with cerebral palsy, and therapists should be aware of the potential need for further screening or assessment in relation to these conditions. For example the high incidence of visual impairment and increased risk of hearing impairments (Reid et al, 2005; Odding et al, 2006) emphasises the need for early screening for these impairments in all children with cerebral palsy.

Early identification (by Dinah Reddihough)
Early identification of cerebral palsy in infants is important. It allows a therapy programme to be started as early as possible in life, and this is crucial for families who are likely to be aware that there is some concern about development.

Clinicians should be particularly vigilant in their monitoring of infants known to be at risk of cerebral palsy, for example, those who have been born extremely preterm and those with a history of neonatal encephalopathy. With increasing use of brain MRI early in life, lesions likely to result in cerebral palsy are often identified, for example, periventricular white matter injury (Woodward et al, 2006).

The diagnosis of cerebral palsy is not always easy. Neurological signs may develop over the first year of life, and conversely, abnormal signs may disappear during this time (Nelson and Ellenberg, 1982). Involuntary movements such as dystonia only appear towards the end of the first or during the second year of life. This is a difficult time for families, who are understandably anxious to know whether their child has cerebral palsy. Multidisciplinary assessment is usually helpful and a period of observation is frequently necessary, especially if there are concerns about the functional well-being of the infant (whether or not they are eventually diagnosed as having cerebral palsy).

Children with cerebral palsy often present with delayed motor milestones, for example, delays in gaining head control and in learning to sit, stand or walk. However, there may be other more non-specific features including feeding problems or irritability. These symptoms should be treated with caution, as there are many causes other than cerebral palsy that may be responsible for them.

Very early physical signs may include hypotonia, sometimes hypertonia (although this is unusual very early unless the motor deficit is severe) and retained primitive reflexes such as the stepping and walking reflexes after the first few months of life. Development of uneven asymmetrical patterns, for example, strong preference for one hand for reaching and grasping in the early months of life, may point to motor problems in the other arm and hand. Hemiplegia may present in this way and the observer may notice intermittent or constant fisting in the involved hand. Similarly, an asymmetric crawl or a 'limp' when the child starts to walk may suggest a diagnosis of cerebral palsy.

There is no single 'test' for cerebral palsy. The diagnosis is made from the history, observing the child and conducting a careful physical examination by people with experience of cerebral palsy. Brain imaging may provide evidence about the timing of the lesion and possible cause, but the diagnosis is ultimately a clinical judgement. Infant motor assessments such as Prechtl's Assessment of General Movements (Einspieler et al, 2004) also have a role to play in predicting atypical motor development that may lead to cerebral palsy (Spittle et al, 2008). A useful decision tree for inclusion and exclusion of cases of cerebral palsy has been developed for clinicians by the SCPE collaborative group (SCPE, 2000).

Gastrointestinal issues
Monitoring and maintaining good nutritional status in children and adults with cerebral palsy is critical to maximizing the individual's growth, health and development. Because of the range of impairments associated with cerebral palsy, children and older individuals with more severe impairments are at particular risk of malnutrition. For more specific information and practical advice readers might find Sullivan's practical guide *Feeding and Nutrition in Children with Neurodevelopmental Disability* of some interest (Sullivan, 2009).

SAFETY AND EFFICIENCY OF EATING AND DRINKING

Oral-motor difficulties range from relatively simple motor incoordination that results in prolonged eating times to complex dysphagia requiring alternative and/or supported eating techniques, specialized food preparation, supplemental nutrition via nasal, gastrostomy or jejunostomy tubes. Physiotherapists and occupational therapists should be able to identify overt signs of aspiration during eating including coughing before, during or after the swallow, voice changes (raspy/noisy breathing), gagging or choking during eating and colour changes (blue lips or face). Coughing in combination with either changes in voice (gurgle, raspy breath sounds) or colour change is highly predictive of aspiration (DeMatteo et al, 2005). Silent aspiration occurs without overt signs, is clinically undetectable and should be considered when there is a history of unexplained spikes of fever plus significant food refusal or in the absence of any other explanatory cause for a significant feeding difficulty. Silent aspiration can only be detected on radiological examination such as by using videofluoroscopy. Referrals to eating specialists, including a speech pathologist, are essential if aspiration is suspected.

One of the consequences of aspiration and/or poor oral-motor control is the risk of failure to thrive and malnutrition. In infants and children who have poor oral-motor control the effort of consuming adequate nutrition to supply the energy needed to grow can easily be compromised. The prevalence of undernourishment in people with cerebral palsy has been reported to be as high as 30% (Odding et al, 2006), with the proportions higher in those children with more severe motor impairments. If undernourishment is suspected in individuals with cerebral palsy, they must have adequate follow-up by nutrition and feeding experts. Provision of supplementary intake either temporarily or permanently through nasal, gastrostomy, or jejunostomy tubes can assist in meeting the nutrition requirements of the child thus reducing the risks to cognitive and physical development that are associated with inadequate intake.

Physiotherapists and occupational therapists may also be involved in assisting with meals and require skills in positioning for safe eating, managing oral tone, abnormal oral reflexes and poor oral coordination where they interfere with function. Eating disorders in people with cerebral palsy can be extremely complex and may require an expert team of specialists including speech pathologist, occupational therapist, dietician/nutritionist, gastrointestinal physician, radiologist, as well as the client's primary physician and carers.

REFLUX AND DIFFICULTIES WITH ELIMINATION

Gastrointestinal disorders in individuals with cerebral palsy are common. Along with the oral-motor difficulties described above, reflux causing pain and oesophagitis, delayed gastric emptying and/or chronic constipation (Sullivan, 2008) are also common. One regional population-based study estimated 59% of children with cerebral palsy aged 4–13 years were constipated, 89% needed help with feeding and 56% choked with food (Sullivan et al, 2000). In individuals with severe impairments the prevalence is higher with one study finding pulmonary aspiration in over 40% and chronic reflux in over 50% (Somerville et al, 2008). The consequences of gastrointestinal problems include malnutrition and poor growth with their associated developmental impacts, pain associated with reflux or constipation and potential for chronic lung disease (Rogers, 2004; Somerville et al, 2008). Careful evaluation and support of the individual's diet, oral feeding practices or alternative method of intake (e.g. percutaneous endoscopic gastrostomy (PEG) feeding tubes) and need for medication are essential for maintaining a healthy gastrointestinal system and for ensuring that the individual's nutritional needs are met and potential constipation managed (Rogers, 2004).

Monitoring of joint range and limb position
The high prevalence of joint deformities in adults with cerebral palsy (Graham, 2004; Hilberink et al, 2007) means that all people with hypertonia require routine screening of joint range of movement and muscle stiffness. Although goniometric measures of individual joint range of movement using strict protocols are still used by clinicians to assess specific joint range of movement limitations, the Spinal Alignment and Range of Motion Measure (SAROMM) (Bartlett and Purdie, 2005) has been developed to provide an overall estimate of flexibility and posture for children with cerebral palsy for the purpose of discrimination (see Appendix, p. 289). It can be used to describe the pattern of movement restrictions across the different regions of the body. Plotting average values, the assessment provides a visual representation of areas that might benefit from therapy to either prevent the development of secondary impairments associated with contractures or minimize the progression of existing limitations. Therapy might include preventative soft tissue stretching exercises and limb positioning using splints, casts or orthoses. All orthotic devices need to be carefully applied and regularly checked for continued good fit, absence of pressure sores and achievement of purpose (McNeill, 2004).

Scoliosis is common in children with spastic quadriplegic cerebral palsy (McCarthy et al, 2006) and it has been observed that development of unilateral hip dislocation often heralds the development of rapidly progressive scoliosis (Graham, 2004). For this reason, hip surveillance in all children in GMFCS levels III –V (Soo et al, 2006; Hägglund et al, 2007) is essential (see below). When the spinal curves are relatively flexible, posterior spinal fusion to the pelvis may be adequate to stabilize the spine. When spinal deformities have become fixed, combined anterior and posterior surgery may be required (Graham, 2004). Deciding to have surgery can be very difficult for the family and child as all surgery carries risk and sometimes the family and child do not want further hospitalizations. Untreated severe scoliosis leads to significant problems with pain, seating, cardiorespiratory compromise and difficulties with caregiving. In adults with even relatively small spinal curves the scoliosis continues to progress after skeletal maturity and must be monitored (Graham, 2004).

Hip surveillance
Many centres around the world have traditionally recommended that the hips of all children with spastic bilateral cerebral palsy (i.e. diplegia or quadriplegia) undergo radiological examination at 12–24 months of age, and at 6 to 12-monthly intervals thereafter with the aim of identifying hip displacement at an early stage (Scrutton et al, 2001; Dobson et al, 2002). Around 80% of children with spastic quadriplegia will develop hip displacement secondary to spasticity and muscle imbalance in the major muscle groups around the hip (Hägglund et al, 2007). This muscle imbalance can lead

to progressive displacement of the hip laterally leading to severe subluxation, secondary acetabular dysplasia, deformity of the femoral head, as well as dislocation and painful degenerative arthritis (Dobson et al, 2002). In the long term, hip dislocation can lead to pain and loss of ability to sit comfortably. Other problems can include difficulty with perineal care and personal hygiene, pelvic obliquity and scoliosis, poor sitting balance and loss of the ability to stand and walk (Bagg et al, 1993).

The aim of the management in children at risk of developing hip displacement is to maintain flexible, well-located and painless hips with a symmetrical range of movement. To achieve this goal, early identification and intervention are necessary because delayed detection can restrict the surgical options. Hip displacement is very strongly related to the GMFCS level of the child (Soo et al, 2006), with its incidence increasing linearly with the severity of disability. A study of over 300 children found that the incidence of hip displacement was

- 0% for children at GMFCS level I;
- 15% for GMFCS level II;
- 41% for GMFCS level III;
- 69% for GMFCS level IV; and
- 90% for those at GMFCS level V (Soo et al, 2006).

Stability of the hip and acetabular development is more certain if the femoral head is well located in the acetabulum before the age of 5 years (Dobson et al, 2002). Hip displacement is silent in the initial stages and is difficult to detect by physical examination alone. It is therefore important to refer children whose hips are at risk for orthopaedic evaluation and management in time to prevent progressive displacement and to centralize the femoral head well before 5 years of age (Dobson et al, 2002). Early detection requires a combination of regular clinical examination of the range of movement of the hip and regular radiographs of the hips (Dobson et al, 2002). This is done by an anterior-posterior pelvic radiograph using standardized positioning. From this radiograph, a migration percentage is calculated (Reimers, 1980). The migration percentage is a measurement of the amount of the ossified femoral head that is lateral to the acetabular margin as measured on an anterior-posterior pelvic radiograph. A migration percentage of greater than 30° is defined as hip displacement and requires an orthopaedic opinion (Soo et al, 2006). The recently published evidence-based *Consensus Statement on Hip Surveillance for Children with Cerebral Palsy: Australian Standards of Care* (Wynter et al, 2008) is available from the following website: http://www.cpaustralia.com.au/ausacpdm/.

Epilepsy
Individuals with cerebral palsy who also have epilepsy have significantly poorer outcomes than those who do not (Himmelmann et al, 2007; Beckung et al, 2008; Carlsson et al, 2008; Venkateswaran and Shevell, 2008). Presence of epilepsy has recently been found to be associated with increased behaviour and psychological difficulties in children with cerebral palsy (Carlsson et al, 2008). Because behaviour

and psychological problems are under-recognized in children with cerebral palsy, this knowledge may assist therapists in early identification and referral to mental health services as needed (McLellan, 2008). Onset of seizure activity can occur throughout childhood although is likely to occur at younger ages in the bilateral forms (Carlsson et al, 2003). Although most families will recognize generalized tonic-clonic seizures, they may not recognize partial seizures, especially as some may mimic other motor disorders, or present as generalized absence seizures. Therapists may be able to assist families in identifying the onset of the more atypical seizures and thus instigate a referral for medical management. The following website provides a good description of the different seizure types: http://www.epilepsy.org.au/epilepsy_explained2.asp#4.

Cognitive and intellectual impairments
In addition to intellectual impairment, which occurs in around 40% of children with cerebral palsy (SCPE, 2000), other cognitive and executive functioning deficits are common, and may exist in the presence of a normal IQ. These deficits include specific learning disabilities, deficits in visuospatial and visual–motor development and impaired short-term and working memory (Lesny et al, 1990; Stiers et al, 2002; Pueyo et al, 2003; Jenks et al, 2007; Pueyo et al, 2009). Disorders of motor memory are also common and have been shown to occur frequently in children with left-sided hemiplegia and diplegia (Lesny et al, 1990). Although difficulties in memory and visual perception occur in all subtypes of cerebral palsy (Stiers et al, 2002), there is some evidence that these abilities are poorer in those with spastic rather than dyskinetic forms (Pueyo et al, 2003) and that the frequency and severity of impairments in executive functioning increase in the presence of epilepsy (Vargha-Khadem et al, 1992). These cognitive issues are critically important to the child's academic development and ability to participate successfully in school, and need to be considered by occupational therapists when planning assessment and intervention (Jenks et al, 2007; Bumin and Kavak, 2008).

General health and well-being
Recent studies of adults with cerebral palsy identify significant gaps in the provision of health care services (Andersson and Mattsson, 2001; Darrah et al, 2002; Ng et al, 2003; Liptak, 2008). Although these gaps often include a cessation of therapy and regular visits to a paediatrician following transition to adulthood, it has also been found that many adults do not receive health and medical checks that would be considered routine in the general population. Women with cerebral palsy also require routine gynaecological health checks, and adults with cerebral palsy, like other adults, are also at risk of cardiovascular disease, cancer, and diabetes, and will experience the effects of ageing. In addition, they are at increased risk of chronic pain, depression, and loss of physical function (Liptak, 2008). Adults with cerebral palsy require regular health checks from a primary physician, preferably someone who has a professional interest in people living with a congenital disability. In addition, it is important for therapists to consider whether changes in functional presentation in an individual are due to another coexisting condition as opposed to cerebral palsy per se.

DENTAL CARE

As well as the need for general medical follow-up, some children and adults with cerebral palsy have significant difficulty with dental hygiene. Without routine dental and orthodontic care, decay and dental misalignment can be a major cause of pain and discomfort, can interfere with eating and ultimately cause serious infections. All children and adults with cerebral palsy require good quality dental health care.

MENTAL HEALTH

Although it is now recognized that children with cerebral palsy are at increased risk of behaviour and psychological problems compared with their peers without disability, these issues remain under-identified. Research using the Strengths and Difficulties Questionnaire with 8- to 12-year-old children with cerebral palsy has found that 25% of parents rated their children's behaviour as abnormal (Parkes et al, 2008) and a further 18% as borderline (Carlsson et al, 2008). The most common problems reported were difficulties with peers, hyperactivity and emotional problems. In addition, conditions such as pervasive developmental disorders including autism can also occur in children with cerebral palsy (Kilincaslan and Mukaddes, 2008). In their study of a large clinical group, Kilincaslan and Mukaddes found that pervasive developmental disorders were more common in children with cerebral palsy who also had an intellectual impairment or epilepsy (Kilincaslan and Mukaddes, 2008). These findings highlight the need for therapists to be aware of the potential for families to require assistance in this area, including providing appropriate referrals to mental health services.

Research into the prevalence of mental health problems in adults with cerebral palsy and other physical disabilities is less clear, because few population-based studies have been carried out in this area and the difficulty of including individuals with complex communication needs in this type of research (Di Marco and Iacono, 2007). There is some evidence of increased depression in adults (Kokkonen et al, 1998) and individuals with cerebral palsy may also experience other mental illnesses such as bipolar disorder or schizophrenia.

References

Andersson C & Mattsson E (2001) Adults with cerebral palsy: a survey describing problems, needs, and resources, with special emphasis on locomotion. *Dev Med Child Neurol*, 43, 76–82.

Bagg MR, Farber J & Miller F (1993) Long-term follow-up of hip subluxation in cerebral palsy patients. *J Orthop*, 13, 32–6.

Bartlett D & Purdie B (2005) Testing of the spinal alignment and range of movement: a discriminative measure of posture and flexibility for children with cerebral palsy. *Dev Med Child Neurol*, 47, 739–43.

Bax M & Brown JK (2004) The spectrum of disorders known as cerebral palsy. In: Scrutton D, Damiano D & Mayston MJ (eds) *Management of the Motor Disorders of Children with Cerebral Palsy*, 2nd edn. London: Mac Keith Press.

Bax M, Tydeman C & Flodmark O (2006) Clinical and MRI correlates of cerebral palsy: the European Cerebral Palsy Study. *JAMA*, 296, 1602–8.

Beckung E, White-Koning M, Marcelli M, McManus V, Michelsen SI, Parkes J, Parkinson K, Thyen U, Arnould C, Fauconnier J & Colver A (2008) Health status of children with cerebral palsy living in Europe: a multicentre study. *Child Care Health Dev*, 34, 806–14.

Blair E & Stanley F (1997) Issues in the classification and epidemiology of cerebral palsy. *Ment Retard Dev Disabil Res Rev,* 3, 184–93.

Blair E, Watson L, Badawi N & Stanley FJ (2001) Life expectancy among people with cerebral palsy in Western Australia. *Dev Med Child Neurol,* 43, 508–15.

Brown K. (2003) Cerebral palsy: Can we prevent it? *Dev Med Child Neurol Suppl,* 45, 30.

Bumin G & Kavak ST (2008) An investigation of the factors affecting handwriting performance in children with hemiplegic cerebral palsy. *Disabil Rehabil,* 30, 1374–85.

Carlsson M, Hagberg G & Olsson I (2003) Clinical and aetiological aspects of epilepsy in children with cerebral palsy. *Dev Med Child Neurol,* 45, 371–6.

Carlsson M, Olsson I, Hagberg G & Beckung E (2008) Behaviour in children with cerebral palsy with and without epilepsy.[see comment]. *Dev Med Child Neurol,* 50, 784–9.

Darrah J, Magil-Evans J & Adkins R (2002) How well are we doing? Families of adolescents or young adults with cerebral palsy share their perceptions of service delivery. *Disabil Rehabil,* 24, 542–9.

DeMatteo C, Matovich D. & Hjartarson A (2005) Comparison of clinical and videofluoroscopic evaluation of children with feeding and swallowing difficulties. *Dev Med Child Neurol,* 47, 149–57.

Di Marco M & Iacono T (2007) Mental health assessment and intervention for people with complex communication needs associated with developmental disabilities. *J Policy Prac Intellec Disabil,* 4, 40–59.

Dickinson HO, Parkinson KN, Ravens-Sieberer U, Schirripa G, Thyen U, Arnaud C, Beckung E, Fauconnier J, McManus V, Michelsen SI, Parkes J & Colver AF (2007) Self-reported quality of life of 8–12-year-old children with cerebral palsy: a cross-sectional European study. *Lancet,* 369, 2171–8.

Dobson F, Boyd R, Parrott GR, Nattrass GR & Graham HK (2002) Hip surveillance in children with cerebral palsy: impact on the surgical management of spastic hip disease. *J Bone Joint Surg Br,* 84, 720–6.

Einspieler C, Prechtl HF, Bos AF, Ferrari F & Cioni G (2004) *Prechtl's Method on the Qualitative Assessment of General Movements in Preterm, Term and Young Infants.* London, Mac Keith Press.

Eliasson AC (2005) Improving the use of hands in daily activities: aspects of treatment of children with cerebral palsy. *Phys Occup Ther Pediatr,* 25, 37–60.

Eliasson AC, Krumlinde-Sundholm L, Rösblad B, Beckung E, Arner M, Öhrvall A & Rosenbaum PL (2006) The Manual Ability Classification System (MACS) for children with cerebral palsy: scale development and evidence of validity and reliability. *Dev Med Child Neurol,* 48, 549–54.

Görter JW, Rosenbaum PL, Hanna S, Palisano RJ, Bartlett DJ, Russell D, Walter S, Raina PS, Galuppi B & Wood E (2004) Limb distribution, motor impairment, and functional classification of cerebral palsy. *Dev Med Child Neurol,* 46, 461–7.

Graham HK (2004) Mechanisms of deformity. In: Scrutton D, Damiano D & Mayston MJ (eds) *Management of the Motor Disorders of Children with Cerebral Palsy,* 2nd edn. London: Mac Keith Press.

Hägglund G, Lauge-Pedersen H & Wagner P (2007) Characteristics of children with hip displacement in cerebral palsy. *BMC Musculoskelet Disord,* 8, 101.

Hemming K, Hutton JL & Pharoah PO (2006) Long-term survival for a cohort of adults with cerebral palsy. *Dev Med Child Neurol,* 48, 90–5.

Hidecker MJC, Paneth N, Kent RD, Lillie J, Johnson B & Chester K (2008) Developing a tool to classify functional communication in individuals with cerebral palsy. *Dev Med Child Neurol Suppl,* 50, 43.

Hilberink SR, Roebroeck ME, Nieuwstraten W, Jalink L, Verheijden JM & Stam HJ (2007) Health issues in young adults with cerebral palsy: towards a life-span perspective. *J Rehabil Med,* 39, 605–11.

Himmelmann K, Beckung E, Hagberg B & Uvebrant P (2006) Gross and fine motor function and accompanying impairments in cerebral palsy. *Dev Med Child Neurol,* 48, 417–23.

Himmelmann K, Hagberg G, Wiklund LM, Eek MN & Uvebrant P (2007) Dyskinetic cerebral palsy: a population-based study of children born between 1991 and 1998. *Dev Med Child Neurol,* 49, 246–51.

Holmefur M, Krumlinde-Sundholm L, Bergström J & Eliasson AC (2009) Longitudinal development of affected hand use in bimanual tasks in children with unilateral cerebral palsy. *Dev Med Child Neurol,* July 3. DOI: 10.1111/j.1469-8749.2009.03364.x [Epub ahead of print].

Howard J, Soo B, Graham HK, Boyd RN, Reid S, Lanigan S, Wolfe R & Reddihough D (2005) Cerebral palsy in Victoria: motor types, topography and gross motor function. *J Paediatr Child Health*, 41, 479–83.

Imms C, Carlin J & Eliasson AC (2009) Stability of caregiver-reported manual ability and gross motor function classification of cerebral palsy. *Dev Med Child Neurol*, May 21. DOI: 10.1111/j.1469-8749.2009.03357.x [Epub ahead of print].

Jahnsen R, Villien L, Stanghelle J K & Holm I (2002) Coping potential and disability – sense of coherence in adults with cerebral palsy. *Disabil Rehabil*, 24, 511–18.

Jahnsen R, Aamodt G & Rosenbaum PL (2006) Gross motor function classification system used in adults with cerebral palsy: agreement of self-reported versus professional rating. *Dev Med Child Neurol*, 48, 734–8.

Jemtå L, Dahl M, Fugle-Meyer KS & Stensman R (2005) Well-being among children and adolescents with mobility impairment in relation to demographic data and disability characteristics. *Acta Paediatrica*, 94, 616–23.

Jenks KM, de Moor J, van Lieshout EC, Maathuis KG, Keus I & Görter JW (2007) The effect of cerebral palsy on arithmetic accuracy is mediated by working memory, intelligence, early numeracy, and instruction time. *Dev Neuropsychol*, 32, 861–79.

Jessen C, Mackie P & Jarvis S (1999) Epidemiology of cerebral palsy. *Arch Dis Child Fetal Neonatal Ed*, 80, F158.

Johnstone BR, Richardson PWF, Coombs CJ & Duncan JA (2003) Functional and cosmetic outcome of surgery for cerebral palsy in the upper limb. *Hand Clin*, 19, 679–86.

Katz RT & Rymer WZ (1989) Spastic hypertonia: mechanisms and measurement. *Arch Phys Med Rehabil*, 70: 144–55.

Kennes J, Rosenbaum PL, Hanna S, Walter S, Russell D, Raina PS, Bartlett DJ & Galuppi B (2002) Health status of school-aged children with cerebral palsy: information from a population-based sample. *Dev Med Child Neurol*, 44, 240–7.

Keogh JM & Badawi N (2006) The origins of cerebral palsy. *Curr Opin Neurol*, 19, 129–34.

Kilincaslan A & Mukaddes NM (2008) Pervasive developmental disorders in individuals with cerebral palsy. *Dev Med Child Neurol*, 51, 289–94.

King GA, Cathers T, Polgar JM, MacKinnon E & Havens L (2000) Success in life for older adolescents with cerebral palsy. *Qual Health Res*, 10, 734–49.

Knox V (2008) Do parents of children with cerebral palsy express different concerns in relation to their child's type of cerebral palsy, age and level of disability? *Physiotherapy*, 94, 56–62.

Kokkonen E-R, Kokkonen J & Saukkonen A-L (1998) Do neurological disorders in childhood pose a risk for mental health in young adulthood? *Dev Med Child Neurol*, 40, 364–8.

Koman LA, Paterson Smith B & Shilt JS (2004) Cerebral palsy. *Lancet*, 363, 1619–31.

Korzeniewski SJ, Birbeck G, DeLano MC, Potchen MJ & Paneth N (2008) A systematic review of neuroimaging for cerebral palsy. *J Child Neurol*, 23, 216–27.

Krägeloh-Mann I & Cans C (2009) Cerebral palsy update. *Brain Dev*, 31: 537–44.

Krägeloh-Mann I & Horber V (2007) The role of magnetic resonance imaging in elucidating the pathogenesis of cerebral palsy: a systematic review. *Dev Med Child Neurol*, 49, 144–51.

Lance JW (1980) Symposium synopsis. In: Feldman RG, Young RR & Koella WP (eds) *Spasticity: Disordered Motor Control*. Chicago: Year Book Medical Publishers.

Lance JW & McLeod JG (1981) *A Physiological Approach to Clinical Neurology*. London: Butterworths.

Lesny I, Nachtmann M, Stehlik A, Tomankova A & Zajidkova J (1990) Disorders of memory of motor sequences in cerebral palsied children. *Brain Devel*, 12, 339–41.

Liptak, GS (2008) Health and well being of adults with cerebral palsy. *Curr Opin Neurol*, 21, 136–42.

Liptak GS, O'Donnell M, Conaway M, Cameron Chumlea W, Worley G, Henderson RC, Fung E, Stallings VA, Samson-Fang L, Calvert R, Rosenbaum PL & Stevenson RD (2001) Health status of children with moderate to severe cerebral palsy. *Dev Med Child Neurol*, 43, 364–70.

Livingston MH, Rosenbaum PL, Russell DJ & Palisano RJ (2007) Quality of life among adolescents with cerebral palsy: what does the literature tell us? *Dev Med Child Neurol*, 49, 225–31.

McCarthy JJ, D'Andrea LP, Betz RR & Clements DH (2006) Scoliosis in the child with cerebral palsy. *J Am Acad Orthop Surg*, 14, 367–75.

McDermott S, Coker AL, Mani S, Krishnaswami S, Nagle RJ, Barnett-Queen, LL & Wuori DF (1996) A population-based analysis of behavior problems in children with cerebral palsy. *J Pediatr Psychol*, 21, 447–63.

McLellan A (2008) Epilepsy: an additional risk factor for psychological problems in cerebral palsy. *Dev Med Child Neurol*, 50, 727.

McNeill S (2004) The management of deformity. In: Scrutton D, Damiano D & Mayston MJ (eds) *Management of the Motor Disorders of Children with Cerebral Palsy,* 2nd edn. London, Mac Keith Press.

Majnemer A, Shevell M, Rosenbaum PL, Law M & Poulin C (2007) Determinants of life quality in school-age children with cerebral palsy. *J Pediatr*, 151, 470–5.

Morris C, Galuppi B & Rosenbaum PL (2004) Reliability of family report for the Gross Motor Function Classification System. *Dev Med Child Neurol*, 46, 455–60.

Morris J (1999) Findings: transition to adulthood for young disabled people with complex health and support needs. York: Joseph Rowntree Foundation.

Nelson KB & Ellenberg JH (1982) Children who "outgrew" cerebral palsy. *Pediatrics*, 69, 529–35.

Ng SY, Dinesh SK, Tay SKH & Lee EH (2003) Decreased access to health care and social isolation among young adults with cerebral palsy after leaving school. *J Orthop Surg*, 11, 80–9.

Nordmark E, Hägglund G & Lagergren J (2001) Cerebral palsy in southern Sweden II. Gross motor function and disabilities. *Acta Paediatr Scand*, 90, 1277–82.

Odding E, Roebroeck ME & Stam HJ (2006) The epidemiology of cerebral palsy: incidence, impairments and risk factors. *Disabil Rehabil*, 28, 183–91.

Palisano RJ, Rosenbaum PL, Walter S, Russell D, Wood E & Galuppi B (1997) Development and reliability of a system to classify gross motor function in children with cerebral palsy. *Dev Med Child Neurol*, 39, 214–23.

Palisano, RJ, Tieman BL, Walter SD, Bartlett DJ, Rosenbaum PL, Russell D & Hanna SE (2003) Effect of environmental setting on mobility methods of children with cerebral palsy. *Dev Med Child Neurol*, 45, 113–20.

Palisano RJ, Rosenbaum PL, Bartlett D & Livingston MH (2008) Content validity of the expanded and revised gross motor function classification system. *Dev Med Child Neurol*, 50, 744–50.

Parkes J, White-Koning M, Dickinson HO, Thyen U, Arnaud C, Beckung E, Fauconnier J, Marcelli M, McManus V, Michelsen SI, Parkinson K & Colver A (2008) Psychological problems in children with cerebral palsy: a cross-sectional European study. *J Child Psychol Psychiatry*, 49, 405–13.

Pharoah PO, Platt MJ & Cooke T (1996) The changing epidemiology of cerebral palsy. *Arch Dis Child Fetal Neonatal Ed*, 75, F169–73.

Pueyo R, Junque C & Vendrell P (2003) Neuropsychologic differences between bilateral dyskinetic and spastic cerebral palsy. *J Child Neurol*, 18, 845–50.

Pueyo R, Junque C, Vendrell P, Narberhaus A & Segarra D (2009) Neuropsychologic impairment in bilateral cerebral palsy. *Pediatr Neurol*, 40, 19–26.

Reddihough D & Collins KJ (2003) The epidemiology and causes of cerebral palsy. *Aust J Physiother*, 49, 7–12.

Reid SM, Lanigan S, Walstab J & Reddihough D (2005) *Third Report of the Victorian Cerebral Palsy Register.* Melbourne, Australia: Murdoch Children's Research Institute & The Royal Children's Hospital.

Reid SM, Lanigan A & Reddihough DS (2006) Post-neonatally acquired cerebral palsy in Victoria, Australia, 1970–1999. *J Paediatr Child Health*, 42, 606–11.

Reimers J (1980) The stability of the hip in children. A radiological study of the results of muscle surgery in cerebral palsy. *Acta Orthop Scand Suppl*, 184, 1–100.

Rogers B (2004) Feeding method and health outcomes of children with cerebral palsy. *J Pediatr*, 145, S28–32.

Rosenbaum PL (2003) Cerebral palsy: What parents and doctors want to know. *BMJ*, 326, 970–4.

Rosenbaum PL, Palisano RJ, Walter S, Russell D, Wood E & Galuppi B (1996) *Development of the Gross Motor Function Classification System: Reliability and Validity Results*. Hamilton, Ontario: Canchild Centre for Childhood Disability Research.

Rosenbaum P, Paneth N, Leviton A, Goldstein M & Bax M (2007a) A report: the definition and classification of cerebral palsy April 2006. *Dev Med Child Neurol Suppl*, 49, 8–14.

Rosenbaum PL, Livingston MH, Palisano RJ, Galuppi BE & Russell DJ (2007b) Quality of life and health-related quality of life of adolescents with cerebral palsy. *Dev Med Child Neurol*, 49, 516–21.

Rosenbaum PL, Palisano RJ, Bartlett DJ, Galuppi BE & Russell DJ (2008) Development of the Gross Motor Function Classification System for cerebral palsy. *Dev Med Child Neurol*, 50, 249–53.

Samson-Fang L, Fung E, Stallings VA, Conaway M, Worley G, Rosenbaum P, Calvert R, O'Donnell M, Henderson RC, Chumlea WC, Liptak GS & Stevenson RD (2002) Relationship of nutritional status to health and societal participation in children with cerebral palsy. *J Pediatr*, 141, 637–43.

Sanger TD, Chen D, Delgado MR, Gaebler-Spira D, Hallett M, Mink JW & Taskforce on Childhood Motor Disorders (2006) Definition and classification of negative motor signs in childhood. *Pediatrics*, 118, 2159–67.

Sanger TD, Delgado MR, Gaebler-Spira D, Hallett M & Mink JW (2003) Classification and definitions of disorders causing hypertonia in childhood. *Pediatrics*, 111, e89–97.

Schaefer GB (2008) Genetics considerations in cerebral palsy. *Semin Pediatr Neurol*, 15, 21–6.

Scrutton D, Baird G & Smeeton N (2001) Hip dysplasia in bilateral cerebral palsy: Incidence and natural history in children aged 18 months to 5 years. *Dev Med Child Neurol*, 43, 586–600.

Somerville H, Tzannes G, Wood J, Shun A, Hill C, Arrowsmith F, Slater A & O'Loughlin EV (2008) Gastrointestinal and nutritional problems in severe developmental disability. *Dev Med Child Neurol*, 50, 712–6.

Soo B, Howard JJ, Boyd RN, Reid SM, Lanigan A, Wolfe R, Reddihough D & Graham HK (2006) Hip displacement in cerebral palsy. *J Bone Joint Surg Am*, 88, 121–9.

Spittle AJ, Doyle LW & Boyd RN (2008) A systematic review of the clinimetric properties of neuromotor assessments for preterm infants during the first year of life. *Dev Med Child Neurol*, 50, 254–66.

Stanley F, Blair EM & Alberman E (2000) *Cerebral Palsies: Epidemiology and Causal Pathways*. London: Mac Keith Press.

Stevenson CJ, Pharoah POD & Stevenson R (1997) Cerebral palsy – the transition from youth to adulthood. *Dev Med Child Neurol*, 39, 336–42.

Stevenson RD, Conaway M, Chumlea WC, Rosenbaum PL, Fung EB, Henderson RC, Worley G, Liptak G, O'Donnell M, Samson-Fang L, Stallings VA & North American Growth in Cerebral Palsy Study (2006) Growth and health in children with moderate-to-severe cerebral palsy. *Pediatrics*, 118, 1010–8.

Stewart D, Law M, Rosenbaum PL & Willms D (2001) A qualitative study of the transition to adulthood for youth with physical disabilities. *Phys Occup Ther Pediatr*, 21, 3–21.

Stiers P, Vanderkelen R, Vanneste G, Coene S, De Rammelaere M & Vandenbussche E (2002) Visual-perceptual impairment in a random sample of children with cerebral palsy. *Dev Med Child Neurol*, 44, 370–82.

Sullivan PB (2008) Gastrointestinal disorders in children with neurodevelopmental disabilities. *Dev Disabil Res Rev*, 14, 128–36.

Sullivan, P. B. (2009) *Feeding and Nutrition in Children with Neurodevelopmental Disability*. London: Mac Keith Press.

Sullivan PB, Lambert B, Rose M, Ford-Adams M, Johnson A & Griffiths P (2000) Prevalence and severity of feeding and nutritional problems in children with neurological impairment: Oxford Feeding Study. *Dev Med Child Neurol*, 42, 674–80.

Surman G, Bonellie S, Chalmers J, Colver A, Dolk H, Hemming K, King A, Kurinczuk JJ, Parkes J & Platt MJ (2006) UKCP: A collaborative network of cerebral palsy registers in the United Kingdom. *J Public Health*, 28, 148–56.

Surveillance of Cerebral Palsy in Europe (SCPE) (2000) Surveillance of cerebral palsy in Europe: a collaboration of cerebral palsy surveys and registers. *Dev Med Child Neurol*, 42, 816–24.

Vargha-Khadem F, Isaacs E, van der Werf S, Robb S & Wilson J (1992) Development of intelligence and memory in children with hemiplegic cerebral palsy. The deleterious consequences of early seizures. *Brain*, 115 Pt 1, 315–29.

Vargus-Adams J (2005) Health related quality of life in childhood cerebral palsy. *Arch Phys Med Rehabil*, 86, 940–5.

Venkateswaran S & Shevell MI (2008) Comorbidities and clinical determinants of outcome in children with spastic quadriplegic cerebral palsy. *Dev Med Child Neurol*, 50, 216–22.

Wake M, Salmon L & Reddihough D (2003) Health status of Australia children with mild to severe cerebral palsy: cross-sectional survey using the Child Health Questionnaire. *Dev Med Child Neurol*, 45, 194–9.

Westbom L, Hägglund G & Nordmark E (2007) Cerebral palsy in a total population of 4–11 year olds in southern Sweden. Prevalence and distribution according to different CP classification systems. *BMC Pediatr*, 7, 41.

Woodward L, Anderson PJ, Austin NC, Howard K & Inder TE (2006) Neonatal MRI to predict neurodevelopmental outcomes in preterm infants. *NEJM*, 355, 685–94.

Wynter M, Gibson N, Kentish M, Love SC, Tomason P & Graham HK (2008) *Consensus Statement on Hip Surveillance for Children with Cerebral Palsy: Australian Standards of Care*. Victoria: CP Australia.

Chapter 3

Understanding the family's perspective: parenting a child with cerebral palsy

Helen Bourke-Taylor

This chapter describes the experience of parents who are raising a child with cerebral palsy. Families that include a member with cerebral palsy are as diverse as those found within any other community and may be bringing up other children in the family as well. The siblings too must be considered within the family dynamics, increasing the responsibilities of and concerns for parents. Professionals, particularly therapists, working with individuals with cerebral palsy should be guided by models that recognize the inextricable influence that family context has on planned interventions. Palisano et al (2004) described three of the most influential models that emphasize family context. They are the person occupation environment (PEO) model, family-centred care (FCC) and the International Classification of Functioning, Disability and Health (ICF).

Family-centred service delivery considers the family as the most important and enduring support system in the child's life and this is fundamental to family satisfaction and efficacy of service delivery (Rosenbaum et al, 1998; Law et al, 2003). Family context has an enormous impact on a child's progress, capabilities and participation in opportunities available to them and this is crucial to the health, development and life success of individuals with cerebral palsy (Law et al, 2004). However, as professionals working with families and individuals with cerebral palsy, we are aware that meeting the day-to-day needs and long-term requirements of a child with cerebral palsy can be a source of challenge for many families. Understanding the perspective of families allows professionals to be more responsive to those needs.

The three subsections in this chapter sketch an overview of the complex journey familiar to many families. The final section connects the information presented to practice.

The objectives of this chapter are to describe

- the experience of mothers as primary carers of children with cerebral palsy;
- the possible effects of a diagnosis of cerebral palsy on families: financial, social, time use;
- the main challenges faced by many families;
- how readers can improve service delivery for families.

Navigating unchartered waters: mastering a different kind of parenting

Parenting a child with a disability is a unique kind of parenting that encompasses many usual childcare practices, plus the need to provide direct assistance in daily living tasks, some medically, educationally and developmentally specialized tasks, as well as the multitude of responsibilities involved with managing the requirements of long-term disability (Nelson, 2002; McGuire et al, 2004; Meester-Delver, 2006). As described in Chapter 2, cerebral palsy is frequently accompanied by other disabilities. Given the range of impairments and medical needs characteristic of this population, families must master a range of specialized and time-intensive tasks that are fundamental to a child's health and development. A diagnosis of cerebral palsy results in forgoing an imagined future for the child, leaving intense feelings of loss and grief (Nelson, 2002; Green, 2007). The expected sequence of developmental, social, educational and other cultural events takes an unpredictable turn. Families are navigating unchartered waters.

> *I also clearly remember, however, the pivotal moment during the first weeks after Amanda's diagnosis at which I moved beyond my sorrow. One moment I was mired in grief and the next moment I thought: 'I can't waste time over the loss of Amanda because Amanda needs her dinner.' While there have been many emotional highs and lows since that day, and the complexity of her care can often seem overwhelming, the experience of raising my daughter has been both positive and powerful.*
>
> *(Green, 2007: p.152)*

Green (2002), a sociologist, provides a first-hand account of mothering her daughter Amanda, who has cerebral palsy. She describes her own profoundly transforming experience and the stages that she grew through as she mastered a different kind of parenting. Adapting to an unfamiliar role and to the child's needs as they grow and develop requires the parent to move through several stages, sometimes concurrently, as described by Green and others. These stages are of interest to health and education professionals as the needs of parents change as they move through different stages.

First, parents enter the stage characterized by shock and intense emotions. Then, the need for knowledge and new skills propels the parent into 'seekership' (Green, 2002). This stage is characterized by rapid knowledge acquisition so that new terms, medical management and therapy options are understood, and so that appropriate services can be located and retained. This stage recurs as the child enters new phases of development such as kindergarten, school and college or adult services.

> *In the early days it was about never doing enough for Andrew. That was. . .before I knew where he'd end up on the scale of disability. When I was really putting in the hard yards and trying to make that first milestone with the movement or whatever and I chased around all the different therapies, gave everything a go.*
>
> *(Alana, mother to Andrew aged 14years[1])*

Following the successful acquisition of the knowledge and skills needed by the child at that stage, the family may move into a 'normalization' stage where they re-focus on other family issues and resumes 'normal' routines and interests. Fortunately most parents shift from a 'disability' focus to a family focus. All phases can recur through the child's life, particularly the initial phase of shock and grief. Some parents feel a sense of 'chronic sorrow' that does not dissipate across the child's life (Nelson, 2002).

> *There are periods of time that I have really had to stop and have a really big cry about different things. It doesn't happen that often. One was when Andrew was given the opportunity to go to a regular kindergarten as a reverse integration thing. I dropped him off and I just cried all day. It was so hard getting into a normal situation, where I'd been in disabled settings. . .There are just different times that it's really hit me. I guess it's just constant now, as he's older, it's a constant sadness to his Dad and I.*
>
> *(Alana, mother to Andrew)*

Health professionals knowledgeable in current theoretical and scientific advances can provide parents with objective resource information during 'seekership' and assist the 'normalization' phase through family-centred practices that reinforce the child's functioning within the family environment, or the environment chosen by the family.

Mothering: responsibilities and effects on health

> *There are so many daily tasks that the mum has to overcome that it's mind boggling . . . [The mothers have a] permanent full time job 24/7.*
>
> *(A paediatrician's response to the workload of mothers with a child with a disability)*

Mothers are usually the primary caregiver, that is, the person most knowledgeable about the child's health and needs (Brehaut et al, 2004; Raina et al, 2004; Crowe and Florez, 2006). Fathers may play a crucial role sharing the responsibilities of caregiving, although they are more likely to be responsible for the child's needs through maintaining the family income (Parish and Cloud, 2006). Some research indicates that couples face additional interpersonal strain when a child has a disability, although these findings are tempered by other couples who believe that their child with special needs strengthens their relationship (Nelson, 2002; Kersh et al, 2006). However, finding time

---

1 Bourke-Taylor HM, (2009) PhD thesis in progress: Study one. All quotations are data collected by the author unless otherwise referenced.

for a couple's relationship outside of childcare responsibilities can be a challenge, especially if the family has no respite care. Paula described her own situation in the following extract.

> We've made sure that Luke's okay, you know the relationships between John and Luke, and me and Luke, are really good. And as a family, we try and go out if there's a long weekend or Easter, and we do things as a family. We have enjoyed that, but the couple relationship has really had to come behind and I'm hoping that in the next few years that's something we can maybe work on it a bit more. I'm hoping that with Luke's school not having to change for another 4 years and hopefully the respite situation being a bit more under control, and next year a house with hoists and everything, that we'll be able to not have to fight the council [for respite workers], and that maybe that's the time for John and I.

As the primary carers, mothers are responsible for a multitude of direct (child is present) and indirect (child is absent) tasks. For many mothers, the types of direct tasks move beyond assisting in self-care, mobility and communication, and into hands-on help to play, socialize and pursue recreational opportunities (Bourke-Taylor et al, 2009). Paula described a gymnastics party that her son Luke attended with school friends, stating: 'And that was full on because I had to be there lifting him in and out, and up on the bars, and down again. And you know, well the other mothers sat there and drank coffee on the side! [Laughs].' Paula also recalled Luke's earlier play experience.

> When he was little he just couldn't amuse himself. So that was a horrible time for John [husband] and I. . .we felt like we had to be there amusing him all the time. Also, he wasn't in a wheelchair. He couldn't get around. So we had to move him and set him up in different activities. Now he's fantastic. He loves reading, he can read independently. He loves the computer, he can get on the computer and do all sorts of things. So it was probably about kinder[garten] year when he really started to get happy to do things on his own. And that's been a major relief.

Indirect care tasks include planning and organizing the child's needs and advocacy tasks that work towards the child's successful integration within school or community. Mothers have successfully advocated for children with disabilities in numerous capacities, to cause positive changes at local community and government levels (Llewellyn et al, 2004). The time and skill involved in direct and indirect caregiving is substantially greater than caring for a typically developing child (Curran et al, 2001; Nelson, 2002; Crowe and Florez, 2006; Gevir et al, 2006). Time use research has revealed that mothers of a child with a disability spend significantly more time performing all childcare tasks. Consequently, they have less time to sleep, socialize, attend to their own health, work for pay and attend to other children and earn a living (Donovan et al, 2005). As Alana stated, 'Andrew comes first and if there's something that I'd like to do, you know, I may very well have to let that go'.

Several studies have investigated the mental and physical health of mothers of children with cerebral palsy or physical disabilities and these studies indicate that mothers may be more susceptible to detrimental health outcomes. This group of mothers consistently reports higher stress and comparatively lower mental, physical and overall health status (Tong et al, 2002; Brehaut et al, 2004; Eker and Tuzan, 2004; Tuna et al, 2004; Raina et al, 2005; Barlow et al, 2006; Singer 2006; Stok et al, 2006). Such findings are a concern for the families themselves, and professionals who seek to address the needs and functioning of children with cerebral palsy.

Mothers have indicated that some of the most difficult aspects of caring for a child with cerebral palsy relate to indirect tasks, rather than direct care tasks (McGuire et al, 2004; Stok et al, 2006; Green 2007). Mothers describe 'fighting, fighting, fighting' to locate and retain professional services for their child and the need constantly to advocate to reduce community barriers of both a physical and attitudinal nature. Some aspects of direct caring also add significant challenges to mothers. They include tasks that are medically difficult, physically difficult (include lifting, holding, stabilizing a heavy child or equipment) and managing challenging behaviour (Thyen et al, 1999; Tong et al, 2002; Raina et al, 2005). For example Paula describes managing lifting in light of her own back injury related to lifting equipment as well as 8-year-old Luke who has spastic quadriplegic cerebral palsy: 'I think the lifting has become a lot more obvious, like even to the point that it's a mental strain. Like in the morning routine. . . it's in my mind. How can I minimize the amount of times I'm manual handling?'

Main challenges associated with parenting a child with cerebral palsy

Caring for a child or family member with cerebral palsy can be difficult, relentless and frequently continues into the parents' retirement years. Adults with cerebral palsy can remain dependent on family well into their adult years because of the lack of adult accommodation and opportunities to become financially independent. Parents love and support their offspring wholeheartedly, and describe absolute joy and an enhanced life-purpose parenting their child (Nelson, 2002). However, parents also describe two main obstacles that interfere with achieving the best outcome for their child and family members. These are financial hardship and social isolation related to perceived stigma.

Special needs are expensive needs

Depending on the health care system families incur excessive costs in the form of specialized therapies and services, adaptive and medical equipment, home and vehicle modifications and other ongoing expenses associated with medical care, medication and caring for the child (Power, 2002; Parish and Cloud, 2006). Costs are estimated to be well beyond raising a typically developing child. Parental employment, whether in single or two-parent families, is crucial to financial well-being, although mothers in such families participate in the workforce less than other mothers (Powers, 2003; Brehaut et al, 2004). Consequently, many families find themselves on a single income, brought in by the father/male adult, or dependant on social supports and payments. The wage-earning parent may find him or herself under considerable pressure to maintain income to support their child with special needs, in addition to family needs. Paula described the stress that her husband was under, stating: 'John's career is heavy. . .I mean that's his career choice but he also makes that choice 'cause he knows we've got Luke, so he needs to earn a good salary.' More frequently, families have lower incomes. Children with disabilities and their siblings are more likely to live in poverty in the UK, USA and Canada (Park et al, 2002; Brehaut et al, 2004; Emerson et al, 2006; Parish and Cloud, 2006). The situation is likely to be similar in other countries.

Social isolation and stigma
Integrating a child into the community's social fabric can be a very harrowing and difficult task for families. Social isolation and stigma compound difficulties experienced by families (Green, 2001, 2003, 2007). Numerous authors have described the isolation mothers feel from others (Nelson, 2002; McGuire et al, 2004; Donovan et al, 2005). Green (2002) describes the enormous support received from other parents of a child with a disability and professionals working with their child. Parents may feel rejected by other people who cannot understand their family situation.

> *People tended to shy away from inviting us. . .they weren't being cruel or anything, but they certainly didn't know how to deal with the Andrew situation. So, we were left off a lot of party lists and wedding lists, lots of different lists. Sometimes I'd think 'Oh, I wonder why I we weren't invited'. . .I guess [we had needed to] hibernate a bit, particularly in the early years. And then, we weren't picked up because we weren't seen and around. We weren't picked up onto lists. That was hurtful.*
>
> *(Alana)*

What do families need from professionals?

Families need assistance from professionals who listen to their perspective, respond to their child's and family's needs and problem solve with them. Families need information about research, new interventions, funding and services that may be appropriate for their family member. Families need their child's services to be family-centred, supportive of inclusion and compatible with the family's cultural perspective. Children with cerebral palsy rely on a capable adult to participate in many required daily tasks, as well as the play, recreation and educational opportunities available to them. In line with family-centred practice, therapists working with the caregiver and child must consider both parties during management planning. Improving a child's capacity to participate in any task should be accompanied by a measurable reduction in the contribution provided by the caregiver during selected tasks (Bourke-Taylor et al, 2009).

Professionals need to be aware of the cultural backdrop of the family, as values about caring and including a child with a disability in family life, beliefs about the cause, cure and need for medical/therapy intervention and customs about childcare all vary in different cultural contexts. While maintaining their duty of care, professionals need to be culturally competent and understand that the family's actions and decisions are tempered by their wish to care for their child within the boundaries of their belief system.

When working with children with cerebral palsy, families do want you to do the following.

- Acknowledge the child's family environment and make all reasonable and possible accommodations to suit the family when providing services.
- Address the needs and goals of the carer and child as 'the client'. Any dependant child is usually a member of a mother–child dyad and this unit becomes central in client-centred/family-centred care planning.
- Understand the culture of the family of the child you are working with. Collaborative goal setting and family-centred care are not possible unless you are a culturally competent professional.
- Work with the child in their real-life environments and assist skill acquisition.
- Consider the mother's (or primary carer's) needs and collaborate to provide services that will reduce the burden of home-based care.
- Prescribe equipment that saves caregivers' backs, necks, knees, arms, hands and mental health after collaborating with family members.
- Advocate on that child's behalf in all contexts – school, community, government, and policy – to better resource families and reduce community barriers.
- Plan ahead for the child's future needs – home modifications, educating the family, funding issues.
- Communicate with colleagues also providing services to improve coordination of care provided for the child and reduce the mother's need to act as coordinator of child's services.
- Resource families with the information that they request and then step back to let the family make an informed choice. Accept that choice.
- Resource families with professionals in the local community who are capable of addressing all family members' issues surrounding disability. The family is the child's support system and everyone matters.
- Celebrate and acknowledge the strengths and talents possessed by children with cerebral palsy and share these with parents.

References

Barlow JH, Cullen-Powell LA & Chesire A (2006) Psychological well-being among mothers of children with cerebral palsy. *Early Child Dev Care*, 769, 421–8.

Bourke-Taylor HM, Law M, Howie L & Pallant JF (2009) Development of the Assistance to Participate Scale (APS) for children's leisure activities. *Child Care Health Dev*, 35, 738–45.

Bourke-Taylor HM, Howie, L & Law M (2009) Impact of caring for a school aged child with a disability: understanding mothers' perspectives. *Aust Occ Therapy J*, October 8. DOI: 10.1111/j.1440-1630.2009.00817.x [Epub ahead of print].

Brehaut J, Kohen D, Raina P, Walter S, Russell D, Switon M, O'Donnell & Rosenbaum P (2004) The health of primary caregivers of children with cerebral palsy: how does it compare with that of other Canadian caregivers? *Pediatrics*, 114, e182–91.

Crowe TK & Florez SI (2006) Time use of mothers with school-age children: a continuing impact of a child's disability. *Am J Occ Ther*, 60, 194–203.

Curran A, Sharples P, White C & Knapp M (2001). Time cost of caring for children with severe disabilities compared with caring for children without disabilities. *Dev Med Child Neurol*, 43, 529–33.

Donovan JM, Van Leit BJ, Crowe TK & Keefe EB (2005) Occupational goals of mothers of children with disabilities: influence of temporal, social and emotional contexts. *Am J Occ Ther*, 59, 249–61.

Eker L & Tuzun EH (2004) An evaluation of quality of life of mothers of children with cerebral palsy. *Disabil Rehabil*, 26, 1354–9.

Emerson E, Hatton C, Llewellyn G, Blacker J & Graham H (2006) Socio-economic position, household composition, health status and indicators of the well-being of mothers of children with and without intellectual disabilities. *J Intellect Disabil Res*, 50, 862–73.

Gevir G, Goldstand S, Weintraub N & Parush S. (2006) A comparison of time use of mothers with and without disabilities. *Occup Ther J Res*, 26, 117–29.

Green SE (2007) "We're tired not sad": benefits and burdens of mothering a child with a disability. *Soc Sci Med*, 64, 150–63.

Green SE (2001) Oh, those therapists will become your best friends: maternal satisfaction with clinics providing physical, occupational therapy and speech therapy services to children with disabilities. *Soc Health Illness*, 23, 796–829.

Green SE (2002) Mothering Amanda: musings on the experience of raising a child with cerebral palsy. *J Loss Trauma*, 7, 21–34.

Green SE (2003) What do you mean 'what's wrong with her?': stigma in the lives of families of children with disabilities. *Soc Sci Med*, 37, 1361–74.

Kersh J, Hedvat TT, Hauser-Cram P & Warfield ME (2006) The contribution of marital quality to the well-being of parents of children with developmental disabilities. *J Intellect Disabil Res*, 50, 883–93.

Law M, Hanna S, King G, Hurley P, King S, Kertoy M & Rosenbaum P (2003) Factors affecting family-centred service delivery for children with disabilities. *Child Care Health Dev*, 29, 357–66.

Law M, Finkelman S, Hurley P, Rosenbaum P, King S, King G & Hanna S (2004) Participation of children with physical disabilites: relationships with diagnosis, physical function and demographic variables. *Scand J Occup Ther*, 11: 156–62.

Llewellyn G, Thompson K & Whybrow S (2004). Activism as a mothering occupation. In: Esdaile S & Olson J (eds) *Mothering Occupations: Challenge, Agency, and Participation*: 282–305. Philadelphia: FA Davis Company.

Lukemeyer A, Meyers MK & Smeeding T (2000) Expensive children in poor families: out of pocket expenditures for the care of disabled and chronically ill children in welfare families. *J Marriage Fam*, 62, 399–415.

McGuire B, Crowe T, Law M & VanLeit B (2004) Mothers of children with disabilities: occupational concerns and solutions. *Occup Ther J Res*, 24, 54–63.

Meester-Delver A, Beelen A, Hennekam R, Hadders-Algra M & Nollet F (2006) Predicting additional care in young children with neurodevelopmental disability: a systematic literature review. *Dev Med Child Neurol*, 48, 143–50.

Nelson A (2002) A metasynthesis: mothering other-than-normal children. *Qual Health Res*, 12, 515–30.

Odding E, Roebreck ME & Stam H (2006) The epidemiology of cerebral palsy: incidence, impairments and risk factors. *Disabil Rehabil*, 18, 183–91.

Palisano R, Snider LM & Orlin MN (2004). Recent advances in physical and occupational therapy for children with cerebral palsy. *Semin Pediatr Neurol*, 11, 66–77.

Parish SL & Cloud JM (2006). Financial well being of young children with disabilities and their families. *Soc Work*, 51, 223–32.

Park J, Turnball AP & Turnball HR (2002) Impacts of poverty on quality of life in families of children with disabilities. *Except Child*, 68, 151–70.

Powers E (2003) Children's Health and maternal work activity: estimates under alternative disability definitions. *J Human Resources*, 3, 522–56.

Raina P, O'Donnell M, Rosenbaum P, Brehaut J, Walter SD, Russell D, Swinton M, Zhu B & Wood E (2005) The health and wellbeing of caregivers of children with cerebral palsy. *Pediatrics*, 115, 626–36.

Rosenbaum P, King S, Law M, King G & Evans J. (1998). Family-centred services: a conceptual framework and research review. *Phys Occ Ther in Peds*, 18, 1–20.

Singer GHS (2006) Meta-Analysis of comparative studies of depression in mothers of children with and without developmental disabilities. *Am J Ment Retard*, 111, 155–69.

Stok A, Harvey D & Reddihough D (2006) Percieved stress, perceived social support, and well being among mothers of school aged children with cerebral palsy. *J Intellect Dev Disabil*, 31, 53–7.

Thyen U, Kuhlthau K & Perrin JM. (1999). Employment, child care and mental health of mothers caring for children assisted by technology. *Pediatrics*,103, 1235–42.

Tong HC, Kandala G, Haig AJ, Nelson VS, Yamakawa KS & Shin KY (2002) Physical functioing in female caregivers of children with physical disabilities compared with female caregivers of children with a chronic medical condition. *Arch Pediatr Adolesc Med*, 156, 1138–42.

Tuna H, Unalan H, Tuna F & Kokino S (2004) Quality of life of primary caregivers of children with cerebral palsy: a controlled study with Short Form-36 questionnaire. *Dev Med Child Neurol*, 46, 646–8.

Chapter 4

Overview of therapy

Karen Dodd, Christine Imms and Nicholas F Taylor

Introduction

This chapter includes brief summaries and descriptions of

- general therapeutic approaches;
- therapeutic interventions more commonly used by occupational therapists and physiotherapists; and
- common medical and surgical procedures for people with cerebral palsy in which physiotherapists and occupational therapists may be involved in providing complementary care.

This chapter does not include descriptions of all therapeutic interventions for people with cerebral palsy. The interventions selected are those with evidence supporting their effectiveness or those that are more commonly practised. Although many of the interventions are appropriate for both children and adults, some were specifically developed for, and only have research evidence relating to, children. The case-based chapters that follow in Parts 2, 3 and 4 expand upon some of the topics introduced in this chapter, providing practical examples of the clinical application of the interventions described. The therapeutic approaches in this chapter are grouped under the three headings 'general approaches to therapy', 'therapeutic interventions' and 'common medical and surgical procedures'. Both 'therapeutic interventions' and 'common medical and surgical procedures' are listed and described in alphabetical order.

General therapeutic approaches

A problem-based clinical reasoning approach

This book has adopted a problem-based approach to planning therapeutic intervention using clinical assessment and reasoning. The model of clinical reasoning is described in Chapter 1 and forms the basis of the case studies described in Parts 2, 3 and 4 of the book. The eight steps of the intervention process model (Canadian Association of Occupational Therapists [CAOT], 2002) used by this book are as follows:

(1) collect initial data;
(2) identify and prioritize concerns;
(3) identify relevant theory;
(4) assess body function and structure, activity and/or participation;
(5) identify contextual factors;
(6) negotiate a management plan;
(7) implement the plan; and
(8) evaluate the outcomes.

One of the key factors underpinning our clinical reasoning approach is the importance of involving the person with cerebral palsy and their family in identifying concerns and negotiating the management plan (Steps 1, 2 and 6). Another key factor is use of an evidence-based approach that helps the clinician to take account of relevant theory and evidence from the literature (Step 3 of the model), and to choose relevant assessment procedures that have evidence of reliability and validity (Steps 4 and 8 of the model). One consequence of taking a person and family-centred approach to therapy within a rigorous clinical reasoning process is that interdisciplinary teamwork and consultation are emphasized.

Although it is recognized that physiotherapy and occupational therapy professions have discipline-based approaches to therapy, we have not attempted to highlight these in the case-based chapters. For example, the occupational approach that is embedded within occupational therapy is supported by at least two theoretical models with growing bodies of evidence to support them: the Canadian Model of Occupational Performance (CAOT, 2002; Townsend and Polatajko, 2007) and the Model of Human Occupation (Kielhofner, 2008). The model of clinical reasoning presented in this book is based on that developed within the Canadian Model of Occupational Performance, and the individual and family-focused approach is compatible with key elements within the Model of Human Occupation, including recognition of the importance of the personal values and goals and the individual's desire or will to engage in activity: their volition (Case-Smith, 2005; Cahill and Kielhofner, 2008). Occupational therapists using the approach outlined in this book will continue to embed their reasoning within an occupation-based paradigm that recognizes the relationship between occupation and health (Wilcock et al 1997; Wilcock, 1998, Townsend and Polatajko, 2007; Kielhofner, 2008,). Thus occupational therapists will continue to focus on how the individual with cerebral palsy can engage in the occupations they need to, want to or have to do, across the many spheres of their lives. Therefore, occupational therapists may use the interventions described in the book as they focus on engagement in school, play and recreation, self-care, work, relationship or community occupations of importance to the individual within the context of their life stage and goals.

Named approaches

Traditionally, a number of named approaches have been advocated for the management of people with cerebral palsy. A difficulty for the clinician is that the common named approaches have adherents yet there is little or no evidence that any of these approaches is superior to another (Mayston, 2004). Another challenge is that these named approaches evolve over time, and may look different at different stages of their evolution despite retaining the same name. Although all approaches use elements of clinical reasoning, a key point of difference is that each of the traditional approaches begins with a theoretical construct, whereas the problem-based clinical reasoning approach used in the book starts with collection of data and evidence through the assessment process. What follows is a brief overview of the most common named approaches to management of people with cerebral palsy.

THE BOBATH APPROACH (NEURODEVELOPMENTAL THERAPY)

The Bobath approach was introduced in the UK in the 1940s and is known as neurodevelopmental therapy (NDT) in some countries. This approach emphasizes the importance of trying to normalize muscle tone and repeating more typical movement patterns as the basis for developing effective movement (Bobath and Bobath, 1984). Therapists use handling, positioning and guiding or facilitating movement to normalize tone and promote optimal participation. A goal of therapy is for the person with cerebral palsy to work actively towards what they can do with little help. These techniques are taught to parents and carers so that they can be used to carry out activities of daily living. The emphasis on positioning and handling is often valued by families. One difficulty with evaluating the approach is that it is not always clear what the Bobath approach really is because it has been adapted by clinicians over time and from person to person and there is considerable variability among proponents about the extent to which other approaches should be incorporated into therapy. Two well-conducted systematic reviews found no strong evidence that the Bobath approach, or NDT, is effective in the management of people with cerebral palsy (Brown and Burns, 2001; Butler and Darrah, 2001). A more recent very small randomized controlled trial showed some support for the value of neurodevelopmental-based trunk co-activation to improve postural control and gross motor skills in infants with posture and movement dysfunction (Arndt et al, 2008).

CONDUCTIVE EDUCATION (PETO)

Conductive education was developed in Hungary in the 1940s (Hari and Tillemans, 1984). Conductive education is usually carried out within group educational settings with a focus on promoting independence. The fundamental philosophy of this approach is that movement problems are viewed as problems of learning. Therefore, proponents argue a learning process should be used to develop independence to the best of the child's ability, without emphasizing movement quality. In therapy a major focus is placed on the child's initiation, practice and participation in daily activities.

Simple plinths, ladder-backed chairs and orthoses are the only equipment used in therapy. Like the Bobath approach, one of the difficulties with evaluating conductive education is that it has been adapted by clinicians over time and from person to person and there is considerable variability among clinicians about the extent to which other approaches should be incorporated into therapy. Effectiveness has been evaluated in four systematic reviews (French and Nommensen, 1992; Ludwig et al, 2000; Pedersen, 2000; Darrah et al, 2004). The overall conclusions of these reviews agree that the number of studies to have evaluated the effectiveness of conductive education is too small, and the quality of those that have been completed is too low, to make conclusions about the effectiveness or lack of effectiveness of conductive education.

OTHER NAMED APPROACHES
There are a number of other lesser known approaches that have been popular such as sensory integration, Vojta and Doman Delacato. Interested readers might find Mayston's (2004) update on treatment approaches a useful summary of other named approaches to therapy for people with cerebral palsy.

Therapeutic interventions

Adaptive equipment and assistive technology
Provision of equipment to enable people to access and use their social and physical environments effectively is a critical component of therapy for many people with cerebral palsy. Technological solutions are most commonly employed to assist people with communication, mobility and to control elements of their environment. Physiotherapists and occupational therapists are likely to be integral to the prescription of mobility and environmental control equipment and assistive technology. For communication systems, they are likely to work closely with speech pathologists when physical impairments place restrictions on the way communication devices are operated. Selection and training in the use of specialized equipment requires knowledge of the individual's goals and desires in regard to the use of the equipment and his or her capacities, as well as regularly updated information on the range of technical solutions available. In addition, therapists will be involved in assisting people with cerebral palsy and their families to access funding to support the purchase of the equipment (see Chapters 12 and 15 for examples).

Many devices are operated by single switches or joysticks and therapists will be involved in selecting appropriate switches and training people in their use. Training of the young child or a child with a cognitive impairment begins with learning simple cause and effect, which can be trained using switch-operated toys and simple computer games. Training using more complex switches and joysticks can also be facilitated through computer games and toys as well as with the equipment that it is intended to operate. The selection of the assistive technology (e.g. type of communication aid, environmental control) is usually based on the cognitive abilities of the individual whereas the device that operates the equipment (e.g. design of single or multiple switch, joystick) is based on hand function. When it is not possible to use the hand alternative body parts such as the leg, head or eyes may be used (Lidstrom and Borgestig, 2008). Selection of the device to control communication systems is critical; if only simple single switch operation is possible the speed and complexity of communication is impacted (Lidstrom and Borgestig, 2008).

ENVIRONMENTAL CONTROL
Environmental controls range from simple low-technology solutions such as reaching sticks to push light switches on or off, to high-technology computerized systems that allow independent control of communication devices, heating and cooling systems, televisions, music systems and telephones through single or multiple switch technology. Microchip technology is a rapidly advancing field and applications that solve complex problems for people with disabilities are constantly emerging. A range of organizations that support the provision of technical solutions, such as the independent living centres (e.g. http://www.ilcaustralia.org/home/default.asp), and technical aids for disabled people (e.g. http://www.technicalaidnsw.org.au/About/tadaust.php), are available in many Western countries.

MOBILITY ASSISTIVE DEVICES
A key indicator of gross motor function for people with cerebral palsy is the way they move about their home, at school and in their community. The usual performance of mobility forms the basis of the Gross Motor Function Classification System (GMFCS) (Palisano et al, 1997, 2008, see Chapter 2). The main discriminators between different levels of the GMFCS are whether the person with cerebral palsy walks with an assistive device or not, or whether they usually mobilize with a wheelchair or not. As well as variability in mobility methods between different levels of the GMFCS, there is also considerable variability within each of the GMFCS levels depending on the environmental context. For example, people in GMFCS level III walk with assistive devices but have difficulty walking outdoors and in the community. Their most common methods of getting about (for children aged 4 to 12 years) is to move about the floor at home, walk with an assistive device at school and to be pushed in a wheelchair when out in the community (Palisano et al, 2003).

Common mobility assistive devices to aid walking include simple canes, forearm crutches, frames and gait trainers. Walking frames come in a wide variety of shapes and forms. There is evidence that the use of a reverse walker (often called a K-walker), which is open at the front and pulled behind, can result in a more upright posture and more energy-efficient walking for children with cerebral palsy, compared with the standard walking frame that is pushed in front (Park et al, 2001). Reverse walkers will often include a mechanism to prevent the frame wheeling backwards away from the person, and can include a range of additional attachments to ensure optimal grip and hip alignment (Thompson-Rangel et al, 1992). One disadvantage of walkers for adolescents and adults with cerebral palsy is that mobility can be limited in confined spaces and steps and stairs cannot be negotiated safely. If independent walking is maintained, the use of single-point forearm crutches is encouraged. Axillary crutches are not appropriate for people with cerebral palsy because of the tendency to lean on the crutch, and because it is difficult to use the hands independently while using the crutch.

Gait trainers are wheeled and framed mobility devices that enable the child with cerebral palsy who is unable to walk to explore their environment in an upright position while providing support even if totally relaxed. Although families often initially view these devices with some enthusiasm, they do not appear to provide therapeutic benefit, and there are safety concerns with their use (Miller, 2005).

Many people with cerebral palsy use wheelchairs to move about. Wheelchairs can be self-propelled, pushed by someone else or be battery powered. The most common way of getting around in the community for children at GMFCS levels III and IV is to be pushed in a wheelchair, with the use of self-propelled wheelchairs and battery powered wheelchairs much less common (Palisano et al, 2003). Multiple factors must be considered when prescribing a wheelchair and expert advice is required to navigate through the choices available. Decisions about the appropriate wheelchair base, frame, seating system, footplate system and trunk and head supports are required. These components will vary according to the functional ability status and age of the person (Miller, 2005). For example, a person with independent walking mobility will require a wheelchair with footrests that flip away to enable transfer to standing and the provision of a crutch holder.

Powered wheelchairs offer the potential for independent mobility for people who are otherwise dependent, but are only appropriate if there is sufficient motor ability, eyesight and cognitive ability to operate the wheelchair safely (Miller, 2005). In addition, contextual factors such as expense and potential difficulties in transportation mean that the decision to use a powered wheelchair is complex and has long-term consequences.

Behaviour management
Recent research has highlighted the relatively high proportion of children with cerebral palsy who present with behaviour problems (Carlsson et al, 2008; Parkes et al, 2008). Therapists require skills in day-to-day management of children's behaviour in therapy as well as in providing support to families and children where significant behavioural difficulties arise (Case-Smith, 2005; Crepeau et al, 2009). Day-to-day management of behaviour in therapy is embedded within the development of a positive therapeutic relationship and requires planning and ongoing clinical reasoning throughout each session. Better behaviour in therapy tends to occur when sessions are well planned. Planning involves determining the structure of the session, grading tasks so the 'just right challenge' is embedded within the session, having a clear beginning and end to tasks and using appropriate prompts and cues to guide the child's responses. During the session, instructions that are clearly articulated at the level of the child's understanding, and feedback that is concrete and specific (e.g. 'good – you looked at the target before throwing the ball', rather than, 'good throw') will help a child stay focused. Clear and specific praise tells the child exactly what they did right so that they can do it again.

Unwanted behaviours are more likely to occur when children do not know what is expected of them, when the task seems never-ending or is too hard or too easy, and when sessions or components of the session are unstructured. Unstructured time often happens when transitioning between activities, so careful preparation and set up is important. Providing children with verbal or visual reminders of the session's activities can assist them to remain focused. Behaviour can break down during a session for many reasons, including fatigue, frustration or anxiety, poor attention or when a child does not know what is expected. Recognizing potential triggers to unwanted behaviour and the body language or actions that forewarn of the impending problem (e.g. yawning, slouching in the chair, looking distracted, fidgeting or rushing through a task) provides the therapist with the opportunity to respond quickly to circumvent behaviour breakdown by changing the task, taking a break, or re-grading the activity difficulty level. Many children have difficulty maintaining their attention and although a distraction-free environment may not be available, removing unnecessary distracters, using the child's name, getting down to their level and providing only one instruction at a time when the child is looking at you, are useful strategies. Sometimes careful use of concrete rewards, such as toys, stickers or access to a favourite activity is a useful motivator within a session or can be used when the therapist observes the child behaving well.

For some children with cerebral palsy psychosocial difficulties are more problematic and therapists may be involved in providing therapy specifically aimed at promoting social competence, self-efficacy and coping skills (Case-Smith, 2005; Kramer and Hinojosa, 2009). Psychosocial approaches to therapy aim to promote positive behaviour, social competence and coping through enhancing the fit between the environment and child. Therapists working within a psychosocial frame of reference may assist families and other service providers in understanding the cause of disruptive behaviour, develop collaborative goals and behavioural management strategies as well as introduce social or life skills groups or other forms of therapy. Where there are significant behaviour problems, families and children may benefit from a referral to a psychologist or paediatric mental health service. In addition, there are resources for both parents and professionals available through programmes such as the *Triple P: Positive Parenting Program* (http://www1.triplep.net/). This site provides books and DVDs for parents, including specific resources for families who have a child with a disability, and information on training programmes for professionals who work with children.

Bimanual upper extremity training
Traditional therapeutic intervention aims to improve a child's ability to use their hands together, especially when children have unilateral impairment or hemiplegia. Little research has focused exclusively on investigating the effectiveness of bimanual interventions, or identified specific intervention strategies and training practices that promote bimanual hand function. However, practice of activities and tasks requiring bilateral hand use is a routine element of therapy (Kaplan and Bedell, 1999; Eliasson, 2007). Charles and Gordon (2006) have developed a bimanual intervention for children with hemiplegia named Hand Arm Bimanual Intensive Training (HABIT). The

principles of the training emerged following the authors' investigation of constraint-induced movement therapy (CIMT) where they proposed that the intensive practice used in CIMT might be the most important element. Hand Arm Bimanual Intensive Training involves providing intensive practice (6 hours per day) of bimanual activities for children with hemiplegia. The choice of activities practised is dependent on the child's movement deficits and the training includes part-task or movement practice as well as whole-task practice. Early results from a small randomized controlled trial have shown promise, with improved quality and frequency of bimanual hand use after implementation of the HABIT protocol (Gordon et al, 2007).

Sheppard et al (2007) have also recently reported on a single-subject design study that investigated the effectiveness of bilateral isokinematic training (BIT) for children with hemiplegia. Sheppard et al's work emerged from early studies of BIT for adults following stroke. The key premise of BIT involves pairing the actions of the impaired upper extremity with the unimpaired upper extremity by having both limbs undertake symmetrical, rhythmical and repetitive movements. Further research evidence is required to support the effectiveness of BIT.

Casts, splints and orthotic applications
Casts, splints, and orthoses are devices designed to hold specific body parts in a particular position. For people with cerebral palsy, casts, splints and orthoses are applied for the following reasons:

- to prevent or correct contractures;
- to provide a base of support;
- to facilitate skills training;
- to reduce spasticity;
- to improve the efficacy of walking or other movements (Condie and Meadows, 1995).

Casts, splints and orthoses are usually used in combination with management strategies such as orthopaedic surgery, anti-spasticity medication and other therapeutic interventions.

Casts, splints, and orthoses work by applying forces to the body. By encompassing parts of the body and preventing movement, muscles and the periarticular structures can be stretched. Many muscles cross two joints (e.g. some of the calf muscles cross both the ankle and knee). To exert a stretch, either the device must hold both joints, or activities that stretch the unfixed joint are encouraged.

Casts are usually made of plaster of Paris, fibreglass or other synthetic material wraps and are designed to fix a limb or limb segment in place. They may be solid or bi-valved (that is, cut in half down the length of the cast to enable the cast to be removed for periods of time). Casts are usually applied for between 2 and 6 weeks. Sometimes they are removed and adjusted to increase the stretch on muscles as the muscles lengthen. This is called serial casting (Teplicky et al, 2003).

The terms *splint* and *orthosis* may be used interchangeably and are typically constructed of low or high temperature thermoplastic material, and wire, leather, Velcro and elastic as needed for the dynamic components or the straps and fasteners. Splints and orthoses may be static or dynamic in their construction and thus used to fix a limb segment or to facilitate movement of a limb segment. The term *splint* usually refers to devices made out of plastics that can be heated and moulded directly onto the body. They can be produced quickly; however, the plastic is often relatively weak. Lower limb splints, therefore, are usually only recommended when the device is needed for a short time (e.g. after surgery), or when there will be little force placed on the material (Teplicky et al, 2003). The term *orthosis* typically refers to custom-made, high-temperature thermoplastic devices that are moulded on plaster models of the client's body. Orthoses are more durable, are used for longer than splints (Teplicky et al, 2003) and are more commonly provided for the lower limb than the upper limb.

Lower limb casts, splints and orthoses can provide stability to help children stand and walk. For example, ankle–foot orthoses (AFOs) can provide a stable base for standing and walking (Morris, 2007). Some splints and orthoses directly influence the alignment of the body segments supported by the device and they can affect lower limb movements, which can lead to more efficient walking patterns. Lower limb devices can also stabilize a part of the body while training is focused on developing other components of a movement or posture (Morris, 2007). For example, if a cast is used to stabilize the ankle joints of a person with cerebral palsy then the therapist could work on strengthening hip and knee extension in standing with the aim of improving upright stance.

There are two key premises underlying the decision to provide an upper limb splint for a child with cerebral palsy: one is biomechanical and the other neurophysiological. The biomechanical rationale for splinting includes promoting joint alignment, providing a long slow stretch to muscles with the goal of minimizing muscle shortening and subsequent joint deformity, and promoting adaptive changes in soft tissues, with the ultimate aim of improving limb position to facilitate functional ability. The neurophysiological rationale relates to the provision of splints to reduce muscle tone or inhibit movement patterns. Although commonly used for people with cerebral palsy there is only a small amount of evidence that splinting can increase passive range in children with cerebral palsy (Autti-Ramo et al, 2006). There is some evidence that the application of a static night splint following botulinum toxin A (BoNT-A) injection in the upper limb assists with maintaining gains made as measured using the Quality of Upper Extremity Skills Test (Kanellopoulos et al, 2009).

Custom-made upper extremity splints include low-temperature thermoplastic resting hand splints for overnight wear to maintain muscle length and provide joint alignment (see example in Chapter 11). Dynamic splints such as neoprene (wetsuit material) thumb abductor wraps are designed to provide a line of pull against mildly spastic thenar muscles and facilitate an open hand for grasp. Although commonly recommended (Granhaug, 2006), there is no research supporting their effectiveness. Lycra garments may be applied to the full body or a body part and are intended to provide dynamic stability by reducing muscle tone and involuntary movements (Nicholson et al, 2001) (see example in Chapter 12). There is little evidence of the effectiveness of Lycra garments, with the few small studies conducted reporting equivocal results (Nicholson et al, 2001; Corn et al, 2003).

Cognitive orientation to daily occupational performance
Originally developed for children with developmental coordination disorder (DCD), cognitive orientation to daily occupational performance (CO-OP) is based on contemporary dynamic systems theories, learning theory and client-centred practice (Polatajko et al, 2001; Mandich et al, 2008). The underlying premise is that the child can learn and use cognitive strategies to enable the learning of activities or tasks that are meaningful and important to the child. As the child learns a global cognitive strategy that is not task-dependent, this intervention promotes transfer and generalization of the strategies required to learn new skills. The process involves eliciting from the child their goal and evaluating the baseline skill to identify what is preventing the successful performance of the task. The child is taught the following global cognitive strategy:

- goal (what do I want to achieve?);
- plan (how will I do it?);
- do (the execution of my plan);
- check (did I follow my plan and did it work?) (Missiuna et al, 2001; Polatajko and Mandich, 2004).

The four steps of the global strategy describe the process the child uses when learning any new task. While learning the desired task, the child is helped to discover specific strategies that solve the problems he or she has with achieving the task. These are called domain specific strategies and may include the use of verbal self-guidance (talking yourself through the task), feeling the movement (attending to the sensation of the movement required) or positioning the body in preparation for a task.

The therapist teaches and reinforces the global strategy throughout therapy, and guides the child to discover for themselves the specific strategies that will enable them to learn their task. Transfer and generalization of task performance and strategy use are promoted throughout the intervention period which is typically 10 weeks (Polatajko and Mandich, 2004). There is emerging evidence of the effectiveness of CO-OP for children with DCD to improve performance of tasks important to the child, and early research describing its use with children with acquired brain injuries (Missiuna, 2006). Currently there is no evidence describing CO-OP's use for children with cerebral palsy, although a pilot study is reported to be under way (Mandich et al, 2008). Conceptually, the intervention holds significant promise. However, because it is a cognitive-based therapy, language and cognitive abilities will influence its successful application and not all tasks will be achievable for people with cerebral palsy. The intervention is applicable for children as young as 3–4 years through to adults.

Constraint-induced movement therapy

Constraint-induced movement therapy (CIMT) has emerged from animal research and subsequent research with adults after stroke (Taub, 1980; Taub et al, 1999). Constraint-induced movement therapy is an upper extremity intervention designed to promote functional use of a hemiplegic or more-impaired arm. Theoretical premises include the notion of a learned non-use of the impaired upper extremity and the need for massed practice to overcome this non-use (Morris and Taub, 2001). In children, learned non-use is theoretically not the same as in adults because children with congenital disabilities do not have underlying motor abilities/behaviours to uncover, but rather must learn new tasks. For this reason, the term developmental disregard has been coined for children (DeLuca, 2002). Regardless of the term, the non-use is thought to be due to behavioural shaping. In other words, the child learns that the hemiplegic limb is not an effective object stabilizer or manipulator and through negative reinforcement gained with failed attempts, gradually learns to ignore the impaired arm and perform most daily activities unilaterally with the more functional limb.

The CIMT intervention is based on two key principles: constraint of the unimpaired upper extremity and intensive practice of the impaired limb. In the paediatric research literature constraint of the limb has been provided in many ways including long or short arm casts, slings, hand splints, mitts or therapist restraint of the limb (Hoare et al, 2007). The length of time the constraint is applied has varied considerably from 24 hours per day to 1 hour. The practice schedule is also variable across studies, ranging from a highly intensive practice schedule of 6 hours per day for 2 weeks (DeLuca, 2002), to 2 hours per day for 8 weeks (Eliasson et al, 2005), to twice weekly therapy for 4 weeks (Naylor and Bower, 2005). Therapy within the practice periods typically is one of two types: behavioural shaping of movement or task practice without shaping. The high variability in provision of this therapy has led to the following three distinct terms:

- CIMT involving constraint and practise for more than 3 hours per day for at least 2 weeks;
- modified CIMT, involving constraint and practice for less than 3 hours per day over 2 months; and
- forced use where only the constraint is applied and no additional therapy is provided.

A systematic review found that the emerging evidence was as supportive of modified CIMT as it was of CIMT with the evidence for forced use compromised by methodological limitations (Hoare et al, 2007). Modified constraint therapy is further described in Chapter 7.

Fitness training

Contemporary therapeutic programmes for adults and children with cerebral palsy often include fitness training. The benefits of fitness training for everyone including people with cerebral palsy include improved cardiovascular functioning, control of body weight and preservation of bone mass (Rimmer, 2005). Fitness training, also known as aerobic training, can therefore help to prevent the long-term health consequences of inactivity to which people with cerebral palsy are susceptible because of the difficulty they often have with movement. Fitness training can be defined as any activity that increases heart rate at a level sufficient to result in physiological change. Adults with disabilities, who are able to, should undertake at least 150 minutes a week of moderate intensity, or 75 minutes a week of vigorous intensity aerobic activity, or an equivalent combination of moderate and vigorous intensity aerobic activity. Aerobic activity should be performed in episodes of at least 10 minutes, and should be spread throughout the week. When possible, children and adolescents with disabilities should also meet these guidelines (US Department of Health & Human Services, 2008).

Fitness training activities for people with cerebral palsy include group exercise classes (including circuit type exercises), brisk walking, swimming and cycling. An additional benefit of fitness training for people with cerebral palsy is that many fitness activities take place in a community setting thereby promoting community inclusion. Despite the clear rationale, fitness training for people with cerebral palsy has rarely been evaluated. A systematic review identified only four studies of reasonable quality, with a combined sample of 58 participants ranging in age from 7 to 22 years completing programmes of duration ranging from 6 weeks to 12 months (Bar-Or et al, 1976; Dresen et al, 1985; van den Berg-Emons et al, 1998; Rogers et al, 2008). These studies provide preliminary evidence that fitness training in young people with cerebral palsy can improve aerobic fitness, and can have a positive effect on body composition, but little is known about the effect of these changes on broader measures of activity and participation.

Functional electrical stimulation
Functional electrical stimulation (FES) is the electrical stimulation of muscles lacking neurological control with the aim of improving useful motor performance (Sujith, 2008). As well as improving motor performance while being stimulated, it has been suggested that FES can lead to long-term benefits through improving muscle strength (Rushton, 2003) and central changes through cortical reorganization in the brain (Liepert et al, 2000).

Much of the literature reports on FES as applied to people with spinal cord injuries and hemiplegia after stroke (Sujith, 2008). Relatively few trials have investigated FES for children with cerebral palsy, and those trials have been characterized by very small sample sizes and non-randomized designs. However, there is some preliminary evidence that FES can lead to immediate benefits in the gait kinematics of children with diplegic and hemiplegic cerebral palsy, such as improved swing phase dorsiflexion and improved initial contact during the gait cycle (Orlin et al, 2005; Postans and Granat, 2005). A trial of FES on eight children with hemiplegic cerebral palsy reported that a daily 30 minute practice session with FES to the affected wrist extensors over 6 weeks led to some sustained improvements in hand function (Wright and Granat, 2000). A recent randomized controlled trial reported that using FES for 8 weeks resulted in immediate benefits, but no long-term benefits compared with controls (Van der Linden et al, 2008).

Most FES systems apply electrical pulses ranging from 20 to 50 Hz, with a pulse width of about 300 µs through surface or percutaneous intramuscular electrodes. One of the problems of FES with current stimulation regimens is that muscles can fatigue very quickly, and children do not always tolerate the intensity of stimulation required. For example, in one of the cerebral palsy trials (Postans and Granat, 2005) 6 of 21 eligible participants were excluded because they did not tolerate electrical stimulation. Another difficulty is that the stimulated movement may not be strong enough to overcome spasticity in the antagonistic muscle group, or the movement may be prevented by joint contractures.

Goal-directed training

Goal-directed training is an activity-based intervention aimed at increasing a client's ability to engage successfully in meaningful daily tasks. The theoretical premise is based on contemporary motor learning theory and dynamic systems theory where motor behaviour is understood to be influenced by factors within the environment, the person and the occupation/task. Four components provide the basis for goal-directed training:

- selection of a meaningful goal;
- analysis of baseline performance;
- intervention/practice regimen; and
- evaluation of outcome (Mastos et al, 2007).

Analysis of baseline performance must include evaluation of the adaptability of the environment and the structure of the task prior to considering the specific client-related personal elements that limit performance. This analysis is conceptually similar to the dynamic performance analysis used within CO-OP. Practice is structured using the principles of motor learning. These include task structure (for example, adaptation of the sequence of the task, equipment, timing or setting), feedback to the client about performance and results (feedback can originate within the client or be provided externally) and frequent repetition (practice of the task). There is evidence that children with cerebral palsy require many repetitions to learn motor skills (Valvano and Newell, 1998; Gordon and Duff, 1999) and therapists and clients need to find ways of ensuring sufficient practice. The intervention is designed so that the client is engaged in the process of solving the problems inherent within their own motor system (Mastos et al, 2007).

The structure of the practice opportunities is adapted depending on the client's stage of motor learning (Fitts and Posner, 1967). The verbal-cognitive stage is where the task or strategies to perform the task are learned; the motor stage is where the task is performed but practice is required to improve the quality of performance; and the autonomous stage is where the task can be performed with consistency and little attention. This intervention is suitable for clients of all ages and abilities, although clients with significant impairments (either cognitive or physical) may not reach the autonomous stage of motor learning (Mastos et al, 2007). Goal-directed training of functional tasks has been shown to be effective for children with cerebral palsy in attainment of meaningful goals and improved self-care and mobility as measured by the Pediatric Evaluation of Disability Inventory (Ketelaar et al, 2001; Ekström et al, 2005). Goal-directed training is further described in Chapter 8.

Handwriting intervention
Intervention for poor handwriting, or to support the acquisition of handwriting skills, is often required for children in MACS levels I and II (DuBois et al, 2004). Children at higher MACS levels may require alternate or augmentative communication devices, including computers for word processing (Murchland et al, 2008). Elements that are required for efficient handwriting include those related to language and symbol reproduction – knowledge of the alphabet, commonly used words and an ability to recall these as needed – as well as the motor elements that support reproduction of legible letters, words and sentences. Handwriting has been taught for generations, but our understanding of how the required elements contribute to handwriting production is incomplete. The gaps in our knowledge affect how remediation is implemented when children have difficulty gaining skills in this area (Ziviani and Wallen, 2006).

Handwriting is a complex skill requiring smooth interaction and coordination between visual, perceptual, cognitive and motor functions. Murchland et al (2008) describe the following four key areas in which cerebral palsy may interfere with handwriting production:

- postural control;
- tool use and fine motor control;
- vision and visual-perceptual skills; and
- cognition, attention and organizational skills.

Therapy for handwriting must include a blend of teaching the rules and procedures for handwriting while assisting the child to find opportunities for practice (Ziviani and Wallen, 2006). Practice is important for all children when learning this complex skill. For children with cerebral palsy the amount of practice needed is likely to be much greater, and skilled therapists will provide learning situations that facilitate the child in learning how they will perform this task and then provide frequent opportunity for practising. For children whose performance of handwriting continues to be highly laboured or illegible, investigation of alternative forms of written communication such as keyboarding are warranted. Computer word processing may facilitate the child's capacity to produce written work, although Ziviani and Wallen (2006) caution that learning the skills of, and becoming proficient in, keyboarding will also require considerable practice.

Home programmes
Home programmes are commonly recommended by therapists and are designed to provide therapeutic activities in the home environment, supervised by parents (Novak et al, 2007). Therapists recommend home programmes to maximize the effect of therapy or in some cases to take the place of therapy when resources are limited

(Novak and Cusick, 2006; Novak et al, 2007). Novak and Cusick (2006) developed a home programme model that they subsequently tested, demonstrating that carefully designed home programmes that address child- and family-centred goals are effective for children with cerebral palsy (Novak et al, 2007; Novak et al, 2009). The model, which is embedded with family-centred care, includes five phases of intervention and describes key inputs and desired outcomes of each phase. The phases are as follows:

- develop a collaborative relationship;
- set mutually agreed goals;
- select therapeutic activities;
- support implementation; and
- evaluate outcomes (Novak and Cusick, 2006: p. 260).

In addition to home programmes that are designed to replace face-to-face therapy, other interventions include home programmes to facilitate the outcomes of therapy. For example modified CIMT or goal-directed training both require intensive practice of skills at home or in the community as well as in specific therapy sessions. It is important to emphasize that people with cerebral palsy need to practise new or emerging skills, and carefully negotiated home programmes that focus on one or two desired goals and identify activity ideas and strategies for practice are one way of enhancing learning opportunities. Home programmes can also be used to embed therapeutic techniques into daily caregiving. This is particularly important in relation to the positioning and handling of young children to maximize positive interactions with their environments (Bower, 2009). Home programmes are used in many of the case-based chapters of this book – see example in Chapter 7.

Learning to play and learning through play
Play is one of the primary occupations of childhood and playfulness and engagement in play, recreation and leisure pursuits continue throughout life. Blanche and Knox (2008) describe how cerebral palsy can impact on the form, function and meaning of play with important consequences for a child's development. The form of play includes how children manage objects and space and the type of play in which they engage, for example, solitary or onlooker play. The function of play relates to its purpose; play is a mechanism through which children learn social roles and develop cognitive and motor skills. The meaning of play relates to the individual's experience of the play, whether they enjoy it and the level of intrinsic motivation for play (Blanche and Knox, 2008). Play is a complex phenomenon that is difficult to define (Parham and Primeau, 1997), because what is considered playful for one person may be considered work for another. In addition, the same individual may consider an activity play or work within different circumstances thus influencing their intrinsic motivation for the activity.

The impairments associated with cerebral palsy can influence the form of play in which the child engages, and subsequently reduce the value of the play in terms of function and meaning for the child (Blanche and Knox, 2008). For paediatric health professionals, play is an important method for engaging children in therapy, and play activities can promote the child's physical, affective (i.e. emotional) and cognitive skills. For occupational therapists, it is critical to ensure that children develop play skills: working with children to promote pretend play, symbolic play, social and object play may be essential goals of therapy. A number of occupational therapy authors have contributed to our understanding of play, play assessment and intervention. This includes, for example Bundy's (2001) work on the Test of Playfulness, Takata's (1974) exposition of play epochs and Stagnitti and Unsworth's (2000) work on child-initiated pretend play. Children with cerebral palsy are at significant risk of reduced ability to develop motor, cognitive and affective skills through play, and of being unable to engage in play sufficiently to develop the skills required to be a successful player either individually or with others. The success or otherwise of play is described by Rigby and Roger (2006) as being dependent on the person–environment–occupation fit. This means that play is promoted in therapy through attention to elements with the environment (social, physical and cultural opportunities or constraints for play), the occupation (play object properties, play set up) and the child (skills, motivation, interest). By attending to each of these elements the therapist can identify where the child's motivation and skill levels lie, guide the selection of appropriate play objects and modify or select the environment as needed to facilitate the play experience and the development of play skills. This framework is applicable to children with cerebral palsy (see example in Chapter 7).

Parent/caregiver education and training
Most health care professionals working with children agree that educating and training the child's parents and other caregivers in the care process is essential and that doing this can also support the therapist to manage their young client's diverse physical, psychological, social and educational problems. Indeed, American survey data suggests that paediatric occupational therapists spend 60–70% of their time educating or training parents or caregivers (Hinojosa et al, 2002). Education and training can include provision of written or verbal information about services, cerebral palsy, intervention choices and techniques, as well as child-specific information such as assessment results. Organizational tools such as *The Kit: Keeping it Together* (available from CanChild http://canchild.ca/en/canchildresources/kityouthkit.asp) provide a mechanism for parents to collect and share information about their child and facilitate communication and interaction between differing agencies. Partnership between parents and service providers lies at the heart of family-centred practice emphasizing parents' joint role in planning, delivering and evaluating their child's health care services. The need for collaboration between health professionals and parents has received ample attention in the literature (Franck and Callery, 2004), with evidence to indicate that family-centred practice enhances outcomes for both children and their families (King et al, 2004).

Positioning and handling
Positioning and handling are core physical techniques primarily aimed at increasing a client's ability to engage safely and successfully in meaningful daily tasks. Occupational therapists and physiotherapists use these techniques, and teach them to parents and caregivers of clients with cerebral palsy, to assist in the performance of everyday tasks.

Positioning refers to activities in which a therapist carefully analyses a client's posture and movement deficits and then works to attain a posture for a client that optimizes their ability to perform everyday activities. Positioning is achieved using the therapist's body or by external devices such as splints and casts, or by specialist equipment or furniture (Colangelo, 1999). For example, to encourage play by a child with poor trunk control and balance in sitting because of hypotonia, the child may be positioned in a chair with a moulded back support, with a firm fitting seat belt across the hips. A stable tray or table in front assists with trunk control and allows the arms and hands to be used to assist with supporting the trunk. The position of the child should be such that their feet comfortably reach the floor with hips and knees in 90° of flexion. In this case, trunk support is largely provided by external equipment providing a stable platform (i.e. posture) from which the child can use their upper limbs to reach and manipulate toys or other objects.

Therapists also use positioning to encourage or assist clients to learn how to change positions by placing them in a posture from which they can more easily move, or be facilitated to move, to another posture. Prevention of secondary complications associated with cerebral palsy such as the development of contractures due to spasticity and general lack of movement is assisted by supporting postures that provide a prolonged stretch to muscles at risk. Positioning a child who has little independent movement in standing can reduce osteoporosis secondary to reduced weight bearing (Caulton et al, 2004; Ward et al, 2004).

Provision of specialist seating to support activity and participation is a key requirement for many people with cerebral palsy. Seating should be prescribed that meets the individual's needs and follows principles associated with management of hypertonia and postural abnormality, prevention of skin breakdown, promotion of visual–motor ability and reduction of pain and fatigue. Novak and Watson's (2005) training CD–ROM assists therapists to learn key principles of assessing abnormal posture and measuring for and prescribing seating. This valuable resource also demonstrates alternative seating solutions using a software wizard, provides case studies and has a quiz to check your learning: http://www.cpinstitute.com.au/publications/seating_positioning.htm.

Handling refers to the way therapists, parents or other caregivers touch and move a client. Handling usually involves specific and individualized strategies that maximize the client's own abilities to move, transfer or maintain a functional posture (Colangelo, 1999; Bower, 2009). Handling may also be used to help a client to learn how to move by providing physical assistance to key points on the body or during critical moments in a movement sequence. For example, for a young child learning to initiate rolling from supine to side-lying, the therapist might assist the movement of hip and knee flexion and early rotation of the trunk to initiate the required movement. Then, using toys or other encouragement, the therapist waits for the child to initiate and complete the remaining movement. Repetitive practice of the movement in relevant contexts, such as during nappy changes or when playing on the floor, encourages the child to learn the movement sequence necessary to achieve this functional activity independently.

Sensory retraining
Children with cerebral palsy are known to be at risk of reduced or altered tactile
sensation in both their dominant and non-dominant hands (Lesny et al, 1993; Cooper
et al, 1995; Eliasson et al, 1995; Arnould et al, 2007). Research has demonstrated
reduced proprioception, two-point discrimination and haptic perception, which is the
ability to retrieve, analyse and interpret tactile properties of objects including texture,
weight and size. In a systematic review, Odding, Roebroeck and Stam (2006) reported
that 44–51% of all children with cerebral palsy have impaired two-point discrimination
and stereognosis. Although it is well recognized that sensation plays a key role in
coordinated hand function, there is little evidence in the literature that sensory
retraining has come under investigation in people with cerebral palsy. Sensory re-
education for adults who have had a stroke is based on the concept of neural plasticity
and the premise that reorganization occurs with repeated use (Bentzel, 2008) and there
is evidence of the effectiveness of training in these adults (Carey and Matyas, 2005).
Theoretically, similar principles apply to children with congenital lesions suggesting that
intense training of tactile discrimination and stereognosis with graded progression,
feedback and repetitive practice might yield positive results. However, investigations of
neural organization of sensory functions in children with cerebral palsy suggest that not
all children are likely to benefit from sensory training (Guzetta et al, 2007). Which
children might benefit and the relationship between improved sensory function and
motor performance for children with varying sensory neural pathways is currently under
investigation.

Sensory processing and modulation
Sensory processing refers to the ability of the person to receive, organize and interpret
sensory inputs (Kramer and Hinojosa, 2009). Information from the environment and the
body is available at all times from all the senses including touch, vision, taste, smell,
hearing, vestibular and proprioceptive senses (Reebye and Stalker, 2008). How an
individual takes in, interprets and responds to sensory information is related to his or her
neurological thresholds, which are defined as the amount of stimulation needed to be
noticed, and his or her self-regulation strategies, which are behavioural responses to
the input (Dunn, 1997). Sensory processing abilities allow individuals to identify
stimuli that require their attention and to accommodate, to tune out or act to remove
irrelevant or distracting sensory input. The ability to manage and integrate sensory input
influences individual's adaptive response to their environment. The ability to respond to
increasingly more complex environments develops over time (Reebye and Stalker, 2008).

Dunn's (1997, 2001) model of sensory processing describes the relationship between
neurological thresholds, which range from high, where an individual is hypo-
responsive, to low where an individual is hyper-responsive, and behavioural responses,
which range from passive to active. The four sensory types that result from the
intersection between these two components of sensory processing are identified as low
registration (the individual does not seek out sensory input and tends not to notice
stimuli), sensory seeking (an active response to a high threshold), sensory sensitivity
(a low threshold but no active avoidance of the stimuli) and sensory avoiding (an active
response to a low threshold). Because sensory processing relates to many senses an

individual may have different sensory thresholds and responses to different stimuli, for example be sensory avoiding, or defensive, for tactile stimuli and seeking of auditory input (Dunn, 1997). The different sensory patterns of response described by Dunn are only problematic if they interfere with the individual's ability to engage appropriately in their environment. The literature suggests that sensory processing patterns do not change developmentally after 5 years of age (Dunn, 1999).

Although many studies have investigated the sensory processing abilities of children with autism or attention-deficit–hyperactivity disorders, for example, very few have examined the abilities of children with a physical disability. Peter (2009) described the sensory processing patterns of a small group of children (*n*=9) with severe intellectual impairment and a physical disability including cerebral palsy and found that more children exhibited patterns of sensory seeking and low registration than sensory avoiding or sensory sensitivity. Therapists may need to consider an individual's pattern of sensory processing and responding when planning therapy. Intervention for those whose responses interfere with their adaptive behaviour includes education and consultation with others to understand the children's sensory processing patterns and to identify strategies to assist them to meet their sensory needs. This might include adaptation of the environment, such as removal or reduction of stimuli, or the integration of activities through the day that provide sought after stimuli (Kramer and Hinojosa, 2009).

Strength training
Strength training, by increasing a muscle's ability to generate force, aims to address the deficit of muscle weakness that is characteristic of many children and adults with cerebral palsy. Strength training programmes were applied to people with cerebral palsy in the middle half of the last century (Healy, 1958), but were infrequently applied in the latter part of the century as a result of concerns that strength training could increase spasticity and reduce range of movement. There is now evidence that strength training programmes can increase muscle strength in people with cerebral palsy, and accumulating evidence that the increased strength can carry over into improved activity (Dodd et al, 2002, Dodd et al, 2003). Strength training appears to be a relatively safe intervention for children (Faigenbaum, 2000) and there is no evidence that strength training programmes have a negative effect on spasticity or range of movement in people with cerebral palsy (Dodd et al, 2002).

The key principles of strength training are as follows:

- the person lifts the weights a relatively small number of times before muscular fatigue;
- sufficient rest is given between exercise sessions to allow for recovery;
- the weight lifted during exercise is progressively increased as the person gets stronger.

For this reason, strength training is also often called progressive resisted exercise. Typical strength training programmes will involve completing one to three sets of a number of exercises working at a maximum intensity of 8–12 repetitions, i.e. only lifting a weight in an exercise that can be lifted 8 to 12 times through the available range with good form. Training occurs two to three times each week for a minimum of 6 weeks. As a result of the effort and adherence required to do a strength training programme some clinicians feel that this type of programme does not work as well with children under the age of 10 years. The exercises included in a strength training programme depend on the specific aim of therapy, and can include gymnasium or home-based exercises. The equipment to provide resistance may include weight machines, elasticized bands, cuff weights and weighted vests. Strength training is described further in the case in Chapter 13.

Treadmill training

Treadmill training programmes, with or without bodyweight support, are increasingly being used to improve the walking performance of people with cerebral palsy. Treadmill training is based on motor learning theory; which suggests that to develop and improve a motor skill such as walking, opportunities for repetitive practice of the skill need to be offered (Shumway-Cook and Woollacott, 2007). Treadmill walking provides increased opportunity to train the whole gait cycle repetitively, facilitate an improved gait pattern and, when a bodyweight support system is used, reduce the impact of poor balance on the person's ability to maintain weight bearing during walking. Some preliminary work suggests partial bodyweight supported treadmill training is feasible in people with cerebral palsy across a wide range of severities and types of disability, and a wide range of ages. Some children with cerebral palsy as young as 15 months have participated in treadmill training programmes, and people who are not yet walking independently have participated successfully (Richards et al, 1997; Dodd and Foley, 2007).

Training is typically conducted two or three times per week, for around 30 minutes each session, for a duration of 6 to 12 weeks. At least one person is required to supervise training sessions and usually this person assists with gait facilitation such as initiation of swing, heel contact, attention to knee extension and prevention of hyper-extension during stance while the person is on the treadmill. Training intensity is increased either by decreasing the amount of bodyweight support provided, increasing the treadmill speed or the time spent walking or a combination of these parameters. The literature suggests that when therapists set the training parameters of treadmill training they should carefully consider matching these parameters with the goals of treatment. Therefore, if the aim of training is to increase a person's walking endurance, over time the programme should increase the amount of time the person spends walking, or if increased walking speed is the aim of the programme the treadmill speed should gradually be increased as the person improves. Under supervision, treadmill training is a safe and feasible intervention for people with cerebral palsy (Dodd and Foley, 2007). Treadmill training is described further in the case in Chapter 13.

Visual–motor skills training
Along with a high incidence of impairments of visual acuity, cognitive and motor performance, children with cerebral palsy are at risk of visual–motor and visual–perceptual impairments. Up to 57% of children without intellectual impairment were found to have visual–perceptual deficits (Kozeis et al, 2006) and in one study of children with intellectual impairment, visual perceptual difficulties over and above that expected with intellectual impairment occurred in 37% (Stiers et al, 2002). Children with periventricular leukomalacia are at particular risk (Jacobson et al, 2002).

Perceptual–motor performance is dependent on the following:

- good quality sensory input (vision and ocular–motor skills);
- processing (cognitive skills to analyse visual information); and
- output (behaviours that rely on visual information – recognition, discrimination, matching and detecting relationships) (Todd, 1999).

Cognitive processing skills include visual attention, visual memory and visual discrimination, which may all be impaired in children with cerebral palsy. Visual–motor skill deficits will affect a person's occupational performance and ability to interact with and learn from their environments from the earliest age and throughout life. It is important to understand where in the visual processing system a person's impairments are and to provide support through adaptation, compensation and training guided by the principles of learning (Todd, 1999). Key learning principles include goal- or task-focused repetition and guided practice with structured feedback. Children with cerebral palsy are likely to require many more repetitions for successful learning than do other children, and building in these opportunities is critical.

Environmental strategies for improving visual attention include modulating arousal levels through lighting, colour, movement or the novelty of stimuli presented, or increasing selective attention and vigilance by decreasing distracting stimuli, grading the complexity of the visual task or providing visual cues. Visual memory is influenced by the ability of the individual to ascribe meaning to the stimuli and to associate new information with old. Scaffolding information and assisting the individual to discover strategies to remember key visual information are useful therapeutic strategies. Visual discrimination is the process of detecting key features and ignoring extraneous features and develops through experience and with age. The four fundamental perceptual components include recognition, matching, categorization and detecting relationships as they relate to visual concepts including increasingly complex shapes (such as letters and words), colour and objects (Todd, 1999).

Common medical and surgical procedures
The following section does not attempt to provide a comprehensive description of all medical and surgical interventions that might be used for people with cerebral palsy. Rather they are a selection of the more common procedures in which physiotherapists and occupational therapists may be involved in providing complementary care.

Botulinum toxin A

Botulinum toxin A (BoNT-A) is a neurotoxin that acts at the neuromuscular junction by inhibiting the release of the neurotransmitter acetylcholine (Graham, 2000). When injected into selected muscles, BoNT-A produces a dose-dependent chemical denervation resulting in reduced muscular activity. The effect of BoNT-A is not immediate; the response delay varies from 12 hours to 7 days (Forssberg and Tedroff, 1997). Clinically useful reduction of muscle activity usually lasts 12–16 weeks. Subsequent sprouting of new nerve terminals leads to re-innervation or restoration of the original terminal and functional recovery of the affected muscles (de Paiva et al, 1999).

Botulinum toxin A has been used as an adjunct to therapeutic techniques to

- reduce focal spasticity and the pain of muscle spasms;
- increase the range of movement;
- improve agonist–antagonist balance; and
- improve function and delay the need for orthopaedic procedures.

It has also been used to support upper extremity surgical planning. Botulinum toxin A is thought to be effective because it allows a prolonged stretch to muscle fibres (by concurrent splinting or active antagonists) that results in the muscle physically lengthening (Wall et al, 1993). This muscle lengthening effect may decrease or delay fixed deformity and thus delay the need for early surgery in children (Kirschner et al, 2001).

Botulinum toxin A is considered safe and effective for children with cerebral palsy although a recent US Food and Drug Administration communication has indicated that botulinum toxins are under review following serious, and in some cases fatal, events following toxin injections (see http://www.fda.gov/Drugs/DrugSafety/Postmarket DrugSafetyInformationforPatientsandProviders/DrugSafetyInformationforHeathcare Professionals/). Local adverse effects of BoNT-A may include pain at the injection site, excessive weakness in the injected muscle or unwanted weakness in the adjacent muscles. Systemic effects, although rare, may include transient flu-like symptoms, dysphagia, anaphylaxis, incontinence, excessive or generalized mild weakness (Carr et al, 1998; Graham et al, 2010). Resistance to BoNT-A, characterized by the absence of any beneficial effect, has occasionally been observed and has been attributed to antibody formation against the toxin (Brin, 1997).

There is evidence to support the effectiveness of BoNT-A in both the lower and upper extremities. In the upper extremity, BoNT-A in conjunction with therapy has been shown to facilitate goal achievement and, in some studies, to improve quality of movement and temporarily reduce muscle tone (Lowe et al, 2006; Wallen et al, 2007). Although the reduction in muscle tone was temporary, studies have shown maintenance of goal achievement up to 6 months following intervention. In the lower extremity, BoNT-A with therapy has been shown to improve the gait pattern, the walking speed, the speed of sit-to-stand transfers and the muscle length of children with spastic cerebral palsy (Papadonikolakis et al, 2003; Park et al, 2006; Scholtes et al, 2007). The use of BoNT-A is described further in the cases in Chapters 8 and 9.

Intrathecal baclofen
Intrathecal baclofen is used to treat severe spasticity or dystonia by delivering very small quantities of the anti-spastic medication baclofen directly to the spinal fluid. A small metal pump and medication reservoir are surgically implanted in the individual's abdomen and a catheter is used to deliver the drug to the intrathecal space in the spine (Royal Children's Hospital, 2007; Hoving et al, 2009). One of the advantages of delivering baclofen in this way is that the side-effects often associated with the higher dosages commonly required in oral delivery of baclofen are minimized. Before a permanent pump is inserted a trial intrathecal injection or the insertion of a temporary intrathecal pump is performed to determine if the medication works for that individual and thus if a pump is appropriate.

People who are suitable and might benefit include those with

- severe spasms that affect the arms, legs or both;
- spasms that interfere with personal care, changing nappies, bathing, or sleep;
- painful spasms;
- enough body mass to support a pump (i.e. the body is big enough to hold the pump) and the person is at least 4 years old (although miniature pumps are now becoming available for younger and smaller people);
- a good response to a trial dose of baclofen;
- intolerance to the higher dose oral medications.

The catheter may become clogged, kinked, disconnected or infected. If this happens, the signs and symptoms include

- redness, pain or swelling of the skin at or near the incision site;
- drainage from the incision;
- a fever higher than 38° Celsius;
- irritability or extreme sleepiness;
- nausea and vomiting;
- repeated headaches;
- little or no effect from the baclofen.

Signs the person is receiving too much baclofen include

- listless or increased sleepiness;
- dizziness;
- lightheaded;
- breathing slowly.

The pump is fitted with an alarm to indicate when the amount of medicine in it gets too low or if the battery is running out. The battery life of a pump is about 5–7 years. A new pump needs to be surgically implanted before the end of the battery life (Royal Children's Hospital, 2007).

Selective dorsal rhizotomy
Selective dorsal rhizotomy is a surgical procedure that aims to improve activity by reducing the effects of spasticity in people with cerebral palsy. The surgical procedure involves exposing the spinal cord and nerve roots in the lumbosacral area by removing a section of bone (laminectomy). Dorsal nerve rootlets that supply sensory inputs to the spinal cord from muscles are evaluated to find which ones are most likely to be contributing to spasticity. A proportion of those rootlets are then sectioned. After the operation an intense period of physiotherapy follows over many weeks to improve strength, restore walking ability and improve motor function. As well as the usual risks of surgery, dorsal rhizotomy can also result in short-term sensory loss to the lower limbs and altered bladder function.

A meta-analysis of three randomized controlled trials with 90 participants with spastic diplegia evaluated at 9–12 months after surgery concluded that selective dorsal rhizotomy was effective in making clinically significant reductions in spasticity, and modest improvements in the Gross Motor Function Measure of about 4% (Steinbok et al, 1997; McLaughlin et al, 1998, 2002). Relatively few adverse events were reported. Longer-term follow-up of up to 5 years confirmed that the benefits were maintained in children with spastic diplegia (Farmer and Sabbagh, 2007). In choosing patients for selective dorsal rhizotomy it is important to determine that spasticity, and not dystonia, is the major movement disorder, and that it is the lower limbs that are mainly affected. The intervention appears to be most effective for children with spastic diplegia aged between 3 and 9 years (Steinbok, 2007). For children with quadriplegia, selective dorsal rhizotomy may be appropriate if lower limb spasticity is disabling and if the relief of upper limb hypertonia is not an important goal (Steinbok, 2007).

Single event multilevel surgery
Although cerebral palsy results from a non-progressive neurological lesion, the secondary musculoskeletal consequences can be progressive with abnormal stresses and forces resulting in bony torsions and joint contractures that progressively affect activity and gait (Graham and Selbar, 2003). Single event multilevel surgery (SEMLS) is the correction of all musculoskeletal deformities in one surgical session, requiring only one admission to hospital and one period of rehabilitation (Graham and Selbar, 2003). Surgical procedures include soft tissue corrections such as lengthening short musculotendinous units and transferring tendons of contracted spastic muscles; and correction of bony deformities through osteotomies and bone stabilization procedures. The surgical corrections are guided by a biomechanical assessment based on instrumented gait analysis. Single event multilevel surgery involves an intense period of post-operative rehabilitation for about 6 months to restore activity and strength. Orthotic management is also important after SEMLS. Most children will use ground

reaction ankle–foot orthoses (GRAFO) after surgery. As recovery continues, they will progress first to solid ankle–foot orthoses (AFOs), and then to hinged AFOs.

Patients' gait function deteriorates after surgery, returning to baseline levels at 12 months and demonstrating improvement at 2 years (Harvey et al, 2007). There is evidence that improvements are maintained 5 years after surgery (Rodda et al, 2006). Single event multilevel surgery has been applied most often to children with spastic diplegia (GMFCS levels II and III) aged from 8 to 14 years. It is thought that SEMLS is most effective after spasticity management in early childhood. A form of SEMLS is also applied to correct fixed deformities of the upper limb in children with spastic hemiplegia, by combining soft tissue lengthening, tendon transfers and spasticity management (Graham and Selbar, 2003). Lower limb SEMLS is described further in the case in Chapter 10.

Upper limb surgical techniques
There is a wide range of techniques designed to improve joint alignment, facilitate functional performance, improve cosmetic appearance and promote ease of skin care and hygiene of the upper extremity. The primary objective of many surgical techniques for the upper limb is to minimize muscle imbalance across joints by reducing the effect of spasticity through muscle releases, supporting weaker muscles with tendon re-routing and, where necessary, release of contractures and joint stabilization (Gschwind 2003; Lawson and Tonkin, 2003; Van Heest, 2003). The specific procedure or group of procedures chosen for any individual is influenced by the severity of impairment and the number of joints targeted. It is common for more than one procedure to be performed; for example Johnstone et al (2003) reported an average 4.5 procedures (range 1 to 12) per surgery.

Groups of procedures described in the literature include correction of thumb-in-palm, (Smeulders et al, 2006), release of flexion contractures of the wrist and fingers (Zancolli, 2003), wrist arthrodesis (Rayan and Young, 1999; Hargreaves et al, 2000) and forearm pronation correction (Gschwind, 2003; Kreulen et al, 2004). Surgery is usually considered for children with primarily spastic motor types in middle childhood or adolescence. Contraindications for surgery, related to issues such as sensation, strength and degree of hand function, all depend on the initial surgical goal.

Two classifications of hand deformity are frequently cited in surgical literature and used to support surgical planning: those of House et al (1981) and Zancolli (1979, 2003). The House classification has demonstrated evidence of good to excellent inter- and intra-observer reliability in adolescents with spastic hemiplegia (Waters et al, 2004).

House et al (1981) classified the thumb-in-palm position of the hand as follows:

- type I: simple metacarpal adduction contracture;
- type II: metacarpal adduction contracture and metacarpophalangeal flexion deformity;

- type III: metacarpal adduction contracture combined with a metacarpophalangeal hyperextension deformity or instability;
- type IV: metacarpal adduction contracture combined with metacarpophalangeal and interphalangeal flexion deformities.

Zancolli (1979, 2003) classified the grasp and release patterns of the wrist and fingers as follows:

- group I: active finger extension with less than 20–30° of active wrist flexion;
- group II: active finger extension with more than 20–30° of active wrist flexion;
- group IIA: active wrist extension with the fingers flexed;
- group IIB: no active wrist extension with the fingers flexed;
- group III: no active wrist or finger extension.

Deformities of the thumb or fingers (swan-neck type) may occur with the wrist and finger deformities. A case describing upper limb surgery is presented in Chapter 11.

Chapter summary

In this chapter we have presented a brief overview of the most frequently used approaches to therapy, and included summaries of some of the more common interventions applied in the management of people with cerebral palsy. The case-based chapters that follow provide descriptions of practical applications of many of these therapeutic interventions, and examples where physiotherapy and occupational therapy are provided in conjunction with the medical and surgical interventions described.

References

Arndt SW, Chandler LS, Sweeney JK, Sharkey MA & McElroy JJ (2008) Effects of a neurodevelopmental treatment-based trunk protocol for infants with posture and movement dysfunction. *Pediatr Phys Ther,* 20, 11–22.

Arnould C Penta M & Thonnard JL (2007) Hand impairments and their relationship with manual ability in children with cerebral palsy. *J Rehabil Med,* 39, 708–14.

Autti-Ramo I, Suoranta J, Anttila H, Malmivaara A & Makela M. (2006) Effectiveness of upper and lower limb casting and orthoses in children with cerebral palsy. *Am J Phys Med Rehabil,* 85, 89–103.

Bar-Or O, Inbar O & Spira R (1976) Physiological effects of a sports rehabilitation program on cerebral palsied and post-polio myelitis adolescents. *Med Sci & Sports,* 8, 157–61.

Bentzel K (2008) Assessing abilities and capabilities: Sensation. In: Radomski, M V & Trombly Latham CA (eds) *Occupational Therapy for Physical Dysfunction,* 6th edn. Baltimore, MD: Lippincott Willliams & Wilkins.

Blanche EI & Knox SH (2008) Learning to play: promoting skills and quality of life in individuals with cerebral palsy. In: Eliasson AC & Burtner P (eds) *Improving Hand Function in Children with Cerebral Palsy: Theory, Evidence and Intervention.* London: Mac Keith Press.

Bobath K & Bobath B (1984) The neurodevelopmental treatment. In: Scrutton D (ed.) *Management of the Motor Disorders of Children with Cerebral Palsy.* London: Spastics International Medical Publications.

Bower E (2009) *Finnie's Handling the Young Child with Cerebral Palsy at Home.* Oxford: Butterworth Heinemann.

Brin MF (1997) Botulinum toxin: chemistry, pharmacology, toxicity, and immunology. *Muscle Nerve Suppl*, 6, S146–55.

Brown T & Burns S (2001) The efficacy of neurodevelopmental treatment in paediatrics: a systematic review. *Br J Occup Ther*, 64, 235–44.

Bundy AC, Nelson L, Metzger M & Bingaman K (2001) Validity and reliability of a test of playfulness. *Occup Ther J Res*, 21, 276–92.

Butler C & Darrah J (2001) Effects of neurodevelopmental treatment (NDT) for cerebral palsy: an AACPDM evidence report. *Dev Med Child Neurol*, 43, 778–90.

Cahill SM & Kielhofner G (2008) Volition: child-oriented intervention for the upper extremity. In: Eliasson AC & Burtner P (eds) *Improving Hand Function in Children with Cerebral Palsy: Theory, Evidence and Intervention.* London, Mac Keith Press.

Canadian Association of Occupational Therapists (CAOT) (2002) *Enabling Occupation: An Occupational Therapy Perspective.* Ottawa, Canada: Canadian Association of Occupational Therapists.

Carey L & Matyas T (2005) Training of somatosensory discrimination after stroke. *Am J Phys Med Rehabil*, 84, 428–42.

Carlsson M, Olsson I, Hagberg G & Beckung E (2008) Behaviour in children with cerebral palsy with and without epilepsy. *Dev Med Child Neurol*, 50, 784–9.

Case-Smith J. (2005) *Occupational Therapy for Children.* St Louis: Elsevier Mosby.

Caulton JM, Ward KA, Alsop CW, Dunn G, Adams JE & Mughal MZ (2004) A randomised controlled trial of standing programme on bone mineral density in non-ambulant children with cerebral palsy. *Arch Dis Child*, 89, 131–5.

Charles J & Gordon AM (2006) Development of hand-arm bimanual intensive training (HABIT) for improving bimanual coordination in children with hemiplegic cerebral palsy. *Dev Med Child Neurol*, 48, 931–6.

Colangelo CA (1999) Biomechanical frame of reference. In: Kramer P & Hinojosa J (eds) *Frames of Reference for Pediatric Occupational Therapy.* Philadelphia, PA : Lippincott, Williams & Wilkins.

Condie DN & Meadows CB (1995) *Report of a Consensus Conference on the Lower Limb Orthotic Management of Cerebral Palsy.* Copenhagen: International Society of Prosthetics and Orthotics.

Cooper J, Majnemer A, Rosenblatt B & Birnbaum R (1995) The determination of sensory deficits in children with hemiplegic cerebral palsy. *J Child Neurol*, 10, 300–9.

Corn K, Imms C, Timewell G, Carter C, Collins L, Dubbeld S, Schubiger S & Froude E (2003) Impact of second skin lycra splinting on the quality of upper limb movement in children. *Br J Occup Ther*, 66, 464–72.

Crepeau EB, Cohn ES & Schell BAB (2009) *Willard and Spackman's Occupational Therapy.* Baltimore: Lippincott, Williams & Wilkins.

Darrah J, Watkins B, Chen L & Bonin C (2004) Effects of Conductive Education intervention for children with a diagnosis of cerebral palsy: an AACPDM evidence report. *Dev Med Child Neurol*, 46, 187–203.

DeLuca SC (2002) *Intensive Movement Therapy with Casting for Children with Hemiparetic Cerebral Palsy: A Randomized Controlled Crossover Trial* (Dissertation). Birmingham: The University of Alabama at Birmingham.

de Paiva A, Meunier FA, Molgo J, Aoki KR & Dolly JO (1999) Functional repair of motor endplates after botulinum neurotoxin type A poisoning: biphasic switch of synaptic activity between nerve sprouts and their parent terminals. *Proc Natl Acad Sci USA*, 96; 3200–5.

Dodd KJ & Foley S (2007) Partial body-weight-supported treadmill training can improve walking in children with cerebral palsy: aA clinical controlled trial. *Dev Med Child Neurol*, 49, 101–5.

Dodd KJ, Taylor NF & Damiano DL (2002) A systematic review of the effectiveness of strength-training programs for people with cerebral palsy. *Arch Phys Med Rehabil*, 83, 1157–64.

Dodd KJ, Taylor NF & Graham HK (2003) A randomized clinical trial of strength training in young people with cerebral palsy. *Dev Med Child Neurol*, 45, 652–7.

Dresen MH, De Groot G, Mesamenor JR & Bouman LN (1985) Aerobic energy expenditure of handicapped children after training. *Arch Phys Med Rehabil*, 66, 302–6.

Dubois L, Klemm A, Murchland S & Ozols A (2004) Handwriting of children who have hemiplegia: a profile of abilities in children aged 8–13 years from a parent and teacher survey. *Aust Occup Ther J*, 51, 89–98.

Dunn W (1997) The impact of sensory processing abilities on the daily lives of young children and their families: a conceptual model. *Infant Young Child*, 9, 23–35.

Dunn W (1999) *Sensory Profile: Users Manual.* San Antonio, TX: Psychological Corporation.

Dunn W (2001) The sensations of everyday life: empirical, theoretical and pragmatic considerations: The 2001 Eleanor Clarke Slagle Lecture. *Am J Occup Ther*, 55, 608–20.

Ekström L, Johansson E, Granat T & Carlberg EB (2005) Functional therapy for children with cerebral palsy: an ecological approach. *Dev Med Child Neurol*, 47, 613–19.

Eliasson AC (2007) Bimanual training for children with unilateral CP: is this something new? *Dev Med Child Neurol*, 49, 806.

Eliasson AC, Gordon, AM & Forssberg H (1995) Tactile control of isometric fingertip forces during grasping in children with cerebral palsy. *Dev Med Child Neurol*, 37, 72–84.

Eliasson AC, Krumlinde-Sundholm, L, Shaw K & Wang C (2005) Effects of constraint induced movement therapy in young children with hemiplegic cerebral palsy: an adapted model. *Dev Med Child Neurol*, 47, 266–75.

Faigenbaum AD (2000) Strength training for children and adolescents. *Clin Sports Med*, 19, 593–619.

Farmer JP & Sabbagh AJ (2007) Selective dorsal rhizotomies in the treatment of spasticity related to cerebral palsy. *Child Nerv Syst*, 23, 991–1002.

Fitts PM & Posner MI (1967) *Human Performance.* Belmont: Brooks/Cole Publishing Co.

Franck LS & Callery P (2004) Re-thinking family centred care across the continuum of children's healthcare. *Child Care Health Dev*, 30, 265–77.

French L & Nommensen A (1992) Conductive education evaluated: future directions. *Aust Occup Ther J*, 39, 17–24.

Forssberg H & Tedroff KB (1997) Botulinum toxin treatment in cerebral palsy: intervention with poor evaluation? *Dev Med Child Neurol*, 39, 635–40.

Gordon AM & Duff SV (1999) Fingertip forces in children with hemiplegic cerebral palsy. I: anticipatory scaling. *Dev Med Child Neurol*, 41, 166–75.

Gordon, AM, Schneider JA, Ashley C & Charles JR (2007) Efficacy of a hand-arm bimanual intensive therapy (HABIT) in children with hemiplegic cerebral palsy: a randomized control trial. *Dev Med Child Neurol*, 49, 830–8.

Graham HK (2000) Botulinum toxin A in cerebral palsy: functional outcomes. *J Paediatr*, 137, 300–3.

Graham HK & Selbar P (2003) Musculoskeletal aspects of cerebral palsy. *J Bone Joint Surg*, 85, 157–66.

Graham HK, Naidu K, Smith K, Brooke A & Yu Z (2010) Systemic events following Botulinum toxin A therapy in children with cerebral palsy. *Dev Med Child Neuro* (forthcoming).

Granhaug K (2006) Splinting the upper extremity of a child. In: Henderson A & Pehoski C (eds) *Hand Function in the Child,* 2nd ed. St Louis: Mosby Elsevier.

Gschwind CR (2003) Surgical management of forearm pronation. *Hand Clinics*, 19, 649–55.

Guzetta A, Bonanni P, Biagi L, Tosetti M, Montanaro D, Guerrini R & Cioni G (2007) Reorganisation of the somatosensory system after early brain damage. *Clin Neurophysiol*, 118, 1110–21.

Hargreaves DG, Warwick DJ & Tonkin MA (2000) Changes in hand function following wrist arthrodesis in cerebal palsy. *J Hand Surg Br*, 25, 193–4.

Hari M & Tillemans T (1984) Conductive education. In: Scrutton D (ed.) *Management of the Motor Disorders of Children with Cerebral Palsy.* London: Spastics International Medical Publications.

Harvey A, Graham HK, Morris ME, Baker R & Wolfe R (2007) The Functional Mobility Scale: Ability to detect change following single event multilevel surgery. *Dev Med Child Neurol*, 49, 603–07.

Healy A (1958) Two methods of weight training for children with spastic type of cerebral palsy. *Res Q*, 29, 389–95.

Hinojosa J, Sproat CT, Mankhetwit S & Anderson J (2002) Shifts in parent-therapist partnerships: twelve years of change. *Am J Occup Ther*, 56, 556–63.

Hoare BJ, Wasiak J, Imms C & Carey L (2007) Constraint induced movement therapy in the treatment of the upper limb in children with cerebral palsy. *The Cochrane Database of Systematic Reviews*, Art. No.: CD004149., DOI: 10.1002/14651858.CD004149.pub2.

House JH, Gwathmey FW & Fidler MO (1981) A dynamic approach to the thumb in palm deformity in cerebral palsy. *J Bone Joint Surg Am*, 63, 216–25.

Hoving MA, Van Raak EP, Spincemaille GH, Palmans LJ, Becher JG, Vles JSH & on behalf of The Dutch Study Group On Child Spasticity (2009) Efficacy of intrathecal baclofen therapy in children with intractable spastic cerebral palsy: a randomised controlled trial. *Eur J Paediatr Neurol*, 240–6.

Jacobson L, Ygge J, Flodmark O & Ek U (2002) Visual and perceptual characteristics, ocular motility and strabismus in children with periventricular leukomalacia. *Strabismus*, 10, 179–83.

Johnstone BR, Richardson PWF, Coombs CJ & Duncan JA (2003) Functional and cosmetic outcome of surgery for cerebral palsy in the upper limb. *Hand Clinics*, 19, 679–86.

Kanellopoulos, AD, Mavrogenis AF, Papagelopoulos D, Mitsiokapa EA, Skouteli H, Vrettos SG, Tzanos G & Papagelopoulos PJ (2009) Long lasting benefits following the combination of static night upper extremity splinting with botulinum toxin A injections in cerebral palsy children. *Eur J Phys Rehabil Med*, 45 (Jan 21) [Epup ahead of print].

Kaplan, MT & Bedell G. (1999) Motor skill acquisition frame of reference. In: Kramer P & Hinojosa J (eds) *Frames of Reference for Pediatric Occupational Therapy*, 2nd edn. Baltimore, MD: Williams & Wilkins.

Ketelaar M, Vermeer A, Thart H, Van Petegem-van Beek E & Helders PJM (2001) Effects of a functional therapy program on motor abilities of children with cerebral palsy. *Phys Ther*, 81, 1534–45.

Kielhofner, G. (2008) *Model of Human Occupation: Theory and Application.* Baltimore, MD: Lippincott Williams & Wilkins.

King S, Teplicky R, King, GA & Rosenbaum PL (2004) Family-centered service for children with cerebral palsy and their families: a review of the literature. *Semin Pediatr Neurol*, 11, 78–86.

Kirschner K, Berweck S, Mall V, Korinthberg R & Heinen F (2001) Botulinum toxin treatment in cerebral palsy: evidence for a new treatment option. *J Neurology*, 248(Suppl 1), 28–30.

Kozeis N, Anogeianaki A, Mitova DT, Anogianakis G, Mitov T, Felekidis A, Saiti P & Klisarova A (2006) Visual function and execution of microsaccades related to reading skills, in cerebral palsied children. *Int J Neurosci*, 116, 1347–58.

Kramer P & Hinojosa J (2009) *Frames of Reference for Pediatric Occupational Therapy.* Philadelphia, PA: Lippincott, Williams and Wilkins.

Kreulen M, Smeulders MJC, Veeger HEJ, Hage JJ & Van der Horst C (2004) Three-dimensional video analysis of forearm rotation before and after combined pronator teres rerouting and flexor carpi ulnaris tendon transfer surgery in patients with cerebral palsy. *J Hand Surg Br*, 29, 55–60.

Lawson RD & Tonkin MA (2003) Surgical management of the thumb in cerebral palsy. *Hand Clin*, 19, 667–77.

Lesny I, Stehlik A, Tomasek J, Tomankova A & Havlicek I (1993) Sensory disorders in cerebral palsy: Two point discrimination. *Dev Med Child Neurol*, 35, 402–5.

Lidstrom H & Borgestig M (2008) Assistive technology devices in computer activities. In: Eliasson AC & Burtner P (eds) *Improving Hand Function in Children with Cerebral Palsy: Theory, Evidence and Intervention.* London: Mac Keith Press.

Liepert J, Bauder H, Wolfgang HR, Miltner WH, Taub E & Weiller C (2000) Treatment-induced cortical reorganisation after stroke in humans. *Stroke*, 31, 1210–16.

Lowe K, Novak I & Cusick A. (2006) Low-dose/high concentration localised botulinum toxin A improves upper limb movement and function in children with hemiplegic cerebral palsy. *Dev Med Child Neurol*, 48, 170–5.

Ludwig S, Leggett P & Harstall C. (2000) *Conductive Education for Children with Cerebral Palsy*, HTA 22. Edmonton: Alberta Heritage Foundation for Medical Research.

Mandich AD, Polatajko H & Zilberbrant A (2008) A cognitive perspective on intervention. In: Eliasson AC & Burtner P (eds) *Improving Hand Function in Children with Cerebral Palsy: Theory, Evidence and Intervention*. London: Mac Keith Press.

Mastos M, Miller K, Eliasson AC & Imms C (2007) Goal directed training as an effective and client centred approach to improving the use of the hands. *Clin Rehabil*, 21, 47–55.

Mayston MJ (2004) Physiotherapy management in cerebral palsy: an update on treatment approaches. In: Scrutton D, Damiano D & Mayston MJ (eds) *Management of the Motor Disorders of Children with Cerebral Palsy*, 2nd edn. London: Mac Keith Press.

McLaughlin J, Bjornson K, Temkin N, Steinbok P, Wright V, Reiner A, Roberts T, Drake J, O'Donnell M, Rosenbaum PL, Barber J & Ferrel A (2002) Selective dorsal rhizotomy: meta-analysis of three randomized controlled trials. *Dev Med Child Neurol*, 44, 17–25.

McLaughlin JF, BJornson K, Astley SJ, Graubert CS, Hays RM, Roberts T, Price R & Temkin N. (1998) Selective dorsal rhizotomy: efficacy and safety in an investigator-masked randomized clinical trial. *Dev Med Child Neurol*, 40, 220–32.

Miller F (2005) Durable medical equipment. In: Miller F (ed.) *Cerebral Palsy: Musculo-Skeletal Management*. Secaucus, NJ: Springer.

Missiuna C, Mandich AD, Polatajko H & Malloy-Miller T (2001) Cognitive orientation to daily occupational performance (CO-OP): Part 1 – theoretical foundation. *Phys & Occup Ther in Pediatr*, 20, 69–81.

Missiuna C, Mandich A, Dematteo C, Law M & Hanna S (2006) Examining cognitive orientation to occupational performance for children with brain injury. *J Can Occup Ther* (Conference supplement), TX.

Morris, C. (2007) Orthotic management of cerebral palsy. *Dev Med Child Neurol* 49, 791–6.

Morris, DM & Taub E (2001) Constraint induced therapy approach to restoring function after neurological injury. *Top Stroke Rehabil*, 8, 16–30.

Murchland S, Lane AE & Ziviani J. (2008) Written communication: clinical decision-making for handwriting in children with cerebral palsy. In: Eliasson AC & Burtner P (eds) *Improving Hand Function in Children with Cerebral Palsy: Theory, Evidence and Intervention*. London: Mac Keith Press.

Naylor CE & Bower E (2005) Modified constraint induced movement therapy for young children with hemiplegic cerebral palsy: a pilot study. *Dev Med Child Neurol*, 47, 356–69.

Nicholson JH, Morton RE, Attfield S & Rennie D (2001) Assessment of upper limb function and movement in children with cerebral palsy wearing lycra garments. *Dev Med Child Neurol*, 43, 384–91.

Novak I & Cusick A (2006) Home programmes in paediatric occupational therapy for children with cerebral palsy: where to start? *Aust Occup Ther J*, 53, 251–64.

Novak I & Watson E (2005) *Seating and Positioning*. Sydney, Australia: CP Institute.

Novak I, Cusick A & Lowe K (2007) A pilot study on the impact of occupational therapy home programming for young children with cerebral palsy. *Am J Occup Ther*, 61, 463–8.

Novak I, Cusick A & Lannin NA (2009) Effectiveness of home program intervention for children with cerebral palsy: A double blind randomised controlled trial. *Dev Med Child Neurol suppl*, 51 13.

Odding E, Roebroeck ME & Stam HJ (2006) The epidemiology of cerebral palsy: incidence, impairments and risk factors. *Disabil Rehabil*, 28, 183–91.

Orlin MN, Pierce SR, Smith BT, Johnston TE, Shewockis PA & McCarthy JJ (2005) Immediate effect of percutaneous intramuscular stimulation during gait in children with cerebral palsy: a feasibility study. *Dev Med Child Neurol*, 47, 684–90.

Palisano RJ, Rosenbaum PL, Walter S, Russell D, Wood E & Galuppi B (1997) Development and reliability of a system to classify gross motor function in children with cerebral palsy. *Dev Med Child Neurol*, 39, 214–23.

Palisano, RJ, Tieman BL, Walter SD, Bartlett DJ, Rosenbaum PL, Russell D & Hanna SE (2003) Effect of environmental setting on mobility methods of children with cerebral palsy. *Dev Med Child Neurol*, 45, 113–20.

Palisano RJ, Rosenbaum PL, Bartlett D & Livingston MH (2008) Content validity of the expanded and revised gross motor function classification system. *Dev Med Child Neurol*, 50, 744–50.

Papadonikolakis AS, Verkis MD, Korompilias AV, Kostas, JP, Ristanis SE & Soucacos PN. (2003) Botulinum A toxin for treatment of lower limb spasticity in cerebral palsy: gait analysis in 49 patients. *Acta Orthop Scand* 74, 749–55.

Parham LD & Primeau LA (1997) Play and occupational therapy. In: Parham LD & Fazio LS (eds) *Play in Occupational Therapy for Children*. St Louis: Mosby.

Park ES, Park CI & Kinm YJ (2001) Comparison of anterior and posterior walkers with respect to gait parametres and energy expenditure of children with spastic diplegic cerebral palsy. *Yonsei Med J*, 42, 180–4.

Park ES, Park CI, Chang HC, Park CW & Lee DS (2006) The effect of botulinum toxin type A injection into the gastrocnemius muscle on sit-to-stand transfer in children with spastic diplegic cerebral palsy. *Clin Rehabil* 20, 668–74.

Parkes J, White-Koning M, Dickinson HO, Thyen U, Arnaud C, Beckung E, Fauconnier J, Marcelli M, McManus V, Michelsen SI, Parkinson K & Colver A. (2008) Psychological problems in children with cerebral palsy: a cross-sectional European study. *J Child Psychol Psychiatry*, 49, 405–13.

Pedersen AV (2000) Conductive education – a critical appraisal. *Adv Physiother*, 2, 75–82.

Peter S (2009) *The Sensory Profile Patterns of Children with a Moderate to Profound Intellectual Disability*. Melbourne: School of Occupational Therapy, Faculty of Health Sciences, La Trobe University.

Polatajko H J & Mandich AD (2004) *Enabling Occupation In Children: The Cognitive Orientation to Daily Occupational Performance (CO-OP) Approach*. Ottawa, ON: CAOT Publications, ACE.

Polatajko H J,Mandich AD, Miller LT & MacNab JJ (2001) Cognitive orientation to daily occupational performance (CO-OP): Part II – the evidence. *Phys Occup Ther Pediatr*, 20, 83–106.

Postans NJ & Granat MH (2005) Effect of functional electrical stimulation, applied during walking, on gait in spastic cerebral palsy. *Dev Med Child Neurol*, 47, 46–52.

Rayan GM & Young BT (1999) Arthrodesis of the spastic wrist. *J Hand Surg*, 24, 944–52.

Reebye P & Stalker A (2008) *Understanding Regulation Disorders of Sensory Processing in Children: Management Strategies for Parents and Professionals*. London: Jessica Kingsley Publishers.

Richards C, Malouin F, Dumas F, Marcoux S, LePage, C & Menier C (1997) Early and intensive treadmill locomotor training for young children with cerebral palsy: feasibility study. *Pediatr Phys Ther*, 9, 158–65.

Rigby P & Rodger S (2006) Developing as a player. In Rodger S & Ziviani J (eds) *Occupational Therapy with Children: Understanding Children's Occupations and Enabling Participation*. Oxford: Blackwell Publishing

Rimmer JH (2005) Exercise and physical activity in persons aging with a disability. *Phys Med Rehabil Clin N Am*, 16, 41–56.

Rodda J, Baker R, Galea M, Nattrass G & Graham HK (2006) The impact of single event multi-level surgery (SEMLS) for severe crouch gait in spastic diplegic cerebral palsy: outcomes at 5 years. *Gait Posture*, 24S, 87–9.

Rogers A, Furler BL, Brinks S & Darrah J (2008) A systematic review of the effectiveness of aerobic exercise intervention for children with cerebral palsy: an AACPDM evidence report. *Dev Med Child Neurol*, 50, 808–14.

Royal Children's Hospital, Department of Developmental Medicine. (2007) *Kids Health Information: Intrathecal Baclofen. Kids Health Information*. Melbourne: The Royal Children's Hospital Mebourne. (http://www.rch.org.au/kidsinfo/handout/index.php?doc_id=11150)

Rushton DN (2003) Functional electrical stimulation and rehabilitation: an hypothesis. *Med Eng Phys*, 25, 75–8.

Scholtes VA, Dallmeijer AJ, Knol DL, Speth LA, Maathuis CG, Jongerius PH & Becher JG (2007) Effect of multilevel botulinum toxin-A and comprehensive rehabilitation on gait in cerebral palsy. *Pediatr Neurol*, 36, 30–9.

Sheppard L, Mudie H & Froude E (2007) An investigation of bilateral isokinematic training and neurodevelopmental therapy in improving use of the affected hand in children with hemiplegia. *Phys Occup Ther Pediatr*, 27, 5–25.

Shumway-Cook A & Woollacott MH (2007) *Motor Control: Translating Research into Clinical Practice*. Philadelphia, PA: Lippincott, Williams & Wilkins.

Smeulders M, Coester A & Kreulen M (2006) Surgical treatment for the thumb-in-palm deformity in patients with cerebral palsy. *The Cochrane Database of Systematic Reviews*, 2005. Issue 4. Art. No: CD004093. DOI: 10.1002/14651858.CD004093.pub2

Stagnitti K & Unsworth C (2000) The improtance of pretend play in child development: an occupational therapy perspective. *Br J Occup Ther*, 63, 121–7.

Steinbok P (2007) Selective dorsal rhizotomy for spastic cerebral palsy: a review. *Childs Nerv Syst*, 23, 981–90.

Steinbok P, Reiner A, Beauchamp R, Armstrong RW & Cochrane DD (1997) A randomized clinical trial to compare selective posterior rhizotomy plus physiotherapy with physiotherapy alone in children with spastic diplegic cerebral palsy. *Dev Med Child Neurol*, 39, 178–84.

Stiers P, Vanderkelen R, Vanneste G, Coene S, De Rammelaere M & Vandenbussche E (2002) Visual-perceptual impairment in a random sample of children with cerebral palsy. *Dev Med Child Neurol*, 44, 370–82.

Sujith OK (2008) Functional electrical stimulation in neurological disorders. *Eur J Neurol*, 15, 437–44.

Takata N (1974) Play as prescription. In: Reilly M (ed.) *Play as Exploratory Learning*. Beverly Hills, CA: Sage Publications.

Taub E (1980) Somatosensory deafferentation research with monkeys: implications for rehabilitation medicine. In: Ince LP (ed.) *Behavioural Psychology in Rehabilitation Medicine: Clinical Applications*. Baltimore: Williams and Wilkins.

Taub E, Uswatte G & Pidikiti R (1999) Constraint-induced movement therapy: a new family of techniques with broad application to physical rehabilitation – a clinical review. *J Rehabil Res Dev*, 36, 237–51.

Teplicky R, Russell D & Law M (2003) *Keeping Current In. . .Alternative and Complementary Therapies: Casts, Splints and Orthoses – Lower Extremity*. Hamilton: Canchild Centre for Childhood Disability Research, McMaster University. (http://www.canchild.ca/en/canchildresources/cso1.asp)

Thompson-Rangel T, Smith SB & Griner DE (1992) Customised walker adaptations for a child with cerebral palsy. *J Assoc Child Prosthet Orthot Clin*, 27, 97–8.

Todd VR (1999) Visual information analysis: frame of reference for visual perception. In: Kramer JF & Hinojosa J (eds.) *Frames of Reference for Pediatric Occupational Therapy*, 2nd edn. Philadelphia, PA: Lippincott, Williams & Wilkins.

Townsend EA & Polatajko HJ (2007) *Enabling Occupation II: Advancing an Occupational Therapy Vision for Health, Well-Being and Justice through Occupation*. Ottawa, Canada: CAOT Publications, ACE.

US Department of Health & Human Services (2008) *Physical Activity Guidelines for Americans*. Washington, DC: US Department of Health & Human Services.

Valvano J & Newell KM (1998) Practice of a precision isometric grip-force task by children with spastic cerebral palsy. *Dev Med Child Neurol*, 40, 464–73.

Van Den Berg-Emons RJ, Van Baak MA, Speth L & Saris WH (1998) Physical training of school children with spastic cerebral palsy: effects on daily activity, fat mass and fitness. *Int J Rehabil Res*, 21, 179–94.

Van Der Linden ML, Hazelwood ME, Hillman SJ & Robb JE (2008) Functional electrical stimulation to the dorsiflexors and quadriceps in children with cerebral palsy. *Pediatr Phys Ther*, 20, 23–9.

Van Heest AE (2003) Surgical management of wrist and finger deformity. *Hand Clin*, 19, 657–65.

Wallen M, O'Flaherty, SJ & Waugh MA (2007) Functional outcomes of intramuscular botulinum toxin type A and occupational therapy in the upper limbs of children with cerebral palsy: a randomised controlled trial. *Arch Phys Med Rehabil*, 88, 1–10.

Wall SA, Chait JA, Temlett B, Perkins B, Hillen G & Becker P (1993) Botulinum A chemodenervation: a new modality in cerebral palsied hands. *Br J Plastic Surg*, 46, 703–6.

Ward KA, Alsop CW, Caulton JM, Rubin C, Adams JE & Mughal ZJ (2004) Low magnitude mechanical loading is osteogenic in children with disabling conditions. *J Bone Miner Res*, 19, 360–9.

Waters PM, Zurakowski D, Patterson P, Bae DS & Nimec D (2004) Interobserver and intraobserver reliability of therapist-assisted videotaped evaluations of upper-limb hemiplegia. *J Hand Surg Am*, 29, 328–34.

Wilcock A (1998) *Health: An Occupational Perspective*. Thorofare, NJ: Slack.

Wilcock A, Chelin M, Hall M, Hamley N, Morrison B, Scrivener L, Townsend M & Treen K. (1997) The relationship between occupational balance and health: a pilot study. *Occup Ther Int*, 4, 17–30.

Wright PA & Granat MH (2000) Therapeutic effects of functional electrical stimulation of the upper limb of eight children with cerebral palsy. *Dev Med Child Neurol*, 42, 724–7.

Zancolli, EA (1979) *Structural and Dynamic Bases of Hand Surgery*. Philadelphia, PA: Lippincott.

Zancolli EA (2003) Surgical management of the hand in infantile spastic hemiplegia. *Hand Clin*, 19, 609–29.

Ziviani J & Wallen M (2006) Development of graphomotor skills. In: Henderson A & Pehoski C (eds) *Hand Function in the Child: Foundations for Remediation*. St Louis, MI: Mosby Elsevier.

Chapter 5

The infant with complex needs

Sarah Foley and Susan Greaves

Case study: Jessica[1]

Jessica is a 6-month-old girl referred from a neonatal intensive care unit (NICU) to our early intervention centre for children diagnosed with neurodevelopmental disabilities, called 'Heidi's'. The steps involved in the clinical reasoning process used in this chapter are summarized in Figure 5.1 and described in Chapter 1.

Stage 1: initial data collection

The referral letter provided the following information.

- Jessica was delivered at term by an emergency caesarean section following fetal distress.
- Jessica remained in hospital for 3 weeks to allow further investigations and to establish feeding. However, feeding difficulties continued and she was discharged being fed nasogastrically. Jessica had recently established oral feeding.
- At 3 months, Jessica was assessed using the General Movements Assessment (Einspieler and Prechtl, 2005; see Appendix, p. 285) and her parents were told she was at risk of having cerebral palsy.
- At 6 months, this diagnosis was confirmed by her paediatrician who told her parents that Jessica had severe spastic quadriplegia (Gross Motor Function Classification System [GMFCS] level V, Palisano et al, 2008; see Box 5.1), with trunk hypotonia.

---

1   Names in this, and all the case-base chapters in the book, have been changed to pseudonyms. Although much of the information in these chapters is based on real individuals and their needs, some aspects have been changed to highlight common issues for individuals with complex disability.

Jessica is Ruth and Peter's first child. Ruth has taken a year's maternity leave from her position as a school teacher. Peter is an accountant. They both attended the initial assessment, looking tired and concerned. The appointment time was offered to coincide with when Jessica would be fed and alert.

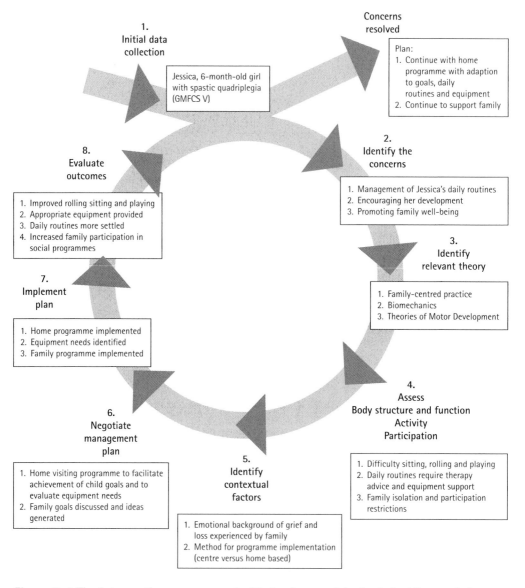

1.
Initial data collection

Jessica, 6-month-old girl with spastic quadriplegia (GMFCS V)

Concerns resolved

Plan:
1. Continue with home programme with adaption to goals, daily routines and equipment
2. Continue to support family

8.
Evaluate outcomes

1. Improved rolling sitting and playing
2. Appropriate equipment provided
3. Daily routines more settled
4. Increased family participation in social programmes

2.
Identify the concerns

1. Management of Jessica's daily routines
2. Encouraging her development
3. Promoting family well-being

3.
Identify relevant theory

1. Family-centred practice
2. Biomechanics
3. Theories of Motor Development

7.
Implement plan

1. Home programme implemented
2. Equipment needs identified
3. Family programme implemented

6.
Negotiate management plan

1. Home visiting programme to facilitate achievement of child goals and to evaluate equipment needs
2. Family goals discussed and ideas generated

5.
Identify contextual factors

1. Emotional background of grief and loss experienced by family
2. Method for programme implementation (centre versus home based)

4.
Assess
Body structure and function
Activity
Participation

1. Difficulty sitting, rolling and playing
2. Daily routines require therapy advice and equipment support
3. Family isolation and participation restrictions

Figure 5. 1 The intervention process used with Jessica: model adapted with permission from the Canadian Occupational Performance Process Model (CAOT, 2002). GMFCS, Gross Motor Function Classification System.

> **Box 5.1 GMFCS level V snapshot[2]**
>
> Proportion of people with cerebral palsy classified as GMFCS level V: 13–16%
>
> Proportion of people classified as GMFCS level V who
>
> - have a severe intellectual disability (IQ <50): about 85%;
> - have a severe visual impairment: about 60%;
> - have epilepsy: about 80%;
> - have behavioural problems: about 10%;
> - have hip displacement requiring surgery: about 65%;
> - use a feeding tube: 42%;
> - who walk alone or with support at home by age 4–12 years: 0%.

Stage 2: identify and prioritize the concerns

Ruth, Peter and Jessica were taken to the assessment room. During the interview, her parents described the traumatic events surrounding Jessica's birth and the stress involved with their stay in the NICU. Although their interview with the paediatrician outlined the initial magnetic resonance imaging (MRI) findings and the diagnosis of cerebral palsy, they were still unsure of what this meant for Jessica's future.

Both parents saw Jessica's sociability as her outstanding asset: for example, she smiled in response to their voices and their faces. They were pleased at being able to access a therapy service close to their home as Jessica was often unsettled after travelling the distance into the hospital. Ruth's mother often accompanied Jessica and Ruth to the hospital. Peter's extended family lived out of state and had little contact with Jessica.

Jessica's parents presented the following issues as their major concerns.

- What were the implications of the diagnosis of cerebral palsy for Jessica's future?
- How could they best manage Jessica's daily routines?
- How could they best promote her development?

Stage 3: identify relevant theory to guide management

Family-centred practice

A family-centred service includes families in decision-making, and recognizes the importance of the well-being of family members, whose health is at risk both physically and psychologically (Rosenbaum et al, 1998; Brehaut et al, 2004; Raina et al, 2005; see Chapter 3).

---

2   See Chapter 2: p. 17 for details of the sources used to derive these data.

Ruth and Peter raised a number of concerns during their initial interview. These included the emotions surrounding the trauma of Jessica's birth, the stress of her time in the NICU, the grief associated with her diagnosis, as well as difficulty communicating Jessica's disability to extended family. These concerns were acknowledged during the interview, and a social worker who was present organized further appointments to continue discussing their concerns.

Ruth and Peter were also facing the day-to-day difficulties of caring for Jessica and managing her special needs. They wanted to give Jessica every opportunity to develop optimally. They requested more information about cerebral palsy, particularly written information to take away and read, and a brochure in parent-friendly language outlining cerebral palsy was provided. They were also directed to informative websites such as the *CanChild* Centre for Childhood Disability Research (McMaster University, Canada) website (http://www.canchild.ca). Ruth and Peter were encouraged to read the information, as well as to continue to ask questions about Jessica's disability and her current and future needs.

Biomechanical frame of reference
The biomechanical frame of reference recognizes that children with cerebral palsy often cannot maintain their posture through normal automatic muscle activity. Consequently, there are two goals of the biomechanical approach to treatment. The first is to enhance the development of postural reactions by reducing the demands of gravity and by better aligning the body. The second is to provide external supports for the child, to reduce demands on postural reactions, and to provide an efficient body position for skilled activity and to improve function (Colangelo, 1999).

The importance of developing postural control and maintaining alignment was reflected in a consensus statement from a recent Mac Keith multidisciplinary meeting (Gericke, 2006). It recommends that children with cerebral palsy receive tailored individual postural management programmes. Programmes may include special seating, night-time postural support, active exercise, orthoses, surgical interventions and individual therapy sessions. The nature of the postural intervention should be guided by the child's GMFCS level. The consensus recommends that children at levels IV and V start a 24-hour postural management programme in lying as soon as appropriate after birth, in sitting from 6 months, and in standing from 12 months. The consensus states that these programmes are helpful for children with bilateral cerebral palsy (usually spastic quadriplegia) to facilitate communication, cognitive and functional skills and enhance participation. They aim to increase the child's comfort and reduce deformity. Hip surveillance is also required (Dobson et al, 2002; see Chapter 2).

Using a biomechanical approach to analyse movement and postural patterns can help identify the impairments, such as spasticity and reduced range of movement, which could be contributing to Jessica's activity limitations. This approach would also evaluate Jessica's postural requirements over 24 hours and provide recommendations for appropriate supportive equipment in different positions/situations, as well as methods for lifting and carrying Jessica.

Theories of motor development

Current theories of motor development and postural control suggest that infants are born with a repertoire of motor behaviours that are refined by experience, and they ultimately select the most efficient motor pattern for a particular task (Hadders-Algra, 2000). Early experience has been shown to alter an infant's brain structure and function (Als et al, 2004).

One of Jessica's main problems was that her motor development was not progressing as fast as that of other children her age. In particular, Jessica was trying to hold her head up to look around but could not substain this. A core skill for therapists is to analyse the components of typical motor development necessary for children to develop their motor skills (Alexander et al, 1994; Bly, 1994), and then use observational analysis of the child's movements to help determine what skills may be emerging and what impairments or activity limitations might be barriers to further skill acquisition. Additionally, other factors that need to be considered when planning therapy interventions to promote motor development include (1) knowledge of the natural history of the movement disorder associated with cerebral palsy based on the GMFM (see Appendix, p. 294) and GMFCS which can predict motor growth (Rosenbaum et al, 2002; see Chapter 2); and (2) describing in detail Jessica's current, individual skill level, including a measure of her intellectual ability.

Stage 4: assessment of body structure and function, activity and participation

Based on the observations collected and analyses in the preceding stage, a schedule for assessment of body structure and function, activity and participation was developed (see Table 5.1).

Table 5.1 Assessments for Jessica

Body structure/function	Activity	Participation restrictions
Spasticity Range of movement	Behavioural regulation Observation of functional motor performance Goal Attainment Scale Gross Motor Function Measure (A & B) Pediatric Evaluation of Disability Inventory	Parent interview

Body structure/body function

SPASTICITY
Spasticity cannot be reliably measured in young infants (Burridge et al, 2005); however, the functional effects of spasticity can be observed and recorded. Jessica had hypotonia in her trunk and neck. Distally she had increased muscle tone. She usually held her arms adducted with elbow, wrist and fingers loosely flexed. Thumbs were across her palms. Her lower limbs were typically in a pattern of hip adduction with internal rotation, knee extension and ankle plantarflexion.

RANGE OF MOVEMENT
When Jessica's upper limbs were moved through passive range, resistance was felt through shoulder elevation, elbow, wrist and finger extension. In the lower limbs there was resistance to hip abduction and knee flexion/extension. However, full passive range of movement was still possible and this was recorded for future reference.

Some spontaneous kicking movements were observed in Jessica's legs, particularly when she was excited; however, little active reach with her arms was observed.

Activity

BEHAVIOURAL REGULATION
An early developmental task for infants is to be able to regulate their behaviour independently, for example to self-calm, go to sleep and maintain alert attention (Gorga, 1989; Gomez et al, 2004). Behavioural regulation is related to the infant's ability to process sensory information. Sensory processing refers to the ability to take in information through our senses (touch, movement, smell, taste, vision and hearing) and to organize and interpret that information, and make a meaningful response. Parents of young children with cerebral palsy can find it difficult to complete standardized assessments of these skills (Dunn, 2002). However, observation of Jessica's reaction to various sensory stimuli was used to guide decisions around management of her daily experiences and routines including handling techniques, choice of toys/objects, bathing, settling to sleep and travel in the car.

Some behavioural responses to sensory stimuli observed included the following.

- Jessica calmed to music or a familiar voice. She enjoyed music. However, loud or sudden noises made her startle and become upset.
- Jessica enjoyed visual stimulation. Ruth and Peter reported that she often turned to the window when it was sunny outside, or looked at the light. Although turning to light can be an almost reflex action, they felt that Jessica reacted positively to their faces or familiar toys by smiling.
- Jessica enjoyed some tactile experiences. Toys did not interest her, but she enjoyed being outside and feeling the sun and the wind on her face. She enjoyed a bath.

OBSERVATIONAL ASSESSMENT FINDINGS

Supine: Jessica usually lay with her head to either side and found it difficult to lift her head off the surface. She could hold her head in midline to look at her parent's face for a few seconds. Her arms were either by her side or loosely flexed, and she did not actively reach for toys. Jessica held her legs in extension usually with adduction. She spontaneously kicked her legs without dissociation, although sometimes reciprocal kicking was observed in outer range.

Prone: when placed in prone (which she disliked), Jessica was able to lift and turn her head to either side. Her arms were usually by her side and Jessica had difficulty using them for active postural support. If her arms were placed under her shoulders she could hold her head up for a short period, but she could not achieve this position herself. She could not reach in prone.

Rolling: Jessica could not roll over from supine to prone or vice versa without assistance. She could not bring her arm across her body or lift her leg across her body to initiate rolling from supine to prone. When placed on her side, Jessica extended her head and upper arm only and 'fell' back into supine. If placed in prone Jessica made no attempt to roll.

Sitting: Jessica required full support at her thoracic level to sit on the floor, and tended to sit with a 'C curve' and posterior pelvic tilt. She could hold up her head for a few seconds to look at a toy. Her legs often fell into a ring-sit position. Her arms were held loosely flexed, with little active movement. Jessica sometimes pushed backwards with her whole body, making it difficult for her parents to carry her.

Playing: When supported in sitting, Jessica made no attempt to reach for toys. If the backs of her hands were stimulated, she made some opening movements of her fingers. If toys were placed in her hands, she was unaware of them and dropped them.

GOAL ATTAINMENT SCALING (GAS)

The Goal Attainment Scale (GAS, see Appendix, p. 292) was used to identify and prioritize areas of Jessica's development that were important to the family. The following areas were identified:

- Jessica was not yet moving. They would like her to learn to roll;
- Jessica was not able to sit on the floor without maximal support. They would like her to gain some head and trunk control in sitting;
- Jessica was not interested in toys. They would like her to begin to play with toys using her hands.

Goals were written using the SMART method (Specific, Measurable, Acceptable, Realistic and Time-specific) (Steenbeck et al, 2008). An example of one goal (sitting on the floor) is provided in Table 5.2.

Table 5.2 Goal Attainment Scale: sitting on the floor

	Goal: sitting on the floor
Setting Task	At home on the floor (carpeted) In 3 months Jessica will be able to control her head and upper trunk when supported at her lower thoracic/waist level when ring sitting
−2, equal to starting level	When supported at the upper thoracic level of the trunk in ring sitting on the floor Jessica can only lift her head for a few seconds to look at a toy
−1, less than expected outcome	When supported at the upper thoracic level of the trunk in ring sitting, Jessica can hold up her head to look at a toy for 20 seconds
0, expected goal	When supported at the upper thoracic level of the trunk in ring sitting Jessica can hold up her head to look at a toy for 1 minute, OR when supported lower at the lower thoracic/waist level, she can maintain head control for 10–20 seconds.
1, more than expected outcome	When supported at the lower thoracic/waist level of the trunk when ring sitting, Jessica can hold up her head to look at a toy for 1 minute
2, much more than expected outcome	When supported at the lower thoracic/waist level of the trunk when ring sitting, Jessica can hold up her head to look at a toy for 5 minutes

GROSS MOTOR FUNCTION MEASURE (VERSION 88)
The GMFM (see Appendix, p. 294) was used to evaluate change in gross motor function over time, and in response to intervention. The GMFM–88 was chosen as it has 22 more items than the GMFM–66, particularly in the descriptions of a child's early motor skills. As Jessica is primarily functioning in the early motor skills dimensions of lying and rolling it was chosen over the GMFM–66. Jessica's results are in Table 5.3.

PEDIATRIC EVALUATION OF DISABILITY INVENTORY (PEDI)
The PEDI (see Appendix, p. 295) interview was used to evaluate Jessica's baseline level of skill and assistance required in daily living tasks. The results are in Table 5.3.

Table 5.3 (a) Results for Jessica aged 6 months – Gross Motor Function Measure (88) scores

Dimension	Raw score	%
A: Lying and Rolling		
1. Supine: head in midline turns head with extremities symmetrical	1[a]	
4. Supine: flexes right hip and knees through full range	1	
5. Supine: flexes left hip and knees through full range	1	
10. Prone: lifts head upright	1	
Total dimension A	4/51	8.0
B: Sitting		
21. Sits on mat, supported at thorax by therapists: lifts head upright, maintains 3 seconds	2[b]	
Total dimension B	2/60	3.0
Total dimension C (crawling and kneeling), D (standing) and E (walking, running and jumping)	0	0
Total score		3.0
Goal total score[c]		6.0

a. Completion of less than 10% of the item.
b. Completion from 10% to less than 100% of the item.
c. Goal areas for Jessica are A and B given her age.

Table 5.3 (b) Results for Jessica aged 6 months – Pediatric Evaluation of Disability Inventory score

Dimension	Functional skills (normative standard score)	Caregiver assistance (normative standard score)
Self-care	22.0	39.4
Mobility	17.6	33.3
Social function	24.2	41.9

Normative standard scores have a mean of 50 and standard error of 10 points. Thus scores between 30–70 are considered to fall in the normal range.

Table 5.3 (c) Results for Jessica aged 6 months –Pediatric Evaluation of Disability Inventory – modified frequencies

Dimension	None	Child	Rehabilitation	Extensive
Self-care (8 items)	6	2	0	0
Mobility (7 items)	4	3	0	0
Social function (5 items)	5	0	0	0

None, no modification required; Child, non-specialized modifications; Rehabilitation, requires rehabilitation equipment; Extensive, requires extensive modifications.

Participation restrictions

PARENT INTERVIEW
Although parent involvement in the goal-setting and therapy provision process is a vital part of family-centred services, attention has often focused on the benefits of this participation from the child's perspective. However, recent research also stresses the need to consider parental needs and functioning as well as the child's needs during this process so that programmes are formulated that are beneficial to both children with chronic disabilities and their families (Jansen et al, 2003; Ahl et al, 2005; Siebes et al, 2007). Discussions with Ruth and Peter highlighted the following difficulties:

● Ruth found car travel difficult as Jessica often became distressed when in her car seat. Consequently, Ruth preferred to stay at home;
● Ruth preferred not to join her local mothers' group as she found the differences in development between Jessica and the other children emotionally difficult. Consequently she felt quite isolated from social contact.

Stage 5: contextual factors: environment and personal

Environmental factors
The home and the family are at the centre of an infant's environment (Rosenbaum, 2007). One facet of family life that changes with the birth of a child with a disability is the family's daily routines; what happens within the family from the time they get up to the time they go to bed. Families often need to make considerable adaptations to sustain their routines (Bernheimer and Weisner, 2007).

As the primary caregiver, Ruth was finding it difficult to complete daily routine tasks such as feeding, bathing and providing appropriate support to Jessica unless Jessica was held. Additionally, Ruth and Peter thought that it would be beneficial for therapy ideas to be considered in the real life environment. A home visiting programme was arranged to further clarify the daily routine difficulties, to assess for possible equipment and modifications that might assist with Jessica's management, and to provide ideas that were relevant to their home environment.

Another accommodation required of Ruth and Peter was to get to know the various therapists and agencies who had become involved with them and their child. Developing trusting relationships with these professionals is important for the therapist and for the family.

Personal factors
Personal factors relate to features of the child that are not part of their health condition such as age and temperament (World Health Organization [WHO], 2001). Although Peter and Ruth found that Jessica had periods of irritability (primarily in the car and when going to sleep), at other times she was too passive.

Stage 6: management plan
The initial visits to Jessica's home were used to clarify difficulties with daily routines and to evaluate environmental issues. Ruth and Peter were then given the option of continuing therapy visits to the house or commencing centre-based services. Flexible and responsive practices that encourage family choices regarding service provision are important considerations for family-centred practice (Hannah and Rodger, 2002; Bernheimer and Weisner, 2007).

Initial home visits allowed clarification of the following environmental and family issues.

Participation restrictions for Ruth and Peter
- Jessica tended to become upset in the car, which often made car travel distressing for Ruth and Peter. Her car seat was still rear-facing and her parents sought advice about the seats most appropriate position in the car, its suitability and ways to help calm Jessica.
- Ruth wanted to attend a mothers' group with children who had similar abilities to Jessica.

Equipment issues
- Bathing: Ruth was finding it difficult to lift Jessica into and out of the bath and support her during bathing.
- Mobility: Jessica tended to slump or extend her legs and slip when she was in her stroller when the stroller was in an upright position. Ruth was using rolled up towels in an attempt to maintain Jessica's body in midline.

Daily routine issues
- Sleeping: Jessica slept poorly and often needed to be carried until she fell asleep. She woke frequently during the night. Her paediatrician recommended reflux medication and placing her in a semi-reclined position during sleep times.

- Feeding: Jessica often took up to an hour to feed orally and then frequently vomited after a feed (reflux). She had not gained as much weight as expected and monitoring on a weight chart showed she had fallen below the third centile.
- Position for play/learning: during the day, Jessica had limited opportunity to interact physically and visually with toys and objects in her environment, and she generally showed little interest in them. She was usually placed on her back on the floor, or seated in a commercially available infant bouncer.

Stage 7: implement plan

Specific child and parent goals

GOAL ONE: ROLLING FOR MOBILITY

Photographs and written descriptions, as well as therapist demonstration and parent practice, are commonly used to teach parents how to assist their baby to learn a motor skill.

The therapist initially highlighted the aspects of rolling Jessica was able to do, such as locating a toy by turning her head and attempting to move to the side leading with her head. The therapist then explained the assistance Jessica needed to progress. Jessica needed to develop flexor control of her head and neck to balance the use of asymmetrical extension she was beginning to use in supine during floor time, and to develop more flexor activity in her abdominal muscles, particularly the oblique abdominals, used in rolling.

Placing a small wedge under Jessica's head and shoulders, combined with light pressure on the sternum, assisted her to 'chin tuck'; using voice, eye contact or toys helped keep Jessica's head in the midline. Abdominals were then activated by tilting the pelvis posteriorly and assisting Jessica's hands forward onto her legs. Rotating her to either side recruited more activity in the oblique abdominals (Figure 5.2).

In side lying both arms were kept forward to assist with head and trunk flexion and to counterbalance Jessica's tendency to extend backwards and fall back into supine. Rolling

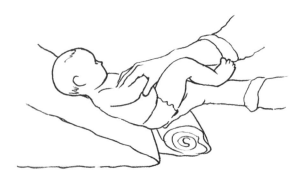

Figure 5.2 The parent assists the baby in supine with chin tuck and posterior pelvic tilt on a wedge. Illustration by Louise Price.

from side lying back into supine was practised first to encourage chin tuck, with assistance given on the ribcage to activate the oblique abdominals (Figure 5.3). As Jessica participated more actively in the rolling task, assistance was reduced.

Rolling into prone is easiest to assist from the pelvis or the legs. Because Jessica adducts and had difficulty with selective leg movement, she was assisted to roll with the top most leg in flexion and the weight-bearing leg in extension so she experienced dissociated leg movement. As she rolled into prone, slight traction was applied to the upper leg which assisted active head extension and lateral righting (Figure 5.4).

Assisting Jessica to shift her weight down to her pelvis in prone makes it easier for Jessica to use her arms for support and to lift up her head and trunk to look around (Figure 5.5). A small wedge or rolled up towel under the axilla can also be used.

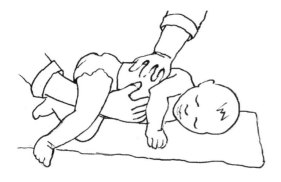

Figure 5.3 The baby is lying on her side, both hands forward, with the therapist's hand assisting over the ribcage. Illustration by Louise Price.

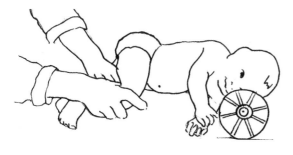

Figure 5.4 Rolling assisted from the leg. Illustration by Louise Price.

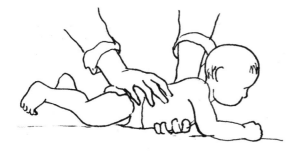

Figure 5.5 Prone lying. Ilustration by Louise Price.

As Jessica could not weight bear through her arms or weight shift her body in prone to initiate rolling, she needed assistance to move from prone to supine. Her weight-bearing arm was placed in a comfortable degree of elevation with her head forward on the arm, and rolling was assisted from the pelvis or legs (Figure 5.6).

Side lying was used as a position for play, with both her arms forward and a rolled up towel at her back to prevent her rolling backwards. Another small towel between her legs controlled hip adduction. Toys were positioned forward and down to encourage head/neck flexion and eye–hand coordination.

Ruth and Peter agreed that suitable times to practise these skills would be nappy changes and when Jessica was playing on the floor.

GOAL TWO: FLOOR SITTING
Jessica's parents were shown how to make it easier for Jessica to sit on the floor and to practise holding her head up actively to look at a toy (Figure 5.7). Jessica's parents practised how much support they needed to give around her trunk so that she could hold her head and trunk with the least amount of assistance. The following aspects were considered:

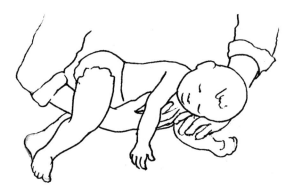

Figure 5.6 Rolling from prone to supine, with arm elevation. Illustration by Louise Price.

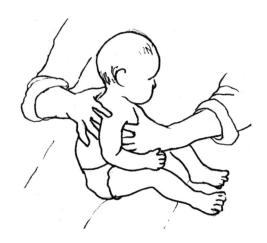

Figure 5.7 Floor sitting. Illustration by Louise Price.

- that the parents were comfortable to play on the floor with Jessica;
- where and how much support Jessica needed;
- the use and choice of a toy to encourage Jessica to hold her head up actively;
- the position of the toy to motivate Jessica's own head and trunk postural activity;
- that the amount of support should be varied so Jessica is an active learner in the task of sitting.

GOAL THREE: HOLDING AND PLAYING WITH TOYS
To help develop play skills two different aspects were considered.

(1) A supported seat option aimed to reduce the demand for postural control during sitting and to provide an efficient body position for skilled upper limb activity. Various infant seats were trialled through Heidi's equipment loan service to evaluate the style and support required. A cut-out table was supplied so that toys were positioned at an appropriate height for reach and play.

(2) Promoting play during her daily routine. Jessica's reaction to different sensory experiences was considered to help find ways to foster her interest in her environment and increase her ability to interact with objects.

Several aspects of the play sessions were considered when setting the session up.

- How far Jessica could reach determined the placement of toys both in height and distance away from her body.
- Jessica's parents were asked to identify which sensory experiences (visual, tactile, auditory etc.) particularly appealed to Jessica.
- The size, shape and properties of the toys were considered and matched to Jessica's current abilities to grasp or interact with toys.
- Jessica's parents sat in front of her during the session so that they could interact with her visually and they could assist her to use her hands.
- Ways to facilitate opening of her hands to grasp, such as a dynamic thumb splint or stimulating the backs of her hands (finger extensors) using vibration or brushing, were trialled.
- Toys that wrapped around her hand (such as beads) were used to encourage Jessica to maintain grasp.

Environmental factors
Mobility: Jessica was referred to a 'stroller/wheelchair clinic' to assess her for a supportive stroller. Information about funding options was given to the family and followed up with appropriate forms and letters of support.

Bathing: the equipment service allowed for evaluation of the most appropriate bathing support for Jessica, which in this instance was a bath support lift. This allowed Jessica to be placed in a mesh 'frame' in a raised position at the top of the bath. Moving a handle/lever on the frame lowered the support into the bath, with Jessica remaining supported in the frame.

Family needs and daily routines

FAMILY PARTICIPATION

(1) Car travel: at this young age, commercially available infant car seats usually provide appropriate support. However, Jessica's car seat was turned around so that she now faced forward, and was placed in maximal recline because of her poor head control. Head support was provided to help keep her head in midline. Jessica's harness was checked to ensure that it held her firmly in the car seat. Ruth and Peter played Jessica's favourite music while travelling.

(2) Ruth was referred to a 'music and movement' playgroup for children less than three years of age with special needs.

(3) Jessica, Ruth and Peter joined an infant swimming programme. Jessica loved being in a swimming pool; her parents felt that this was the time that she moved and responded to her environment the most.

DAILY ROUTINES

(1) Feeding: many children with severe cerebral palsy have feeding issues such as oro-motor dysfunction, food refusal, vomiting, gastrointestinal problems (including reflux), aspiration of food, failure to thrive and chronic undernourishment (Reilly et al, 1996; Sullivan et al, 2000). Assessments by Jessica's speech pathologist (including observation of feeding in the home environment), dietician and paediatrician enabled them to develop an individualized feeding programme aimed to ensure adequate and safe nutritional intake.

(2) Carrying: Ruth and Peter were shown new ways to carry Jessica, which were more comfortable for both Jessica and themselves (for one example see Figure 5.8).

(3) Sleeping: variations to Jessica's sleeping routine, her environment and her position in the cot were considered. Some ideas that were trialled included raising the cot at one end to help with her reflux, a warm bath and massage before bedtime, a night light and relaxing music, firm wrapping in a muslin wrap.

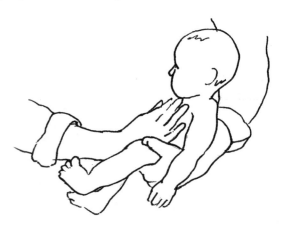

Figure 5.8 Carrying.
Illustration by Louise Price.

Stage 8: evaluate outcomes

A family meeting was scheduled 6 months after the initial contact to monitor progress and assess the need for changes in Jessica's programme. Reassessment showed the following.

Body structure and function and activity performance

- Passive range of movement continued to be full. However, given the risk of hip subluxation, a referal was made to the orthopaedic clinic for hip radiograph, and the protocol for hip surveillance was explained to Jessica's parents (Wynter, 2008).
- GMFM scores had improved. Dimension A: lying and rolling 15%; dimension B: sitting 10%.
- PEDI was not reassessed at this time but would be repeated annually.
- GAS: Jessica had reached the expected outcome (level 0) for rolling and playing with a toy, and more than expected (Level 1) for sitting. Ruth and Peter were pleased with progress and decided to continue with the sitting goal but to re-set the desired outcome and levels. In addition, the following goals for the next 6 months were added:
    - for Jessica be able to activate a simple cause and effect toy using her hands;
    - for Jessica to stand in a prone standing frame for half an hour each day.

Environmental factors

- Mobility: Jessica attended the wheelchair clinic and was given a supportive stroller that allowed her to sit upright without falling to the side or extending. Parents often describe getting their child's first wheelchair/stroller as one of the most confronting and highly emotional early experiences. It is confronting because getting a wheelchair often highlights the severity of their young child's disabilities, and can in the parents' minds mark the loss of hope that their child will be like everybody else. Because of this, the therapists broached the possibility of prescribing a wheelchair when both parents were present and spent considerable time providing information and listening to Ruth and Peter express how they felt about Jessica needing a wheelchair/stroller. These conversations occurred over several home visits. Once Ruth and Peter decided that a more suitable means of mobility would be beneficial, the physiotherapist offered to go with the parents to the wheelchair clinic to provide support and advice.
- Bathing: the new bath aid had decreased the lifting and transferring burden for Ruth and Peter and Jessica continued to enjoy bath time.

Family factors

- Car travel: Jessica enjoyed facing forwards in her car seat and was more settled. Jessica preferred a mobile hung from the window than music playing in the car. The harness and head support maintained Jessica in an appropriate position.
- Ruth joined a local music and movement programme and although she initially found it confronting to see other children with disabilities, she found it beneficial to be able to talk to other mothers in a similar situation. Ruth also felt that talking to families of older children gave some insight into Jessica's future needs.

- Ruth and Peter continued taking Jessica to the pool and in the summer months also took her to the beach. Jessica enjoyed feeling the sand as well as the movement of the waves.

Daily routines
- Feeding: Jessica's weight and growth continued to be monitored. After two chest infections requiring hospitalization, a video fluoroscopy was performed to evaluate for aspiration of food and drink. Nothing conclusive was found. The speech pathologist continued to see Jessica at home.
- Sleeping: raising one end of her bed and her resolving reflux problem meant that Jessica was more settled at night. Jessica responded well to the night light and calming music, but did not like to be wrapped. A sleep system for night-time positioning was trialled successfully.

Box 5.2 Key clinical messages

- Intervention with young infants is inextricably linked to the baby's family and their well-being.
- Principles of family-centred practice are integral to every aspect of therapeutic intervention.
- Parents often require extra support following initial diagnosis.
- Effective interventions are those that are successfully incorporated into the baby's daily routines.

References

Ahl LE, Johansson E, Granit T & Carlberg EG (2005) Functional therapy for children with cerebral palsy: an ecological approach. *Dev Med Child Neurol*, 47, 613–19.

Alexander R, Boehme R & Cupps B (1993) *Normal Development of Functional Motor Skills: The First Year of Life.* Tucson, AZ: Therapy Skill Builders.

Als H, Duffy, McAnulty GB, Rivkin MJ, Vajapeyam S, Mulkern RV, Warfield SK, Huppi PS, Butler SC, Conneman N, Fischer C & Eichenwald EC (2004) Early experience alters brain structure and function. *Pediatrics*, 113, 846–57.

Bernheimer LP & Weisner T S (2007) "Let me just tell you what I do all day. . ." The family story at the centre of intervention research and practice. *Infants Young Child*, 20, 192–201.

Bly L (1994) *Motor Skills Acquisition in the First Year: An illustrated Guide to Normal Development.* San Antonio, TX: Psychological Corporation.

Brehaut J, Kohen D, Raina P, Walter S, Russell D & Switon M (2004) The health of primary caregivers of children with cerebral palsy: How does it compare with that of other Canadian caregivers? *Pediatrics* 114, 182–91.

Burridge JH, Wood DE, Hermens HJ, Voerman GE, Johnson GR, Van Wijck F, Platz T, Gregoric M, Hitchcock R & Pandyan AD (2005) Theoretical and methodological considerations in the measurement of spasticity. *Disabil Rehabil* 27, 69–80.

Canadian Association of Occupational Therapists (CAOT) (2002) *Enabling Occupation: An Occupational Therapy Perspective.* Ottawa: Canadian Association of Occupational Therapists.

Colangelo, CA (1999) Biomechanical Frame of Reference. In: Kramer P Hinojosa J (eds) *Frames of Reference for Pediatric Occupational Therapy*: 257–322. Philadelphia: Lippincott, Williams & Wilkins.

Dobson F, Boyd R, Parrott J, Nattrass GR & Graham HK (2002) Hip surveillance in children with cerebral palsy. *Dev Med Child Neurol*, 36, 386–96.

Dunn W (2002). *The Infant Toddler Sensory Profile*. San Antonio, TX: Psychological Corporation.

Einspieler C & Prechtl HF (2005) Prechtl's assessment of general movements: a diagnostic tool for the functional assessment of the young nervous system. *Ment Retard Dev Disabil Res Rev*, 11, 61–7.

Gericke T (2006) Postural management for children with cerebral palsy: a consensus statement. *Dev Med Child Neurol*, 48: 244.

Gomez CR, Baird S & Jung L(2004) Regulatory disorder identification, diagnosis, and intervention planning: untapped resources for facilitating development. *Infants Young Child*, 17, 327–39.

Gorga D (1989) Occupational therapy treatment practices with infants in early intervention. *Am J Occup Ther*, 43, 731–6.

Hadders-Algra M (2000) The neuronal group selection theory: promising principles for understanding and treating developmental motor disorders. *Dev Med Child Neurol*, 42: 707–17.

Hannah K & Rodger S (2002) Towards family-centred practice in paediatric occupational therapy: A review of the literature on parent-therapist collaboration. *Aust Occup Ther J*, 49, 14–24.

Jansen LMC, Ketelaar M & Vermeer A (2007) Parental experience of participation in physical therapy for children with physical disabilities. *Dev Med Child Neurol*, 45, 58–69.

Palisano RJ, Rosenbaum PL, Bartlett D & Livingston MH (2008) Content validity of the expanded and revised gross motor function classification system *Dev Med Child Neurol*, 50, 744–50.

Raina P, O'Donnell M, Rosenbaum P, Brehaut J, Walter SD, Russell D, Swinton M, Zhu B & Wood E (2005) The health and wellbeing of caregivers of children with cerebral palsy. *Pediatrics*, 115, 626–36.

Reilly S, Skuse D & Poblete X (1996) Prevalence of feeding problems and oral motor dysfunction in children with cerebral palsy: a community survey. *J Pediatr*, 129, 877–82.

Rosenbaum P (2007) The environment and childhood disability: opportunities to expand our horizons. *Dev Med Child Neurol*, 49: 643.

Rosenbaum P, King S, Law M, King G & Evans J (1998) Family-centred services: a conceptual framework and research review. *Phys Occup Ther Pediatr*, 18, 1–20.

Rosenbaum P, Walter S, Hanna S, Palisano R, Russell D, Raina P, Wood E, Bartlett D & Galuppi B (2002) Prognosis for gross motor development in cerebral palsy. *JAMA*, 288, 1357–63.

Siebes RC, Ketelaar M, Görter JW, Wijnroks L, De Blecourt ACE, Reinders-Messelink HA, Van Schie PEM & Vermeer A (2007) Transparency and tuning of rehabilitation care for children with cerebral palsy: a multiple case study in five children with complex needs. *Dev Neurorehabil*, 10, 193–204.

Steenbeek D, Ketelaar M, Galama K & Görter JW (2007) Goal attainment scaling in paediatric rehabilitation: a critical review of the literature. *Dev Med Child Neurol*, 49, 550–6.

Sullivan PB, Lambert B, Rose M, Ford-Adams M, Johnson A & Griffiths P (2000) Prevalence and severity of feeding and nutritional problems in children with neurological impairment: Oxford feeding study. *Dev Med Child Neurol*, 42, 674–80.

World Health Organization (2001) *International Classification of Functioning, Disability and Health (ICF)*. Geneva, WHO.

Wynter M, Gibson N, Kentish M, Love SC, Thomason P & Graham HK. *2008 Consensus Statement on Hip Surveillance in Cerebral Palsy. Australian Standards of Care*. Victoria: CP Australia. (http://www.cpaustralia.com.au/ausacpdm/).

Chapter 6

Early steps

Karen J Dodd and Susan Greaves

Case study: Benjamin
Benjamin is 2 years and 7 months old and has been referred by a large metropolitan tertiary hospital to the local community paediatric early intervention centre. The centre offers a range of services to children with developmental disabilities from birth to 6 years of age and their families. The referral focused on the provision of occupational therapy and physiotherapy, and so the occupational therapist and physiotherapist arranged a joint initial meeting with the family. The steps involved in the clinical reasoning process used in this chapter are summarized in Figure 6.1 and described in Chapter 1.

Stage 1: initial data collection
The referral letter provided the following information.

- Benjamin was delivered at 27 weeks' gestation, birthweight 805 grams, as a result of maternal cervical incompetence. He had an uncomplicated postnatal period.

- He has had no seizures and was on no medications.

- He had no cognitive or communication problems.

- At 4 months, Ben was assessed using the General Movements Assessment (Einspieler and Prechtl, 2005; see Appendix, p. 285) and his parents were told he might have cerebral palsy.

- At 8 months, this diagnosis was confirmed by his neonatologist who said Ben had severe spastic diplegia (Gross Motor Function Classification System [GMFCS] level III to IV, Palisano et al, 2008, see Box 6.1 and Box 6.2). An MRI scan showed bilateral periventricular leukomalacia (PVL).

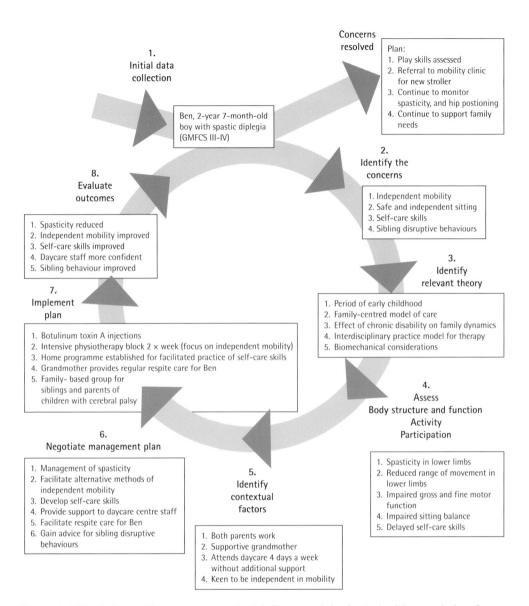

Figure 6.1 The intervention process used with Ben: model adapted with permission from the Canadian Occupational Performance Process Model (CAOT, 2002). GMFCS, Gross Motor Function Classification System.

Ben is Karyn and Cameron's second child. Karyn works part time (4 days a week) as a university lecturer in economics, and Cameron works full time as an accountant. Ben and his parents attended the initial assessment; Karyn and Cameron looked tired and concerned. The appointment time coincided with when Ben's 6-year-old brother Michael was at school.

Box 6.1 GMFCS level III snapshot[1]

Proportion of people with cerebral palsy classified as GMFCS III: 8–12%

Proportion of people classified as GMFCS level III who

- have a severe intellectual disability (IQ <50): about 30%;
- have a severe visual impairment: about 20%;
- have epilepsy: about 25%;
- have behavioural problems: less than 5%;
- have hip displacement requiring surgery: about 18%;
- use a feeding tube: 4%;
- walk alone at home by age 4–12 years: about 10%;
- walk with support at home by age 4–12 years: 36%.

Box 6. 2 GMFCS level IV snapshot

Proportion of people with cerebral palsy classified as GMFCS IV: 9–15%

Proportion of people classified as GMFCS level IV who

- have a severe intellectual disability (IQ <50): about 25%;
- have a severe visual impairment: 25–37%;
- have epilepsy: about 50%;
- have behavioural problems: less than 5%;
- have hip displacement requiring surgery: about 45%;
- use a feeding tube: 11%;
- walk alone at home by age 4–12 years: 0%;
- walk with support at home by age 4–12 years: 7%.

Stage 2: identify and prioritize concerns

Karyn and Cameron were particularly concerned about how Ben's impairments might affect his ability to walk, sit alone and perform everyday tasks such as dressing and washing.

Ben's primary method of self-mobility was to commando crawl with his trunk in contact with the floor. He began commando crawling at about 2 years of age. In the last month he had begun to pull-to-stand independently against the coffee table and he could cruise

---

1 See Chapter 2: p. 17 for details of the sources used to derive these data.

one or two steps along stable surfaces. Karyn and Cameron said they were becoming increasingly worried that Ben might not be able to walk independently. Karyn and Cameron also said it was hard for Ben to sit on the floor unless he 'W' sat (sitting between flexed and internally rotated hips and knees). He could roll independently into prone and get himself up into 'W' sitting.

Ben could perform few self-care activities. He lay down to be dressed and it was difficult to get his shoes and pants on because his legs were so stiff. On questioning it became clear that Ben did not try to assist with dressing, had difficulty sitting in the bath and did not attempt to wash himself. He could feed himself finger foods, but had difficulty learning to use a fork or a spoon. Karyn said that because Ben took so long to complete self-care activities, it was easier and quicker for either Karyn or Cameron to do them for him. Toilet training had not yet been attempted.

Karyn and Cameron said that when Ben was first diagnosed with cerebral palsy they had been shocked and upset, but Ben was a happy and sociable child and they had resolved to overcome any problems they encountered. Ben's neurologist and previous therapists had been unable to tell them definitely whether Ben would walk or not, nor could they tell them specifically what other things he might not be able to do. Cameron said that until recently they had hoped that if they continued intensive therapy (primarily physiotherapy and occupational therapy) at the tertiary hospital where specialist services were located then Ben would be 'OK'. For this reason they had until now refused referral to the local community paediatric early intervention centre, because they thought the centre would have fewer resources to help Ben. However, because Ben was becoming older, it was becoming clearer that rather than getting 'better' the severity of Ben's impairments and the level of his disabilities were becoming more obvious. Therapy, although helpful, was not 'curing' him and both parents were getting very tired going into the city to attend therapy sessions each week. Ben also attended a local daycare centre 4 days a week when Karyn was at work, and fitting therapy visits into a busy week was becoming increasingly difficult.

Ben's 6-year-old brother, Michael, was also causing his parents concern because he was becoming increasingly disruptive at home and at school. Karyn and Cameron had recently been called to see his school teacher about his behaviour as he had been breaking objects, and bullying some children in his class.

For these reasons they had decided to accept the referral to the local occupational therapy and physiotherapy services.

The most important concerns identified during the interview were as follows:

- Ben's problems moving independently around the house, and inside and outside at the daycare centre;
- Ben's difficulty sitting independently and safely on a stool or chair while at daycare for mealtimes and for some table play sessions with the other children;

- Karyn and Cameron's increasing realization that Ben was getting older and yet he was still unable to independently feed himself, help dress or wash himself, and he was not toilet trained;
- Michael's behavioural problems at home and school.

The therapists realized that it was going to be very important to gain the trust and confidence of Ben's family. Karyn and Cameron would need considerable emotional support during this time when their hopes for a 'cure' were diminishing, there was uncertainty as to Ben's level of disability as he got older, and Michael's behaviour was becoming more disruptive.

The therapists also thought a wider range of input might assist this family. It had become clear from this first meeting that occupational therapy and physiotherapy were important but, provided Karyn and Cameron agreed, other members of the community early intervention team such as the child and family psychologist and the special education preschool teacher might also offer resources of benefit.

Stage 3: identifying relevant theory

The period of early childhood

The transition from infancy to early childhood occurs at around 2 years of age. Early childhood (usually considered as being from around 2 to 6 years of age) is characterized by the development of increasing independence. For this reason early childhood is considered an important stage for providing therapy to children with cerebral palsy. This period is usually when the rapid development of locomotor skills such as walking, running and stair climbing, as well as the development of increasingly sophisticated communication skills enable the child to start to assert their independence. It is also a period when children without impairment start to learn self-care skills such as how to dress independently, use utensils at mealtimes and become toilet trained, and when they start to socialize with other children, follow instructions and learn to hold a crayon and scribble.

Family experience of living with a child with disability

Caregiving is a normal part of parenting a young child. However, parental expectations of caregiving change when a child is diagnosed with cerebral palsy. A recent study (Schuengel et al, 2009) of 255 parents of children with cerebral palsy showed that although a diagnosis of cerebral palsy is a distressing event for any parent, parents of children with more severe forms of cerebral palsy (GMFCS levels IV–V) are at greater risk of exhibiting prolonged unresolved reactions to a diagnosis of cerebral palsy than parents of children with less severe forms. Unresolved reactions can lead to feelings of sorrow and anxiety that in turn can negatively impact on the parents' ability to care effectively for their child, and can in some cases impair attachment with the child (Schuengel et al, 1999).

Parenting children with cerebral palsy often requires extraordinary physical, emotional, social and financial resources. In addition to being responsible for the physical care of their child, parents must coordinate their child's numerous and multifaceted medical, education and developmental interventions while balancing competing family needs (Silver et al, 1998). Parents are often daunted by caring for a child with complex disabilities at home, and this can impact negatively on the physical health and the psychological well-being of parents (Raina et al, 2005). Therefore, therapists working with families of children with cerebral palsy should consider strategies for optimizing parents' physical and psychological health. This might include providing support for behavioural management and daily functional activities as well as introducing strategies to help parents manage stress and improve feelings of self-efficacy (Raina et al, 2005).

Parenting a child with a chronic disability also impacts on other family relationships. Parents of children with cerebral palsy commonly describe feeling uncertain and sometimes guilty about how well they meet the needs of other family members, such as their spouse, other children in the family and even extended family such as the child's grandparents (Murphy et al, 2006). Parents typically spend time with other family members only after the needs of the child with disabilities are satisfied (Murphy et al, 2006). Many families describe having a child with cerebral palsy as a positive experience, and believe that they have become more compassionate and 'more accepting and open to other people' (Murphy et al, 2006). Other families who have a child with a chronic disability experience increased family tension, marital breakdown and behavioural problems in siblings (Murphy et al, 2006).

The well-being of the siblings of children with a disability is an important consideration for therapists. Siblings of children with a disability have been shown to have significantly more adjustment difficulties, emotional symptoms and problems with peers compared with their peers (Giallo and Gavidia-Payne, 2006). Additionally, siblings may experience problems with depression, anxiety and externalizing behaviours (Summers et al, 1994; Rossiter and Sharpe, 2001; Sharpe and Rossiter, 2002). High levels of parent stress, poor family communication and problem-solving and limited time spent together as a family have been shown to be predictive of sibling adjustment problems (Giallo and Gavidia-Payne, 2006).

Importance of timely prognostic information
Information about the most likely motor outcome for their child with cerebral palsy is very important for most families. The uncertainty around the child's future abilities can be a source of stress, particularly up to the age of 3–4 years when the likely motor outcomes become clearer. The ability to predict prognosis also helps clinicians make decisions about the appropriateness of interventions, and allows service providers to plan for future resource requirements at home, at school and in the community.

Biomechanical considerations
Ben has gross motor abilities somewhere between GMFCS level III and IV. Gross motor curves for each GMFCS level have been developed (Rosenbaum et al, 2002) and at this age Ben should be on the upswing of the gross motor curve and ready to make rapid

progress. His motor skills are more likely to progress if spasticity can be managed and an appropriate therapy programme implemented. Spasticity management options include the use of anti-spasticity agents such as oral baclofen, multilevel injections of botulinum toxin A (BoNT-A), selective dorsal rhizotomy (SDR) or an intrathecal baclofen pump (ITB). The advantages and disadvantages of each of these approaches depend on different factors which have been discussed in recent review articles (Farmer et al, 2007, Novacheck and Gage, 2007; see Chapter 4).

One aim in the pharmacological management of spasticity is to prevent the development of fixed contractures (Graham and Selber, 2003). Botulinum toxin A injections are indicated primarily in children aged between 2 and 6 years (Cosgrove et al, 1998; Graham et al, 2000). An important aim of early effective spasticity management is to defer the need for more extensive deformity correction until the child is at an optimal age of around 8 to 10 years when the greatest benefits are obtained from surgical intervention (Bache et al, 2003; see Chapter 10).

Stage 4: assessment of body structures and function, activity and participation

Based on initial observations of Ben and the information and concerns expressed by his parents, a list of assessments of body structure and function, activity and participation was developed (Table 6.1).

Body structures and function
Table 6.2 summarizes the body structures and function assessment findings.

Table 6.1 Assessments for Ben

Body structures and function	Activity and participation
Spasticity: modified Tardieu scale Range of movement: goniometry	Overall gross motor function: Gross Motor Function Measure-66 (GMFM–66) Sitting balance: Sitting Assessment for Children with Neuromotor Dysfunction (SACND) Clinical observations of sitting (floor, stool and chair), pull-to-stand and walking Fine motor performance: Peabody Developmental Motor Scales–2 (grasping and visual motor integration domains) Self-care performance: Pediatric Evaluation of Disability Inventory (PEDI): self-care functional skills and caregiver assistance scores Clinical observations during a visit to Ben's daycare centre

Table 6.2 Assessment findings for the tests of body structures and function

	Assessment findings	
	Right side	Left side
Spasticity Modified Tardieu test		
Hip: abduction	R2–R1: 30° (X=2)	R2–R1: 20° (X=2)
extension	R2–R1: 10° (X=1)	R2–R1: 15° (X=1)
flexion	R2–R1: 40° (X=2)	R2–R1: 30° (X=2)
Knee: extension	R2–R1: 30° (X=1)	R2–R1: 20° (X=1)
Ankle: dorsi-flexion	R2–R1: 30° (X=2)	R2–R1: 20° (X=2)
Range of movement Goniometry[a]		
Hip: abduction	40°	50°
extension	15°	20°
flexion	45°	50°
Knee: extension	–5°	0°
Ankle: dorsi-flexion	+20°	+20°

R1, joint angle of muscle reaction (catch) at a V3 (as fast as possible) speed; R2, full passive range of movement (R2) at a V1 (as slow as possible) speed; X, the intensity and duration of the muscle reaction (the resistance felt when muscle is passively stretched).

a. All range of movement measures were assessed at V1 which is the slowest velocity of passive movement.

SPASTICITY AND RANGE OF MOVEMENT

As Table 6.2 shows, the severity and quality of Ben's spasticity was assessed using the modified Tardieu scale (see Appendix, p. 289). Hip abductor, extensor and flexor muscle length, as well as hamstring and ankle plantar-flexor muscle length were assessed using goniometry. As Ben shows diffuse spasticity in his lower limb muscles and cannot walk independently, he is at significant risk of spastic hip dislocation (Soo et al, 2006). Ben is on a hip surveillance programme at the tertiary hospital, being radiographed every 6 months. Thus far hip subluxation is minimal, with hip migration of 10° on the right and 5° on the left.

Activity

GROSS MOTOR FUNCTION

Ben's overall gross motor ability was assessed using the Gross Motor Function Measure (GMFM–66; Russell et al, 2000, see Appendix, p. 294). The GMFM–66 total score of 39 indicate that Ben is significantly limited physically, particularly in higher-level activities such as sitting, standing and walking and provide confirmation that his gross motor abilities are somewhere between GMFCS level III and IV.

Sitting: the following areas were highlighted.

- Floor sitting: Ben can pull himself into a 'W' sitting posture when on the floor. He cannot assume any other floor sitting position such as side sitting or ring sitting (i.e. sitting on the floor with bilateral hip flexion, external rotation and abduction and knee flexion), and when placed in these positions he either loses his balance or quickly becomes uncomfortable. Ben does not effectively use his upper limbs to help with balancing or to save himself.

- Stool/chair sitting: the Sitting Assessment for Children with Neuromotor Dysfunction (SACND; Reid, 1995; see Appendix, p. 295) was used to assess Ben's sitting balance when sitting on a bench. His score of 30 (14 on the rest module and the maximum 16 on the reach module) confirmed his poor sitting balance.

- Clinical observations were that Ben could sit when placed on a bench with no arm or back support, but that his balance was unreliable and after approximately 5 minutes he would start to extend his hips which would make him lose balance. He could not effectively use his arms to reach without requiring minimal support from Karyn. These results explained why Ben did not like to sit on stools in unsupported sitting, and he became anxious and would not use his hands to play, eat or do any other activities while sitting on a stool.

- When Ben was placed on a chair with side and back supports he was more confident in using his hands for play and other activities, but after approximately 15 minutes his hips would start to extend requiring him to assume an uncomfortable flexed trunk position to maintain his sitting posture and he would want to get off the chair.

Pull-to-stand: Ben could pull-to-stand independently using his arms. When he did this both lower limbs became very stiff, his hips and knees maintained a bilateral semi-flexed posture and his ankles became strongly plantar-flexed. There was no dissociation between his lower limbs and he did not push through his legs or fully weight bear on his feet when he was standing upright. He could not safely sit down from standing, and frequently he would either fall or cry for his parents to help him sit down.

Independent mobility: Spastic diplegia results in a generalized lower limb spastic hypertonia and during standing the lower limbs are usually held in a posture of hip adduction, flexion and internal rotation, knee flexion and ankle plantar flexion. Because of this posture the child cannot achieve an adequate base of support in standing and will have difficulties stepping. Ben could take one or two steps while holding on to a stable surface, but his lower trunk remained in contact with the stable surface, his steps were small and there was a tendency for him to take weight through the balls of his feet because his ankles remained in some degree of plantar-flexion.

Ben was keen to walk, energetically trying to step when held by both hands. However, his lower limbs felt 'tight' and his legs crossed as he stepped, one foot catching on the other. He was unable to get his feet flat on the floor and could not stand or walk independently.

Ben predominately used commando crawling to move around at home and at daycare. This meant he could not easily move around outside and in the playground at the daycare centre, and other children were in danger of tripping over him. His legs remained stiff with little reciprocal leg movements during commando crawling.

Assisted mobility: Ben's mother transported him in a standard infants' stroller, which he was rapidly outgrowing, for all outdoor and some indoor mobility. The stroller provided minimal postural support. When not in the stroller, Ben was often carried by his parents. He needed to be lifted in and out of the bath, his bed and car seat. Ben sometimes sat in his stroller during mealtimes.

FINE MOTOR FUNCTION

Although young children with spastic diplegia present primarily with difficulty in gross motor skills, their ability to use their upper limbs for handling and manipulating toys and for functional everyday tasks can also be compromised (Himmelmann et al, 2006; Nunes et al, 2008; See Chapter 11).

Ben's fine motor skills were assessed using the Peabody Developmental Motor Scales–2 (Wang et al, 2006; see Appendix, p. 294). This is a standardized norm-referenced test designed to measure the motor skills of children from birth to 6 years. In this instance only the fine motor subtests (grasping and visual motor integration) were used. Ben's raw scores on these two subtests were 40 and 82 respectively. These scores indicate that Ben is working at an age-equivalent of 14 months for grasping, and 19 months for visual motor integration, with corresponding centile rankings of sixteenth and fifth. Observations of Ben's fine motor skills during testing showed the following.

- When Ben was seated using a small supportive chair and table he was able to hold and manipulate objects optimally. When he was less supported in sitting he had greater difficulty holding and playing with objects/toys.
- Although Ben could easily grasp a variety of objects including using a pincer grip for small objects, he held a crayon using an immature upright grasp (palmar supinate).
- Ben could complete familiar actions such as building a tower of blocks and turning the pages of a book, and could complete actions that he imitated such as copying the therapist draw a line. However, he had difficulty with new tasks such as

snipping with scissors, threading beads, unscrewing the lid of a bottle and inserting shapes into a form board.

These findings suggested that as well as his neuromotor disorder, Ben might also have difficulties with motor planning. Motor planning is the ability to conceive of, organize and perform a sequence of unfamiliar actions involved in learning new skills. It requires the person to draw on past experiences of movement and apply this knowledge when planning and executing a new activity (Golisz and Toglia, 2003).

Some indicators that a child with cerebral palsy may have motor planning problems include the following:

- they find it difficult to complete tasks (especially if they are novel) even when they are physically capable. For example they can stack blocks, but find copying a block design difficult;
- they have numerous attempts to do the task, but their choice of an inappropriate 'plan' makes it difficult for them to complete it, or they may take a longer time than would typically be expected;
- simple physical guidance or verbal input helps the child achieve the task.

SELF-CARE ACTIVITIES

Ben's baseline self-care skills were assessed using the Pediatric Evaluation of Disability (PEDI; see Appendix, p. xx). Only the self-care domains for functional skills and caregiver assistance were scored. The expected mean score for these domains is 50 with a standard error of 10 points; Ben's raw scores of 16 and 1 converted to normative standard scores of 14.7 and less than 10 respectively. This showed Ben was having considerable difficulty completing self-care tasks as compared with other children of a similar age, and that Karyn and Cameron provided a great deal of assistance. The interview helped identify particular areas of difficulty for Ben and his parents, which were dressing, mealtimes, bathing and toilet training.

Dressing: Ben was dressed lying on the floor as a result of his poor balance in sitting and standing. He did not assist. Karyn and Cameron said it was particularly difficult getting his shoes and lower limb garments and nappy on as they could not easily move his legs apart.

Mealtimes: Ben still ate most of his meals in his high chair or sometimes his stroller as he needed the support they provided. Karyn and Cameron found that getting Ben into and out of his high chair was difficult as he kept his legs extended, and when he was there he tended to slump backwards (push his bottom forward). He could finger feed and he drank from a spouted beaker. However, Karyn fed him food from a spoon for most of his meals.

Bathing: as Ben's sitting balance was poor, he either had a bath with a parent (who held him) or he lay down in a very shallow bath of water. He was getting heavier to lift into and out of the bath.

Toileting: Ben was not toilet trained during the day, and he had no toileting programme. He experienced constipation about once a week.

Participation

DAYCARE
Ben enjoyed his time at the daycare centre. However, a visit to the centre by the special education preschool teacher and the occupational therapist identified the following issues.

- The chairs and tables at the daycare were not suitable for Ben. He tended to push his bottom forward and slide out of them or slump to the side. He needed someone to be with him when he sat at a table for play or mealtimes.
- Ben required assistance for mealtimes. He could feed himself finger foods, but needed the assistance of a staff member when eating foods off a spoon or fork.
- When Ben was on the floor he usually commando crawled with his stomach on the floor and the staff found this difficult to manage with the other children.
- During story-time, Ben lay on the floor or used 'W' sitting.
- The staff found it difficult for Ben to be outside with the other children as he was unable to move from place to place independently, nor could he use the outdoor play equipment. This made him isolated from his peers for much of the time.
- Ben was still in nappies and so a staff member was required to change him frequently.
- The staff were unsure about Ben's potential abilities and the things that they should be encouraging.

There is currently no provision of extra assistance for Ben at daycare.

Stage 5: contextual factors: personal and environmental

Personal factors
Ben is generally a happy child who enjoys interacting with others. He particularly enjoys music and water play. He has no cognitive or communication difficulties and is keen to be mobile and independent of adult assistance for mobility.

Ben was in a period of development when, due to natural history, rapid change in physical, social and psychological skills might be expected even without extensive therapy intervention. Intervention at this time was directed at optimizing Ben's natural development.

Environmental factors
Ben attends long hours (8.00 am to 6.00 pm) of daycare four days a week and he is expected to attend a mainstream preschool with his age peers. Ben's family have not accessed any respite care for him, even from close family members. Karyn's mother

Janet lives relatively close by and she is willing and even enthusiastic about becoming involved in his care by minding Ben on a regular basis.

Ben's precarious mobility is making it difficult for him to move independently around the daycare centre and access the playground at daycare. The family is financially secure.

Stage 6: negotiate the management plan

To avoid overwhelming Karyn and Cameron with too much information and by introducing too many new things at this early stage, the therapists worked with Karyn and Cameron to prioritize their intervention goals for the next 3 months. The team agreed that a review at 3 months would allow them to assess progress. The following issues were prioritized:

(1) spasticity management;
(2) facilitation of alternative methods of safe, independent mobility for home and daycare;
(3) development of self-care skills, particularly to provide ideas and suggestions for bathing, dressing, toileting and play positions;
(4) support for daycare centre staff;
(5) negotiate regular respite support for Karyn and Cameron through other family members (e.g. Ben's grandmother) or more formal respite services;
(6) provide advice and resources to assist with sibling disruptive behaviours at school and at home.

Stage 7: implement plan

(1) Spasticity management
The physiotherapist first referred Ben back to the tertiary referring hospital for advice about spasticity management, specifically suitability for injections of BoNT-A. A decision was made to inject sites in gastrocnemius, the hip adductors and the hamstrings bilaterally.

Fourteen days after the BoNT-A injections the local community physiotherapist completed a home visit and implemented a programme. Frequency of physiotherapy was increased to twice weekly at this time and continued at this intensity for 6 weeks. Frequency of physiotherapy should increase after BoNT-A injections to take advantage of the reduction of spasticity to improve range of movement and promote functional gains. Frequency should be determined on an individual basis and will depend on the child's age, functional level, compliance and family factors as well as therapist availability and funding.

(2) Facilitation of alternative methods of independent mobility
Photographs and written descriptions, as well as therapist demonstration and parent
practice, are commonly used to teach parents how to assist their young child learn a
motor skill. In the intensive physiotherapy period after the BoNT-A injections the
physiotherapist focused on facilitation of Ben's independent pull-to-stand and stepping,
walking with a walking assistance device, crawling rather than commando crawling and
sitting on the floor and on a chair.

The therapist initially highlighted the aspects of the pull-to-stand activity that Ben was
able to do, such as using his arms to help pull himself up to standing and using his arms
to stabilize and balance himself during this activity. The therapist then explained the
assistance Ben needed to progress. Because spasticity had been reduced significantly
with the BoNT-A injections, with assistance Ben could now move from sitting to kneel
stand, to half kneel stand and then pushing up through his lower limbs stand against a
stable surface, taking most of his body weight through his plantigrade feet. Once in
standing, Ben was encouraged to hold the stable surface and step sideways along it.
Karyn and Cameron were shown how the pull-to-stand and cruising activities could be
facilitated with good handling, and with repeated practice Ben would learn to perform
these activities independently. Ben's parents agreed to help Ben practise these activities
during floor play time. In addition, to facilitate better standing, Ben was given a
standing frame to enable him to have periods of time each day weight bearing through
his feet with hip and knee extension.

The reduced spasticity in his legs also helped Ben to use four-point crawling as a
means of floor mobility rather than commando crawling on his tummy. Ben's
parents were shown how to facilitate transitions into crawling from the floor, and
transitions from crawling into and out of long sitting through rotation and side
sitting. This also facilitated Ben's use of his arms for postural support and balance
while in sitting. Once in long sitting, Ben's parents practised how much trunk support
he needed to enable him to sit with the least amount of assistance, and they were
shown how to flex his hips adequately so that his trunk was relatively straight. This
freed his arms for play.

For greater independent mobility outside at home and at daycare Ben was provided with
an adapted tricycle. The tricycle was equipped with a lap belt, a modified supportive
saddle seat, and adapted Velcro fasteners to help maintain his feet on the pedals. The
tricycle enabled Ben to move relatively quickly in outside areas, made him more upright
to encourage interaction with the other children at daycare, and also facilitated range of
movement and reciprocal movements of his lower limbs.

Ben was also provided with a posterior walker (a K-walker) to encourage him to begin
to walk independently. Karyn and Cameron were shown how to encourage Ben not to
walk too fast and therefore start to drag his legs, and the family agreed to supervise his
practice for 20–30 minutes each day.

(3) Development of self-care skills
One of the most important things the therapists did to facilitate Ben's self-care skills was to help Karyn and Cameron understand the importance of teaching Ben to assist with self-care and feeding and to give him time to practise these new skills. A home visiting programme was implemented that addressed the following issues.

DRESSING
Dressing practice before and after Ben's nightly bath was considered the most suitable time because they had more time. Ben sat on a small bench seat pushed up against a wall and Karyn/Cameron knelt in front of him to provide assistance. Different ideas were tried to help Ben dress/undress himself. These included the following.

- As undressing is easier than dressing, Ben was encouraged to try this first and he was provided with less assistance in these tasks.
- Looser upper body clothing was used as they were easier for Ben to get into/out of. Elastic waists are good for trousers/jeans/pyjama bottoms rather than buttons/zips.
- Ben was helped to learn to undress/dress by using the same method every time. For example, some children find it easier to take off upper body garments over their head, whereas other children find it easier to pull an arm out first, then over their head and then the other arm. Ben was also guided verbally and physically through the easiest method, but only provided with the assistance that was needed. Ben was encouraged to do part of the task for himself right from the beginning. These strategies helped address Ben's motor planning difficulties associated with the skill of dressing.

MEALTIMES
A Tripp Trapp® high chair (manufactured by Stokke®, Ålesund, Norway) was modified for Ben. The seat base and foot rest were adjusted for his size, side support was provided, non-slip matting was placed on the seat base and the footplate, and a firm pelvic strap was fixed to the chair to prevent Ben's pelvis sliding forward. This chair enabled Ben to sit up at the table with the family during mealtimes. Ben's food was cut up, but he was encouraged to feed himself (initially only part of the meal) using child sized cutlery (spoon and fork).

TOILETING
Young children can be quite variable in their motivation and interest in toilet training. As Ben was only two and a half, toilet training was planned for the upcoming spring/summer when it would become warmer. In preparation, a supportive potty chair was bought for both home and daycare. It was decided that when he began toilet training a toilet timing programme (regularly putting Ben on the toilet especially after meals) would be implemented rather than expecting Ben to indicate when he wanted to go to the toilet.

Like many children with cerebral palsy Ben had experienced regular bouts of constipation and although it was not a high priority at this time the therapists provided the following general suggestions for how constipation can be managed.

- The use of a supportive potty seat is considered very important. Children with constipation need to feel secure and safe during toileting so they feel they can 'let go'. The occupational therapist accompanied Ben and his parents to a local baby store to see if a suitable supportive potty chair could be purchased. Figure 6.2 shows an example of a stable and supportive chair.

- Adequate opportunities should be given to go to the toilet, such as that provided by a toilet timing programme.

- Maintaining a high fibre diet and maintaining adequate fluid levels can be important.

- Increasing the time the child spends in more upright postures (including sitting) and being mobile can improve bowel activity.

- Discussing constipation with the child's paediatrician is also recommended because medication may be required for some children.

BATHING
A bath chair was required to give Ben sufficient postural control to sit in the bottom of the bath and play (Figure 6.3).

POSITIONING FOR PLAY
A number of play positions were encouraged besides 'W' sitting, which had become Ben's favoured position. The therapists explained that it was important to encourage alternative positions because Ben was becoming stuck in the 'W' sitting posture and he couldn't easily move in and out of it, making him relatively immobile. When on the floor, Ben's parents were shown how to help and encourage Ben to transition from crawling into long sitting to play with toys. Ben was encouraged to do some simple play activities in standing, in a standing frame he was given. For some of the time Ben used a small adapted chair and table. An example of a suitable chair is seen in Figure 6.4. To help maintain adequate hip flexion and discourage the tendency for Ben to extend his

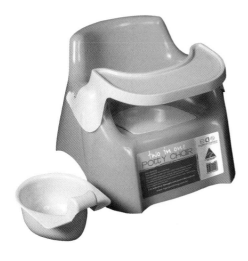

Figure 6.2 Two in one potty chair (Roger Armstrong Nursery Furniture, Victoria, Australia).

Figure 6.3
This low-backed bath
support is an example
of a suitable bath
support to trial with Ben
(Columbia Medical, Santa
Fe Springs, CA, USA).

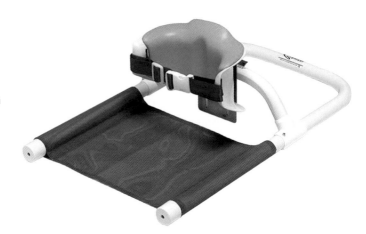

Figure 6.4 K1 Kinder chair
(Kaye Products Inc, Hillsborough,
NC, USA).

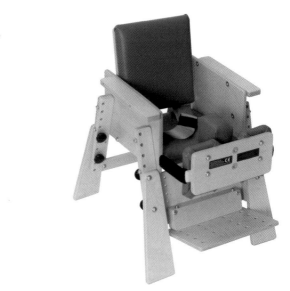

hips, the chair was fitted with a pelvic strap which fastened securely around his hips and a padded bilateral knee block. The height of the table was just above waist level so that Ben could use his arms and hands optimally.

(4) Daycare centre staff support
Disability awareness training for the daycare centre staff was instigated. This included visits by the physiotherapist, occupational therapist and special education preschool teacher to the daycare centre to discuss alternate mobility, show staff how to help Ben dress and go to the toilet, demonstrate positions Ben could use for play, and discuss which play and fine motor activities to encourage.

Appropriate equipment was also provided for Ben's use at daycare. This included a Kaye Kinder chair (adjusted to an appropriate height for the tables in the daycare centre) and a potty training chair similar to the equipment used at home. Karyn and Cameron brought in Ben's adapted tricycle and left it at the daycare centre during the week so that he could use it during the day when he was not tired. Ben's posterior K-walker was also brought in every day.

(5) Organize regular respite care for Ben
Ben's grandmother, Janet, was very keen to have Ben to visit on a regular basis (once a fortnight over night), which enabled Karyn and Cameron to spend 'special' time with their other son, Michael, as well as time with each other.

(6) Assistance with sibling disruptive behaviours at school and at home
The special education teacher assessed Michael's disruptive behaviour as being his attempts to gain attention. Karyn, Cameron and Michael were referred to a family-based group for young siblings and parents of children with a disability that was run in the local community health centre by a child psychologist, and the special education teacher.

The programme ran for six 1-hour sessions and was divided into sessions for parents and sessions for siblings. The aims of the group were to assist families in developing better coping skills to deal with daily stress, assist parents strengthen parenting skills supportive of siblings, and to help families to strengthen their communication and problem-solving skills, routines and time spent together as a family (Giallo and Gavidia-Payne, 2008).

Parent-based sessions covered topics such as stress in the family, dealing with children's behaviour, managing family times and routines, communication in the family and dealing with problem behaviours. Sibling sessions covered topics such as coping with stresses, getting along with others and dealing with problems. Families were also given written information and telephone support.

Stage 8: evaluate outcomes
At the 3-monthly review Karyn and Cameron reported they were pleased with the progress that had been made in a number of areas.

Spasticity management
The severity of Ben's lower limb spasticity and joint range of movement were reassessed (Table 6.3). As the table shows, the BoNT-A injections had reduced the spasticity in Ben's lower limbs.

Facilitation of alternative methods of independent mobility
As a result of the reduced spasticity and the intensive physiotherapy sessions, Ben could now move independently and safely from sitting on the floor to standing through half kneel stand, and he could walk along a stable surface with his trunk slightly away from the surface with light support from his hands to assist balance. He was also beginning to lower himself safely from standing to sitting, but he still sometimes fell. Ben could

Table 6.3 Reassessment findings for the tests of body structures and function

	Assessment findings	
	Right side	Left side
Spasticity Modified Tardieu test Hip: abductors extensors flexors	R2–R1: 15° (X=1) R2–R1: 10° (X=1) R2–R1: 20° (X=1)	R2–R1: 10° (X=1) R2–R1: 15° (X=1) R2–R1: 20° (X=1)
Knee: extensors	R2–R1: 20° (X=1)	R2–R1: 10° (X=1)
Ankle: dorsi-flexion	R2–R1: 10° (X=1)	R2–R1: 10° (X=1)
Range of movement Goniometry[a] Hip: abduction extension flexion	60° 30° 65°	70° 30° 90°
Knee: extension	0°	0°
Ankle: dorsi-flexion	+40°	+40°

R1, joint angle of muscle reaction (catch) at a V3 (as fast as possible) speed; R2, full passive range of movement (R2) at a V1 (as slow as possible) speed; X, the intensity and duration of the muscle reaction (the resistance felt when muscle is passively stretched).

a. All range of movement measures were assessed at V1 which is the slowest velocity of passive movement.

walk independently slowly with the assistance of his posterior walker a distance of about 75 metres.

Although Ben could crawl better with his trunk held off the floor, it was noticed that when he wanted to move quickly across the floor he was starting to bunny hop (both lower limbs remained flexed at the hips and knees and they were hopped through without any reciprocal leg movements). Because repetition of this flexed posture and movement tends to make standing and walking more difficult, and because his peer group no longer used floor mobility as their primary means of locomotion, a decision was made to limit mobility on the floor; instead Ben was encouraged to use his tricycle and the posterior walker more for independent mobility.

Ben still predominately used the 'W' sitting position, but if he was asked he could maintain a ring sitting position for floor play and he was able to move quickly and safely from the floor to sitting and back again. Reassessment of the SACND (see Appendix, p. 295) to assess Ben's sitting balance when sitting on a bench revealed a score of 26 (12 on the rest module and 14 on the reach module). This confirmed that his sitting balance was still poor when sitting independently on a bench, but it had improved over the previous 3 months.

Development of self-care skills
Ben's self-care skills had also improved markedly over the 3 months. He had learned to feed himself cut-up foods using both finger feeding and his spoon and fork. He was also feeding himself at the daycare centre. The bath chair enabled Ben to sit independently in the bath, and Ben was beginning to take off easy items of clothing independently before the bath and help with dressing after the bath. The dressing programme was also extended to weekends when there was more time available. The toilet timing programme had not yet commenced.

Support for daycare centre staff
The daycare staff were feeling more comfortable with providing Ben with an appropriate programme to encourage his independence, promote his motor and cognitive development and to foster his participation in the centre's daily activities. Provision of equipment helped to support these aims.

Regular respite care for Ben
Ben had been staying overnight with his grandmother on a regular fortnightly basis during the weekend. This had worked well for Ben, his grandmother Janet and the rest of Ben's family. However, Janet had recently experienced a fall and had fractured her wrist and so was not able to care for Ben for the next 3 months. Karyn and Cameron decided that rather than exploring other respite care options they would wait until Janet was well and could once again care for Ben on a regular basis.

Sibling disruptive behaviours at school and at home
Cameron and Karyn reported they enjoyed the parent and sibling group and that Michael's behaviour at school had improved considerably. Fitting family activities into their busy lifestyle and following up some of the other recommendations was sometimes difficult. However, Karyn and Cameron recognized the importance of following through with the ideas that had been generated from the sessions.

Next steps
Karyn and Cameron reported that they felt more in control and confident about how things were going to develop in the next few years.

New directions for intervention were also negotiated with Karyn and Cameron. These included the following:

- assessment of Ben's play skills both at home and within the daycare setting;
- incorporating ideas to encourage the development of his fine motor skills into his daycare programme;

- referral to a mobility clinic where Ben would be assessed and provided with an appropriate adapted stroller so that Karyn and Cameron would not need to carry him around as much and they could more easily take him to community venues. For example, he could more easily go shopping or to the picture theatre with the family;

- an application for funding was submitted to provide an additional 8 hours (2 hours a day for 4 days per week) of assistance for Ben while he was at daycare;

- ongoing assessment of Ben's level of spasticity;

- assessment of Ben's need for lower limb splints/orthoses;

- ongoing and regular hip surveillance (see Chapter 2);

- commencement of Ben's toilet training programme.

Box 6.3 Key clinical messages

- Effective support of the young child with cerebral palsy involves assisting the child's support network, such as their family members and daycare staff.

- Utilizing the skills of a range of health professions working in a multidisciplinary team can be the most effective way of managing the array of needs of children with cerebral palsy and their families.

- Limitations in mobility can reduce a child's access to opportunities for social engagement and participation in other daily living activities that can in turn limit their opportunity to learn these skills.

References

Bache CE, Selber P & Graham HK (2003) The management of spastic diplegia. *Curr Orthop*, 17, 88–104.

Canadian Association of Occupational Therapists (CAOT) (2002) *Enabling Occupation: An Occupational Therapy Perspective*. Ottawa: Canadian Association of Occupational Therapists.

Cosgrove AP, Corry IS & Graham HK (1998) Musculoskeletal modelling in determining the effect of Botulinum toxin on the hamstrings of patients with crouch gait. *Dev Med Child Neurol*, 40, 622–5.

Einspieler C, Prechtl HF (2005). Prechtl's assessment of general movements: a diagnostic tool for the functional assessment of the young nervous system. *Ment Retard Dev Disabil Res Rev*, 11, 61–7.

Farmer J-P & Sabbagh AJ (2007) Selective dorsal rhizotomies in the treatment of spasticity related to cerebral palsy. *Childs Nerv Syst*, 23, 991–1002.

Giallo R & Gavidia-Payne S (2006) Child, parent and family factors as predictors of adjustment for siblings of children with a disability. *J Intellect Disabil Res*, 50, 937–48.

Giallo R & Gavidia-Payne S (2008) Evaluation of a family-based intervention for siblings of children with a disability or chronic illness. *Aust e-J Adv Mental Health (AeJAMH)*, 7, 1–13.

Golisz K & Toglia J (2003) Section II: Perception and cognition. In: Crepeau E, Cohn E & Schell B (eds) *Willard and Spackman's Occupational Therapy*: 395–416. Philadelphia, PA: Lippincott, Williams & Wilkins.

Graham HK, Aoki KR, Autti-Rämö I, Boyd RN, Delgado MR, Gaebler-Spira DJ, Gormley ME, Guyer BM, Heinen F, Holton AF, Matthews D, Molenaers G, Motta F, García Ruiz PJ and Wissel J (2000)

Recommendations for the use of botulinum toxin type A in the management of cerebral palsy. *Gait Posture*, 11, 67–79.

Graham HK & Selber P (2003) Musculoskeletal aspects of cerebral palsy. *J Bone Joint Surg Br*, 85, 157–66.

Himmelmann K, Beckung E, Hagberg G & Uvebrant P (2006) Gross and fine motor function and accompanying impairments in cerebral palsy. *Dev Med Child Neurol*, 48, 417–23.

Murphy NA, Christian B, Caplin DA. & Young PC (2006) The health of caregivers for children with disabilities: caregiver perspectives. *Child Care Health Dev*, 33, 180–187.

Novacheck TF, Gage JR (2007) Orthopedic management of spasticity in cerebral palsy. *Childs Nerv Syst*, 23, 1015–31.

Nunes G, Braga LW, Rossi L, Lawisch VL, Nunes LGN & Dellatolas G (2008) Hand skill assessment with a reduced version of the Peg Moving Task (PMT–5) in children: normative data and application in children with cerebral palsy. *Arch Clin Neuropsychol*, 23, 87–101.

Palisano RJ, Rosenbaum PL, Bartlett D & Livingston MH (2008) Content validity of the expanded and revised gross motor function classification system. *Dev Med Child Neurol*, 50, 744–50.

Raina P, O'Donnell M, Rosenbaum P, Brehaut J, Walter SD, Russell D, Swinton M, Zhu B, Wood E (2005) The health and well-being of caregivers of children with cerebral palsy. *Pediatrics*, 115, e626–36.

Reid D, Schuller R & Billson N (1995) Reliability of the SACND. *Phys OccupTher Pediatr*, 16, 23–32.

Rosenbaum P, Walter S, Hanna S, Palisano R, Russell D, Raina P, Wood E, Bartlett D & Galuppi B (2002) Prognosis for gross motor function in cerebral palsy. *JAMA*, 288, 1357–63.

Rossiter L & Sharpe D (2001) The siblings of individuals with mental retardation: a quantitative integration of the literature. *J Child Fam Stud*, 10, 65–84.

Russell DJ, Avery LM, Rosenbaum PL, Raina PS, Walter SD & Palisano RJ (2000) Improved scaling of the gross motor function measure for children with cerebral palsy: evidence of reliability and validity. *Phys Ther*, 80, 873–85.

Schuengel C, Rentinck ICM, Stolk J, Voorman JM, Loots GMP, Ketelaar M, Görter JW, Becher JG (2009) Parents' reactions to the diagnosis of cerebral palsy: associations between resolution, age and severity of disability. *Child Care Health Dev*, 35, 673–80.

Schuengel C, Backermans-Kranenburg MJ, Van Ijzendoorn MH (1999) Frightening maternal behavior linking unresolved loss abd disorganized infant attachment. *J Consult Clin Psychol*, 67, 54–63.

Sharpe D & Rossiter L (2002) Siblings of children with a chronic illness: a meta-analysis. *J Pediatr Psychol*, 27, 699–710.

Silver EJ, Westbrook LE, Stein RE (1998) Relationship of parental psychological distress to consequences of chronic health conditions in children. *J Pediatr Psychol*, 23, 5–15.

Soo B, Howard JJ, Boyd RN, Reid SM, Lanigan A, Wolfe R, Reddihough D & Graham HK (2006) Hip displacement in cerebral palsy. *J Bone Joint Surg Am*, 88, 121–9.

Summers C, White K & Summers M (1994) Siblings of children with a disability: a review and analysis of the empirical literature. *J Soc Behav Pers*, 9, 169–84.

Wang HH, Liao HF & Hsieh CL (2006) Reliability, sensitivity to change, and responsiveness of the Peabody developmental motor scales-second edition for children with cerebral palsy. *Phys Ther*, 86, 1351–9.

Chapter 7

Modified constraint–induced therapy for young children

Margaret Wallen and Christine Imms

Play-based intervention during the toddler and preschool years offers many opportunities for therapists to engage children in meaningful and therapeutic interactions. Exploiting this stage when children's play repertoires are rapidly expanding provides the vehicle for implementing motivating therapy and optimizing the learning environment.

Case study: Callum

Callum is a 2-year-old boy with a right-sided spastic hemiparesis (unilateral cerebral palsy). Callum's mother requested occupational therapy support to carry out modified constraint-induced therapy (modCIT), an intervention she had read about on the Internet. Callum's parents were exploring modCIT and botulinum toxin A (BoNT-A) injections as options for improving Callum's ability to use his affected arm in everyday activities. Chapter 3 discusses the concept of 'seekership' whereby families of children with disabilities gather knowledge of appropriate interventions, strategies and services to assist them in making decisions about their child's management. The steps involved in the clinical reasoning process used in this chapter are summarized in Figure 7.1 and described in Chapter 1.

Stage 1: initial data collection

Callum attended an initial occupational therapy assessment with his parents, Sonja and Andrew. A medical history was gathered as a basis for understanding Callum's disability.

Callum was born at full term after an uneventful pregnancy and birth. In the 24 hours following birth he experienced seizures. Magnetic resonance imaging (MRI) revealed an infarct in the left middle cerebral artery region. Callum has since been free of seizures, but a right-sided hemiplegia has persisted. On assessment at 24 months of age, Callum

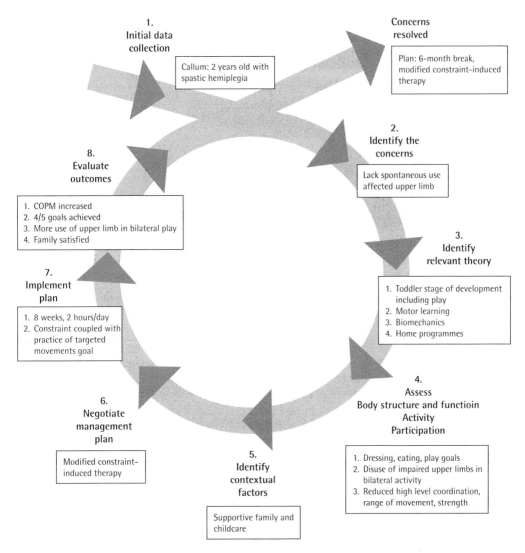

Figure 7.1 The intervention process used with Callum: model adapted with permission from the Canadian Occupational Performance Process Model (CAOT, 2002). COPM, Canadian Occupational Performance Measure.

had normal hearing and vision, and typically developing left, dominant unilateral hand skills, verbal communication and cognition. Callum's gross motor skills were mildly delayed. He was classified as level I on the Gross Motor Function Classification System (GMFCS, Palisano et al, 2008; see Chapter 2 and Box 7.1) but was too young to be classified on the Manual Ability Classification System (MACS, see www.macs.nu, Eliasson et al, 2006).

Box 7.1 GMFCS level I snapshot[1]

Proportion of people with cerebral palsy classified as GMFCS I: 32–48%

Proportion of people classified as GMFCS level I who

- have a severe intellectual disability (IQ <50): about 5%;
- have a severe visual impairment: less than 10%;
- have epilepsy: about 10%;
- have behavioural problems: less than 5%;
- have hip displacement requiring surgery: less than 1%;
- walk alone at home by age 2–3years: 90%;
- walk alone at home by age 4–12 years: 99%.

Stage 2: identify and prioritize concerns

Consistent with a family-focused care framework for practice, involvement began with identifying Sonja and Andrew's priorities for intervention and determining with them whether modCIT was an appropriate intervention for Callum and the family unit (see Chapter 4 for an overview of constraint-induced movement therapy). Sonja and Andrew had read that modCIT involved constraining Callum's unimpaired hand to encourage him to use his impaired hand. Their primary concern was that Callum avoided involving his right upper limb in activity despite potentially adequate motor ability and they thought modCIT might work for him. Sonja and Andrew identified dressing, eating and play activities that they believed Callum should be completing more independently. They predicted that Callum's performance on many essential preschool activities, such as drawing and ball skills, would not reach potential because of his limited capability to engage in bimanual hand use. Detailed discussion ensued about the nature of modCIT, the rationale behind this intervention, the intensity of its implementation and the amount of support provided by therapists. Sonya and Andrew agreed they were committed to undertaking therapy and would like to pursue modCIT. Callum was informally assessed to ascertain that he would be able to cooperate with therapy and had some voluntary movement in his shoulder, elbow, wrist and fingers that would allow him to stabilize an object on a tabletop or against his body even if he was, as yet, unable to do so. These are minimum criteria for a child to participate in modCIT.

Stage 3: identify relevant theoretical foundations involved in working with Callum

Developmental stage: toddlerhood and play

Play is a particularly important developmental domain in toddlerhood. Children with cerebral palsy, who have limitations in their ability to interact with their world,

---

1   See Chapter 2: p. 17 for details of the sources used to derive these data.

may need play to be both the medium and a desired outcome of therapy (Humphry, 2002; see Chapter 4). Therapists working with children need to attend to the social and environmental opportunities for (and constraints on) play in addition to child-centred elements such as skill development (Humphry and Wakeford, 2006).

The sensorimotor stage of play is in evidence until about 2 years of age. Children engage widely in play that is exploratory – of themselves, their environment and the objects within it (Cronin and Mandich, 2005). Children begin to move into the preoperational play stage from approximately 2 years of age, in which play becomes more symbolic, including simple make-believe, use of everyday objects in play and construction games (Parham and Primeau, 1997). Knowledge of the child's play strengths, age-specific developmental motivators and the next stages of play development allows play to be integrated as both a means and an end to therapy. There are a number of sources of information on the developmental characteristics of being two (Gething et al, 1995; Cech and Martin, 2002; Case-Smith, 2005).

Using motor learning principles with modCIT

Motor learning principles can be used with constraint of the unaffected arm in hemiplegia to achieve movement goals. During the period in which the unaffected hand is constrained, therapy activities are selected that elicit many self-generated voluntary repetitions (that is, involve practice) of the required movements (Valvano, 2004; Eliasson, 2005). Activities can be used in which the unaffected arm is used as an assisting arm, within the limits of the constraint. Children are likely to require several different activities to provide adequate repetition of target movements rather than simply repeating one activity. Sufficient repetition may be difficult to achieve but the priority is to facilitate active, spontaneous and voluntary movement. Activities must be fun and motivating to engage the child fully and maximize learning. Activities that are suitably challenging and carefully graded will capture the child's attention and maintain motivation. Feedback, whether verbal, manual or using rewards, is also critical to the therapeutic process.

Attention to the child's stage of motor learning is important. During the verbal cognitive stage a child learns to solve a movement problem to achieve the task and will require careful support from the therapist. In the motor stage, repetition is important for task learning and in the automatic phase the child's motor behaviour becomes smooth and flexible (Fitts and Posner, 1967). Not all children will reach the automatic phase of motor learning and those with more severe impairments, or with cognitive impairments, will require longer periods of time and more support in the earlier stages.

Motor learning is supported by the use of demonstration, imitation, manual guidance and strengthening. Demonstration of movement patterns that are object-related, followed by a child's attempts to imitate the action, may assist a child to learn that movement (Buccino et al, 2006). Manual guidance can give a child the sense of a required movement without compensatory patterns.

Biomechanical considerations

Hypertonia, which may be accompanied by spasticity (Lin, 2004), can mechanically hinder function (Dunne et al, 1995). Constraint-induced therapy may be effective in combination with BoNT-A injections particularly for children with more severe impairments. Callum's family decided, however, to delay consideration of BoNT-A, despite his potential eligibility, in favour of the less invasive modCIT.

Reduced strength is common in cerebral palsy. Upper limb strength is necessary for sustaining a desired movement and achieving resisted movement, for example, grasping to stabilize a piece of lego, pulling down pants or pushing off a shoe. Movement against resistance is essential for developing strength (Damiano, 2004) and can be built into therapy activities.

Home programmes

Modified constraint-induced therapy relies on the family providing daily therapy to maximize outcomes for the child. Novak and Cusick (2006) propose that an effective home programme is founded on a collaborative relationship with the family. Mutually agreed goals are generated and therapeutic activities collaboratively determined. These activities are demonstrated and documented with accompanying diagrams and photos where possible, and families are offered a variety of strategies or a 'library of ideas' from which to select suitable tasks. Important components of home programme implementation are to review the programme regularly, including parent and child performance, and to evaluate outcomes with the family. Novak et al (2007) have demonstrated positive outcomes for children with cerebral palsy using their model of home programme implementation (see Chapter 4).

Stage 4: assessment of participation, activity and body structure and function

Participation-focused and family-centred frameworks (see Chapter 3) provided the foundation for interaction with Callum and his family. The first step in the assessment process involves families identifying participation restrictions or activities and tasks that their child struggles to complete in daily life. The Canadian Occupational Performance Measure (COPM, Law et al, 2005) is an appropriate assessment for this purpose (see Appendix, p. 291). The next step is to complete a task analysis of the areas identified as being high priorities. For Callum, this had the following two objectives:

- to determine Callum's current level of ability as a baseline for setting goals;
- to identify deficient movement patterns to target using motor learning principles.

Further assessment is also useful to identify strengths and weaknesses of performance as they relate to the achievement of the goals identified. The Assisting Hand Assessment (AHA, Krumlinde-Sundholm and Eliasson, 2003; Krumlinde-Sundholm et al, 2007; see Appendix, p. 291) provided a structured means for understanding Callum's bimanual performance. His AHA score of 69 (possible range 22–88, with 88 indicating a high level of bimanual ability) was 71% of the total. Callum's successful and independent bimanual task performance was mildly affected by his hemiplegia. He consistently involved his affected hand in stabilizing objects, often using grasp, although there was a slight delay in initiating use. Callum's main limitations were associated with fine manipulative grasping and releasing. In addition, Callum did not use his affected hand to obtain objects when they were in his affected body space but reached long distances to obtain them with his non-affected hand.

Other potentially useful assessments include the Pediatric Evaluation of Disability Index (Haley et al, 1992); the Melbourne Assessment of Unilateral Upper Limb Function (Randall et al, 1999); the Quality of Upper Extremity Skills Test (DeMatteo et al, 1991); and the Pediatric Motor Activity Log (Taub et al, 2004; Wallen et al, 2008a). Assessments of spasticity (for example the modified Tardieu scale) and range of movement could also be considered although modCIT does not target, nor is it expected to effect change, in these impairments.

Finally, Goal Attainment Scaling (GAS, Kiresuk et al, 1994) can be used to formulate specific goals for intervention (see Appendix, p. 292). Callum's goals reflected three aspects of the assessment: priorities identified by his family when completing the COPM, Callum's upper limb abilities as identified using the AHA; outcomes of the task analysis of the activities identified as priorities for intervention. Callum's goals and the selected movements to target using modCIT are listed in Table 7.1.

Stage 5: contextual factors: environmental factors

Support and relationships
Sonja's mother was involved with the family and offered to be available three times a week to assist by either working with Callum or supervising his sister Lilly. Callum's daycare centre was willing to allocate one staff member to work with Callum for 30 minutes each day he attended.

Stage 6: management plan

Summary of assessment findings
Completing the COPM identified five meaningful goals for intervention. Task analysis identified a number of movement strengths and limitations that could be targeted during modCIT. The AHA provided specific opportunity to observe bilateral play and confirmed Callum's parents' impression that he avoiding using his affected upper limb in bilateral activity. Importantly these assessments can also be used to evaluate the impact of intervention.

Negotiated treatment plan
Sonja and Andrew agreed that Callum would wear a mitt for 2 hours per day, for 8 weeks in minimum blocks of 30 minutes. Time spent discussing Callum's daily routine helped identify the optimum times for mitt wear around his meals and his

Table 7.1 Functional and movement goals identified for intervention

COPM identified areas	Desired outcome for each functional goal	Target movements
Pulling pants down for toileting	Before going to the toilet, and wearing elastic top shorts that his helper has taken past his bottom, Callum will use both hands to pull the pants down to his knees each occasion within 8 weeks	Grip strength Elbow extension and strength
Holding paper for drawing	Sitting in appropriate size furniture at home, and using A4 paper and thick textas to draw, Callum will stabilize the paper with his right arm for 25 to 50% of the time of the drawing task without prompting, within 8 weeks	Stabilizing with downwards pressure using open hand Massed practice to encourage more spontaneous involvement[a]
Catching a ball	Callum will catch a 25 cm ball, thrown at his chest from 1.5 m away, 3 to 5 times out of 10 attempts within 8 weeks	Supination Speed of movement
Taking off T-shirt	Callum will remove his right arm from the sleeve of a loose fitting short-sleeve T-shirt within 5 seconds of starting the task 51 to 75% of the time, within 8 weeks	Shoulder extension and abduction/adduction
Holding a drink bottle to open	Callum will hold his drink bottle in his right hand and successfully open the bottle with his left hand on the first attempt, 26 to 50% of the time, within 8 weeks	Grip strength and sustained grasp with forearm in mid-position

COPM, Canadian Occupational Performance Measure.

a. Massed practice is where use of the affected upper limb is encouraged without specific regard to targeted movement goals. The aim of massed practice is to increase the recruitment and general use of the affected hand and arm in all functional tasks.

sleep routines. It was agreed that one 30-minute session per day could be nested within a daily routine (for example, meal or bath times) without necessarily targeting movement goals. The family would complete a logbook of time spent wearing the mitt, the activities completed and Callum's motor and behavioural responses. The family would attend an appointment with the occupational therapist once a week. Plans were also made with Sonja and Andrew to re-evaluate Callum's progress at the end of the 8-week intervention to determine goal achievement and plan future intervention.

Stage 7: implement plan

Modified constraint-induced therapy

The modCIT (see Chapter 4 for overview) used with Callum was adapted from work by Eliasson and colleagues (2005). It differs from traditional constraint-based therapies, which involve 24-hour per day constraint and intense therapy for several hours during the day for 2 to 3 weeks. Modified constraint-induced therapy is more family focused (Wallen et al, 2008b) as mitt wearing times can be integrated into family and child routines and accommodate the individual needs of the child. In particular, modCIT may be more appropriate for children with severe impairments, as reduced time in constraint can limit the potential frustration experienced. The shorter period of wear per day, which theoretically is counterbalanced by the longer duration of therapy (i.e. 8 weeks), is likely to be better tolerated by children and be more achievable for families.

Modified constraint-induced therapy is essentially a unilateral intervention. We rely on the assumption that improving movement through targeted practice will generalize to the functional bimanual activities that are the intervention goals. This assumption has yet to be proven. Occupational therapists do not usually use one model of intervention in isolation, tending to employ a combination of approaches to meet the individual needs and goals of their client. Pragmatically therapists might choose to supplement modCIT with other techniques such as splinting (Copley and Kuipers, 1999) or goal-directed training (Mastos et al, 2007). Posturing of the thumb-in-palm is a common problem in young children with hemiplegia, and a neoprene thumb abductor splint or strapping to assist the child to maintain an open thumb web space can be used.

THE MITT

The aim of the mitt is to prevent grasp and release. The mitt that Callum wore had a solid volar insert and a fastening at the wrist to prevent removal (Figure 7.2). Wrist, elbow and shoulder movements are unimpeded so the constrained arm can still be used as an assisting arm to stabilize objects during manipulation by the affected arm. This model allows experience of bimanual activity with the mitted hand used as a stabilizer and may also reduce frustration from attempts to master tasks unilaterally with an affected hand. In addition, wearing the mitt does not prevent the unaffected arm being used for balance and to protect against falling (Wallen et al, 2008b).

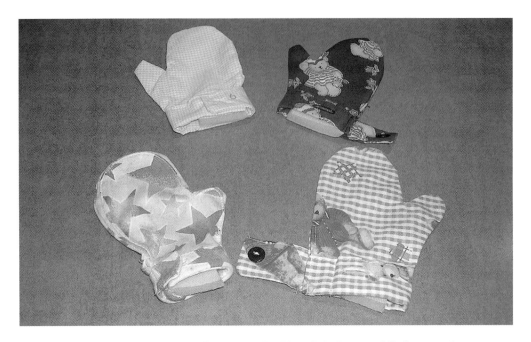

Figure 7.2 Examples of mitt used for unimpaired hand during modified constraint-induced therapy.

OCCUPATIONAL THERAPY AND MOTOR LEARNING PRINCIPLES

Families have reported that weekly therapy sessions provide critical support for the implementation of modCIT (Wallen et al, 2008b). Callum and his parents attended occupational therapy once a week although some families may require support more frequently. The therapy sessions were used to monitor Callum's progress, assist in identifying motivating activities and upgrade the difficulty of tasks as improvements occurred. Each week a therapy plan was developed that specified activities to target movement goals (Table 7.2).

A weekly written home programme was given to the family providing reminders of general principles of therapy and several activity ideas (Figure 7.3) along with demonstrations and explanations of activities and rationales for their selection (Novak and Cusick, 2006). Sonja and Andrew were advised to continue encouraging Callum to use both hands in everyday activities during the periods he was not wearing the mitt. They also followed strategies devised to assist Callum in achieving his activity goals. These strategies included assisting Callum to learn the requirements of the task and providing opportunities for practice. For instance, each time Callum was required to remove a T-shirt, specific strategies were used to improve his ability to remove his affected arm from the sleeve.

Motor learning principles were used to identify and implement activities that would achieve the nominated movement goals. The movement goals and the rationale for their

Table 7.2 Extract from a therapy plan for Callum

Activity	Movement goals	Implementation
Making slice (mix dry ingredients with melted ones and press into a tin)	1. Massed practice	1. Use all aspects of activity e.g. count marshmallows into measuring cup (could place these on a higher surface to encourage shoulder and elbow extension, hand them to Callum asking him to supinate his hand), press microwave buttons, pour each jug of (cooled) ingredients into bowl, place cut slice into container to take home
	2. Grip strength	2. Grasp built up handle of a wooden spoon to stir mixture and to spoon into slice tin Use hand to squish mixture together
	3. Downward pressure with hand open	3. Use flat hand to push down and smooth mixture into tin

---

A few ideas for Callum
Week 3

🚒 Remember to use the clean up as part of mitt time, i.e. wipe down table, wash hands, place garbage in bin, wash sponges and squeeze out and lay out to dry etc.

🚒 Painting with sponges (use different items from home, eg cotton balls, dishcloths cut into interesting shaped pieces). Put paper on wall to encourage shoulder movement as well as on table-top to push down onto. Offer some sponges to Callum so he must turn his palm up to grasp them.

🚒 Skittles/10-pin bowling – rolling a ball into empty water bottles, or stacks of blocks. The important part of this game is for Callum to build the blocks or set up water bottles. Water bottles encourage Callum to turn his palm around and precise release, as well as extending his elbow.

Figure 7.3 Extract from Callum's home programme.

importance were explained so that Sonya would understand why particular activities were selected. She could then modify, adapt or identify other activities to supplement those suggested by the therapist. For instance, Callum's therapist demonstrated handing game pieces to Callum at different heights to achieve a wide range of shoulder motion including functional ranges such as on the top of his head, over the opposite shoulder and towards the floor.

Feedback is a critical component of motor learning. Callum responded to verbal guidance to assist him to complete activities. The feedback was positively framed; for example, 'let's see if you can do it this way', 'turn your hand around a little more', 'come just a bit closer', 'let go now' etc, rather than correcting or criticizing. Callum responded well to feedback, either verbal or other forms (cheering, clapping or contact), that rewarded small approximations of success.

PLAY ACTIVITIES AND MATERIALS
Sonja kept a 'magic basket' of special and motivating toys that were only used during mitt time to enhance Callum's engagement while wearing the mitt. Sonja was encouraged to search her cupboards and budget merchandise shops for cheap and readily available activity options. Modifying some items with larger handles, for instance, paint brushes and wooden spoon handles, enhanced success. See Figure 7.4 for an example of the logbook Sonja kept of Callum's participation in modCIT.

A critical component of successful adherence to modCIT and achievement of motor learning is that the activities the child completes are fun and highly motivating (Figure 7.5). Activities that engage the child completely will maximize the time the child spends in activities and will promote the repetition of movement required for learning. Knowledge of Callum's stage of play development and his play preferences enabled both the therapist and his parents to select engaging activities. A helpful resource for promoting play in children aged 1 to 6 years is the Symbolic and Imaginative Play Developmental Checklist (Stagnitti, 1998). Stagnitti identifies developmental levels for symbolic and imaginative play in areas such as the child's ability to relate to objects, sequence play actions, role play and use a doll or teddy within play (Stagnitti, 1998). For example, for 2-year-old Callum, imaginative play scenarios that are common to his daily life (Stagnitti, 1998), such as preparing food and eating, caring for his sister Lilly, gardening and shopping were appropriate. Thus, dolls and teddies, blankets, cars, kitchen toys, household and shopping items can become part of play during mitt time.

SUGGESTIONS FOR FACILITATING IMPLEMENTATION
Sonja found it useful to plan a weekly timetable. On Sunday evenings, she mapped out the week ahead, selecting optimal time slots for Callum to wear the mitt. She would list the activities for each session, attempting to achieve a balance of activities to target each movement goal. Advanced planning allowed Sonja to prepare a variety of activities and manage particular busy days with simpler sessions that did not require preparation or cleaning up.

Date: July 20th		
Place	**Time**	**Activities and Comments**
Home	7.45am, 35 mins	Playdough – squashed flat, pushed in pegs and rolled up playdough, pulled out pegs. Enjoyed wearing the mitt, opening and closing hand more to grasp toys, reached to other side to pick up pegs. Also ate vegemite toast, handed toast to get him to turn palm up more with flat hand.
Nannas	12.30pm, 45 mins	Batted balloon all through hallways and used paper towel roll to bat ball. This was hard but fun. Callum got all Grandpa's socks from drawer and put in container. Nanna hid them for Callum to find and replace in drawer, happy doing this for a long while. Ate cheese and apple chunks.
Home	5.45pm, 40 mins	With Dad – rolled golf balls across table and down cardboard tubes, gave balls to Callum up high, to the side, down low, palm up etc. Bath with foam shapes, stuck to tiles, caught them and put them in containers. Bath time great for mitt wear.

Figure 7.4 Excerpt from the log book from Callum's modified constraint-induced therapy programme.

Although rarely reported in the literature (Eliasson et al, 2005; Wallen et al, 2008b), children and families sometimes find it difficult to maintain their participation in a negotiated modCIT programme. Occasionally children reject the mitt and family stressors (not all of which are predictable but may include ill health, moving house, change of work status) play a role in a family's ability to complete a programme. In addition, it appears that some families find it difficult, about 5 to 6 weeks into the 8-week block of intervention, to sustain the level of intensity required. Factors influencing this difficulty seem to be related to both the child's engagement and the family's time.

Support for families to find strategies to facilitate participation is critical if they wish to persevere with modCIT. Families can be assisted to develop a timetable of activities, and can be provided with an array of options for therapeutically and developmentally appropriate activities that are also motivating and sufficiently challenging. Increased frequency of contact with the therapist or a home visit may be used to demonstrate how to identify and adapt activities to be used in novel and diverse ways. Therapists can also help families find a variety of activities, for instance borrowing from relatives, therapist, friends and toy libraries and purchasing inexpensive resources from budget shops.

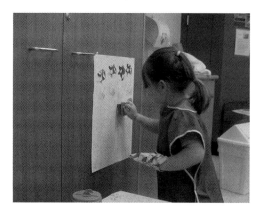

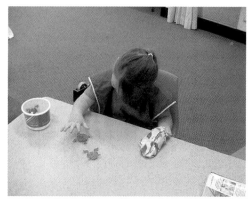

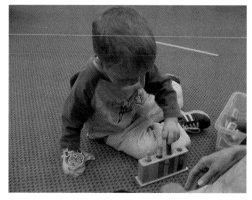

Figure 7.5 Examples of play activities used with different children during modified constraint-induced therapy. Please note: the mitt is worn on the unimpaired hand.

Meaningful encouragement and rewards may be suggested. Caregivers can be encouraged to seek assistance from the extended family or daycare centres to contribute to the modCIT programme. A review of the child's progress may also provide some motivation to continue with modCIT.

Ultimately, the welfare of the child and family is paramount and a decision to cease modCIT should be respected. Offering families the opportunity to continue with an alternative intervention for the remainder of the negotiated 'block' can minimize any sense of guilt or failure and optimize the therapy that has been completed. The nature of the intervention can be determined collaboratively with the family with the aim of achieving the goals established for therapy.

Stage 8: evaluate outcomes
Callum wore the mitt an average of 1 hour and 40 minutes per day over the 8-week intervention period. He demonstrated meaningful and substantial improvements when retested on each outcome measure at the completion of the intervention. His parents' average ratings on the COPM increased by 4.8 on the Performance Scale and 4.2 on the Satisfaction with Performance Scale, representing clinically meaningful changes on both scales (Law et al, 2005).

Callum improved on four of his five GAS goals. Based on his level of disability and progress over the previous months, this is substantially better progress than would be expected in an intervention-free period of similar length.

- Callum made much greater than expected improvement by independently stabilizing the paper while drawing on almost every occasion.
- He achieved a better than expected outcome by being able to catch a ball 6 to 8 times out of 10.
- He achieved the goal of pulling his affected arm out of a T-shirt sleeve 51–75% of occasions.
- He improved, but less than expected, on pulling down his pants for toileting as he could pull his pants from below his bottom to his knees about half the time.
- Callum did not improve in his ability to open his drink bottle.

Callum's AHA scores improved from 69 to 79 points, a clinically important increase of 13%.

- His ability to complete bimanual tasks easily and fluently improved.
- Callum was able to grasp objects of different sizes and shapes with ease.
- His ability to use appropriate force, to orient objects for action by the unaffected side and the precision of coordination between his hands also improved.
- Callum still avoided using his affected side to obtain an object even when it was the closer hand.

Sonja and Andrew reported that Callum appeared more aware of his affected arm and that his affected arm was 'much' better following intervention. Callum used his arm more spontaneously and effectively in play and daily activities. As the family definitely wanted to be involved in modCIT again, plans were made for recommencing modCIT in 6 months time. A reassessment would determine maintenance of the progress made during the initial block of modCIT and plan the goals for the subsequent intervention. Callum's progress through the intervention cycle described in this chapter is presented in Figure 7.1.

Box 7.2 Key clinical messages

- ModCIT is a unilateral intervention for children with hemiplegia that involves constraining the unimpaired hand and using principles of motor learning to facilitate intense practice for the hemiplegic hand.
- Structuring sufficient practice to achieve family-focused outcomes, and which maintains the motivation of the child, requires a committed therapist and family, careful planning and availability of a high degree of support for families who undertake home programmes.

References

Buccino G, Solodkin A & Small SL (2006) Functions of the mirror neuron system: Implications for neurorehabilitation. *Cogn Behav Neurol*, 19, 55–63.

Canadian Association of Occupational Therapists (CAOT) (2002) *Enabling Occupation: An Occupational Therapy Perspective*. Ottawa: Canadian Association of Occupational Therapists.

Case-Smith J (2005) *Occupational Therapy for Children*. St Louis, MO: Elsevier Mosby.

Cech DJ & Martin S (2002) *Functional Movement Development Across the Life Span*. Philadelphia, PA: WB Saunders Company.

Copley J & Kuipers K (1999) *Management of Upper Limb Hypertonicity*. San Antonio, TX: Therapy Skill Builders.

Cronin A & Mandich MB (2005) *Human Development and Performance throughout the Lifespan*. New York, NY: Thomson: Delmar Learning.

Damiano DL (2004) Physiotherapy management in cerebral palsy: moving beyond philosophies. In: Scrutton D, Damiano DL & Mayston MJ (eds) *Management of the Motor Disorders of Children with Cerebral Palsy*, 2nd edn. London: Mac Keith Press.

DeMatteo C, Law M, Russell D, Pollock N, Rosenbaum PL & Walter S (1991) *QUEST: Quality of Upper Extremity Skills Test Manual*. Hamilton ON: McMaster University.

Dunne JW, Heye N & Dunne SL (1995) Treatment of chronic limb spasticity with botulinum toxin A. *J Neurol Neurosurg Psychiatry*, 58, 232–5.

Eliasson AC (2005) Improving the use of hands in daily activities: aspects of treatment of children with cerebral palsy. *Phys Occup Ther Pediatr*, 25, 37–60.

Eliasson AC, Krumlinde-Sundholm L, Shaw K & Wang C (2005) Effects of constraint induced movement therapy in young children with hemiplegic cerebral palsy: an adapted model. *Dev Med Child Neurol*, 47, 266–75.

Eliasson AC, Krumlinde-Sundholm L, Rösblad B, Beckung E, Arner M, Öhrvall A & Rosenbaum PL (2006) The Manual Ability Classification System (MACS) for children with cerebral palsy: Scale development and evidence of validity and reliability. *Dev Med Child Neurol*, 48, 549–54.

Fitts PM & Posner MI (1967) *Human Performance*. Belmont CA: Brooks/Cole Publishing Co.

Gething L, Papalia DE & Olds SW (1995) *Life Span Development*. Sydney: McGraw-Hill.

Haley S, Coster W, Ludlow L, Haltiwanger J & Andrellos P (1992) *Pediatric Evaluation of Disability Inventory (PEDI). Version 1. Development, Standardization and Administration Manual*. Boston MA: New England Medical Centre Hospitals.

Humphry R (2002) Young children's occupations: explicating the dynamics of developmental processes. *Am J Occup Ther*, 56, 171–9.

Humphry R & Wakeford L (2006) An occupation-centred discussion of development and implications for practice. *Am J Occup Ther*, 60, 258–67.

Kiresuk TJ, Smith A & Cardillo JE (1994) *Goal Attainment Scaling: Applications, Theory and Measurement*. Hillsdale, NJ: Lawrence Erlbaum Associates.

Krumlinde-Sundholm L & Eliasson AC (2003) Development of the Assisting Hand Assessment: a Rasch-built measure intended for children with unilateral upper limb impairments. *Scand J Occup Ther*, 10, 16–26.

Krumlinde-Sundholm L, Holmefur M, Kottorp A & Eliasson AC (2007) The Assisting Hand Assessment: Current evidence of validity, reliability and responsiveness to change. *Dev Med Child Neurol Suppl*, 49, 259–64.

Law M, Baptiste S, Carswell A, McColl M, Polatajko H & Pollock N (2005) *Canadian Occupational Performance Measure*. Ottawa, ON: CAOT Publications, ACE.

Lin JP (2004) The assessment and management of hypertonus in cerebral palsy: A physiological atlas ('road map'). In: Scrutton D, Damiano DL & Mayston MJ (eds) *Management of the Motor Disorders of Children with Cerebral Palsy*, 2nd edn. London: Mac Keith Press.

Mastos M, Miller K, Eliasson AC & Imms C (2007) Goal-directed training: linking theories of treatment to clinical practice for improved functional activities in daily life. *Clin Rehabil*, 21, 47–55.

Novak I & Cusick A (2006) Home programmes in paediatric occupational therapy for children with cerebral palsy: where to start? *Aust Occup Ther J*, 53, 251–64.

Novak I, Cusick A & Lowe K (2007) A pilot study on the impact of occupational therapy home programming for young children with cerebral palsy. *Am J Occup Ther*, 61, 463–8.

Palisano RJ, Rosenbaum PL, Bartlett D & Livingston MH (2008) Content validity of the expanded and revised gross motor function classification system. *Dev Med Child Neurol*, 50, 744–750.

Parham LD & Primeau LA (1997) Play and occupational therapy. In: Parham LD & Fazio LS (eds) *Play in Occupational Therapy for Children.* St Louis, MO: Mosby.

Randall M, Johnson L & Reddihough D (1999) *The Melbourne Assessment of Unilateral Upper Limb Function: Test Administration Manual.* Melbourne: The Royal Children's Hospital.

Stagnitti K (1998) *Learn to Play: A Practical Program to Develop a Child's Imaginative Play Skills.* Melbourne: Co-ordinates Publications.

Taub E, Landesman Ramey S, DeLuca SC & Echols K (2004) Efficacy of constraint-induced movement therapy for children with cerebral palsy with asymmetric motor impairment. *Pediatrics*, 113, 305–12.

Valvano J (2004) Activity-focused motor interventions for children with neurological conditions. *Phys Occ Ther Pediatr*, 24, 79–107.

Wallen M, Bundy A, Pont K & Ziviani JM (2008a) Psychometric properties of the Pediatric Motor Activity Log (PMAL). *Dev Med Child Neurol*, 51, 200–8.

Wallen M, Ziviani JM, Herbert RD, Evans R & Novak I (2008b) Modified constraint-induced therapy for children with hemiplegic cerebral palsy: A feasibility study. *Dev Neurorehabil*, 11, 124–33.

Chapter 8

Goal-directed training of activity performance

Brian Hoare and Christine Imms

Case study: Travis

An occupational therapist working in a metropolitan paediatric hospital received a referral for an opinion of the potential benefit of further upper limb botulinum toxin A (BoNT-A) injections in a 4-year-old child with right-sided spastic hemiplegia (unilateral cerebral palsy). The referral also requested assistance with facilitating the child's transition to primary school next year. The steps involved in the clinical reasoning process used in this chapter are summarized in Figure 8.1 and described in Chapter 1.

Stage 1: initial data collection

Travis and his family regularly attended the cerebral palsy clinic and he had previously received upper limb intervention following three separate BoNT-A injection sessions beginning at 18 months of age. Travis' disabilities were classified as level I on both the Gross Motor Function Classification System (GMFCS; Palisano et al, 2008; see Box 8.1) and on the Manual Ability Classification System (MACS; Eliasson et al 2006; see Chapter 2).

Travis was born following an uncomplicated pregnancy and birth but experienced a single neonatal seizure at 2 days. At 5 months of age, Travis' mother Sally observed asymmetrical upper limb posturing and movement. Magnetic resonance imaging (MRI) at 7 months of age indicated a periventricular lesion.

Travis attends preschool and has funding that provides an additional childcare worker for 5 hours per day. He receives fortnightly community-based occupational therapy and physiotherapy services and regularly attends the cerebral palsy clinic where he is reviewed by a specialist multidisciplinary team. Travis' mother, Sally works 3 days per week and David, his father, works full time. David shares the responsibilities of

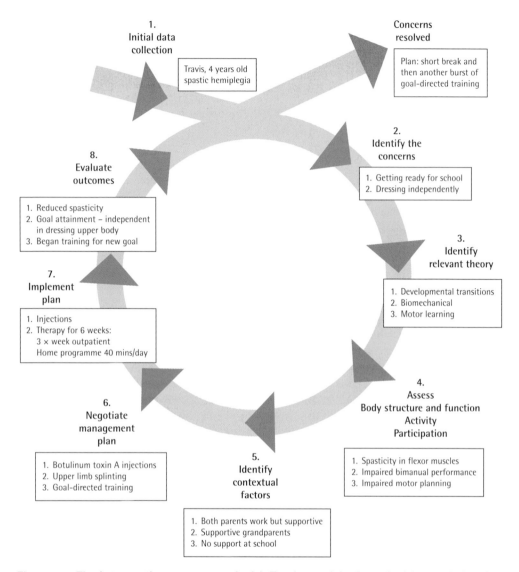

Figure 8.1 The intervention process used with Travis: model adapted with permission from the Candian Occupational Performance Process Model (CAOT, 2002).

caregiving when at home. Travis's grandparents are supportive and often transport him to appointments.

Stage 2: identify and prioritize concerns

During the initial interview, Sally expressed concerns about Travis commencing school the next year without any additional assistance in the classroom or playground. She felt

> **Box 8.1 GMFCS level I snapshot[1]**
>
> Proportion of people with cerebral palsy classified as GMFCS I: 32–48%
>
> Proportion of people classified as GMFCS level I who
>
> - have a severe intellectual disability (IQ <50): about 5%;
> - have a severe visual impairment: less than 10%;
> - have epilepsy: about 10%;
> - have behavioural problems: less than 5%;
> - have hip displacement requiring surgery: less than 1%;
> - walk alone at home by age 2–3 years: 90%;
> - walk alone at home by age 4–12 years: 99%.

he was struggling with personal care and preschool activities. She had concerns that he would need to be able to perform these independently and feared this might negatively affect his self-esteem and confidence.

To further identify and prioritize Sally's goals for Travis, the therapist used the Canadian Occupational Performance Measure (COPM) (Law et al, 2005; see Appendix, p. 291) with Sally and Travis together. The outcome is detailed in Stage 4.

Stage 3: identify relevant theory

Developmental stage: preschool
Transition to primary school is a challenging period where children are expected to complete classroom-based and self-care tasks independently in a busy environment. For some children with cerebral palsy, there may be no additional physical assistance (such as an integration aide), environmental modifications, specialized equipment or school-based therapy services. Primary school transition is often the first experience of 'nomalization' (see Chapter 3) for a child with a disability and their family. Following years of navigating disability services, and acquiring knowledge of early intervention options and medical services, this is a period where a family can refocus on other family issues and resume 'normal' routines and interests. Focusing therapeutic intervention on improving independence for a child with cerebral palsy assists parents to increase time spent in socialization, relationships and attending to other siblings. A therapist's support during this period can assist parents with indirect care tasks such as advocating for the child and family to reduce potential barriers of both a physical and attitudinal nature in the school environment.

---

1   See Chapter 2: p. 17 for details of the sources used to derive these data.

Biomechanical considerations

Upper limb hypertonicity results in abnormal posturing during performance of tasks. The resistance in the spastic muscles often restricts full range of active movement, leading to muscle stiffness and shortening. Shortening of the pronators and wrist/digit flexors alters the length–tension relationship resulting in grip strength weakness (Richards et al, 1996; Vaz et al, 2006). Coupled with other sensorimotor deficits, poor motor control and mirror movements (Kuhtz-Buschbeck et al, 2000), this weakness results in clumsy and inefficient movement significantly limiting a child's ability to perform daily tasks independently. One option for managing hypertonicity is the use of anti-spasticity agents such as BoNT-A (see Chapter 4). In the upper extremity, BoNT-A in conjunction with occupational therapy to train hand function in the weeks following injection has been shown to be effective in reducing spasticity and increasing goal achievement (Hoare and Imms, 2004; Lowe et al, 2006; Wallen et al, 2007).

Motor skill acquisition

MOTOR LEARNING

Motor learning is a process that results in a change in motor behaviour or acquisition of a skill, through active problem-solving and the formulation, practice and repetition of successful strategies (Eliasson, 2005). The clinical utility of task-based approaches for people with neurological impairments has been demonstrated (Valvano, 2004; Eliasson, 2005; Mastos et al, 2007).

MOTOR PLANNING

Children may have the sensorimotor abilities to execute a task, but the planning, organization and sequencing of movements may limit performance (Steenbergen and Gordon, 2006; Steenbergen et al, 2007). Recent findings suggest intensive practice of functional tasks improves motor planning abilities in children with hemiplegic cerebral palsy (Duff and Gordon, 2006).

MOTOR CONTROL

Children with hemiplegic cerebral palsy often experience reduced selective motor control; which refers to 'the impaired ability to isolate the activation of muscles in a selected pattern in response to demands of a voluntary posture or movement'(Sanger et al, 2006: 2162). Several factors influence these difficulties including the presence of mirror movements. These occur when repetitive voluntary movements of one hand are accompanied by involuntary mirrored movements of the other hand (Kuhtz-Buschbeck et al, 2000). As a result of ipsilateral cortical reorganization in some children with hemiplegic cerebral palsy, mirror movements are observed to be more pronounced or are prolonged and result in impaired bimanual coordination (Kuhtz-Buschbeck et al, 2000). This is because the two hands are often required to perform asymmetrical actions in most activities of daily living. Clinical assessment of mirror movements (Woods and Teuber, 1978; see Appendix, p. 287) should be considered when planning intervention and if appropriate, strategies to avoid their influence during bimanual tasks need to be implemented.

SENSATION

Children with hemiplegic cerebral palsy experience both motor and sensory deficits in their affected limbs. One study (Krumlinde-Sundholm and Eliasson, 2002) demonstrated a strong correlation between tactile sensation and dexterity, but not bimanual performance. By age 4 to 5 years, children may be able to report perceptions of sensation reliably and formal assessment should be considered.

Advances in neuroimaging of children with hemiplegic cerebral palsy have provided important insights into the organization of sensory and motor pathways. Unlike motor function, which is often reorganized to the unaffected cerebral hemisphere or a combination of both affected and unaffected hemispheres, sensory function is consistently reorganized in the affected hemisphere (Guzetta et al, 2007). This results in inter-hemispheric differences between motor and sensory pathways (Thickbroom et al, 2001). Compared with children with hemiplegia without dissociation of motor and sensory functions, the quality of motor function is usually affected more in children with dissociated motor and sensory pathways, irrespective of the degree of the sensory impairment (Guzetta et al, 2007).

Behaviour, cognition and learning

Although about 10% of children with hemiplegia will have a severe cognitive impairment (Himmelmann et al, 2006), many more are at risk of impairments of executive functioning, including poor selective attention and memory and the presence of specific learning disabilities (Lesny et al, 1990; Stiers et al, 2002; Jenks et al, 2007). Learning of new tasks requires children to develop and retrieve memories of past performance, including motor images of movement plans (Cech and Martin, 2002; Steenbeek et al, 2007), as well as other cognitive skills related to anticipation of events, planning, and integration and interpretation of multiple sensory inputs (Kantak et al, 2008). The cognitive effort required in learning new tasks is thought to be related to the success of skill acquisition and retention (Sherwood and Lee, 2003). Children with hemiplegia and impaired higher cortical functioning are likely to require increased support for learning of new tasks, especially as specific difficulties with memory and perceptual motor deficits are common (Kantak et al, 2008).

Although the age at onset for most children with cerebral palsy who have epilepsy is typically less than 4 years (Carlsson et al, 2003), the presence of a neonatal seizure in Travis alerted the therapist to consider the possibility of further issues in this area. Children with cerebral palsy who also have epilepsy have poorer behavioural and cognitive outcomes (Carlsson et al, 2003, 2008, see Chapter 2) and typically require much more support with learning new tasks and with integration into school.

Behavioural problems may stem from difficulties with selective attention, frustration resulting from an inability to perform as expected, fatigue which is commonly associated with epilepsy, as well as difficulties with making judgements and decisions about suitable behaviours and responses in complex social environments. Parents who have questions about managing the behaviour of their children may benefit from resources available through programmes such as the Triple P: Positive Parenting

Program (http://www1.triplep.net/). This international, evidence-based programme provides resources for parents and practitioners.

Stage 4: assessment of body structure and function, activity and participation

Based on the initial discussion with Sally and Travis a list of assessments was developed (Table 8.1). Although alert to the possibility of executive dysfunction or learning disability, the therapist did not formally assess this area as Sally did not report any concerns with Travis.

Impairment

SPASTICITY AND RANGE OF MOVEMENT

The modified Tardieu scale was used to provide a clinical measure of spasticity (Boyd and Graham, 1999; see Appendix, p. 289). When assessing Travis' upper limb, a goniometer was used to measure the joint angle of muscle reaction (catch or R1) at a V3 (as fast as possible) speed and the full passive range of movement (R2) at a V1 (as slow as possible) speed in the elbow flexors, forearm pronators and wrist flexors. During this time, the quality and intensity of the muscle reactions (X) were also graded (Table 8.2). The same method was used to assess the level of spasticity in Travis' long finger flexors and thumb however, a goniometer was not used. Importantly, the four fingers were assessed as a whole, while the wrist was held in extension. A consistent catch was evident at the proximal interphalangeal joint (V3) indicating spasticity in flexor digitorum superficialis. The thumb rested in an adducted position and Travis was unable to abduct and extend his thumb fully and actively at the metacarpophalangeal joint. This indicated spasticity in the adductor pollicis and opponens pollicis muscles.

Table 8.1 Assessments for Travis

Body function and structure	Activity[b]	Participation
Spasticity, passive range of movement (PROM) Modified Tardieu scale Mirror movements[a]	Bimanual performance Assisting Hand Assessment	Parent interview
	Activity level goal setting Canadian Occupational Performance Measure Goal Attainment Scaling	

a. Woods and Teuber, 1978.
b. In this case, the Canadian Occupational Performance Measure was used to measure Travis' activity performance rather than his participation.

Table 8.2 Assessment findings for the modified Tardieu scale

Elbow	Pronators	Wrist
R1: 130° R2: 180° X: 2	R1: 45° R2: 90° X: 2	R1: 0° R2: 70° X: 1
R2–R1: 50°	R2–R1: 45°	R2–R1: 0°

R1, joint angle of muscle reaction (catch) at a V3 (as fast as possible) speed; R2, full passive range of movement (R2) at a V1 (as slow as possible) speed; X, the intensity and duration of the muscle reaction (the resistance felt when muscle is passively stretched).

MIRROR MOVEMENTS

Presence of mirror movements was evaluated using the protocol developed by Woods and Teuber (1978) (see Appendix, p. 287). Results are reported in Table 8.3.

SENSATION

A three-test approach has demonstrated validity in the assessment of the different aspects of tactile sensibility in children with hemiplegia using two-point discrimination, stereognosis of familiar objects and the Pick-up Test (Krumlinde-Sundholm and Eliasson, 2002). Following prioritization of outcomes and information required for intervention planning, a decision was made to administer only the Pick-up Test (Krumlinde-Sundholm et al, 1988) with and without vision (see Appendix, p. 289). Travis was asked to pick out ten 10 millimetre (mm) wooden cubes from a box (120 × 120 × 40 mm) as quickly as possible. Using his affected hand, Travis required 16 seconds to complete the task with vision and 20 seconds without vision.

Table 8.3 Assessment findings for the mirror movements

	Mirroring hand	
	Right	Left
Finger tapping	1	1
Fist rotation	1	1
Finger alternation	2	2

1, barely discernible repetitive movement; 2 slight but unsustained repetitive movement.

Activity performance

BIMANUAL UPPER LIMB PERFORMANCE
The Assisting Hand Assessment (AHA, see Appendix, p. 291) was used to understand how Travis typically used his hemiplegic upper limb in bimanual tasks. Travis scored 55 on the AHA, which is equivalent to a scaled score of 50%. The videotaped play session of the AHA was also used to observe how Travis' spasticity influenced his upper limb performance and assisted in identifying specific muscles for possible injection of BoNT-A.

GOAL SETTING
Areas of performance difficulties identified using the COPM in the initial session were prioritized and rated by Sally (Table 8.4)(Law et al, 2005).

Issues prioritized using the COPM were then set as goals and scaled using the Goal Attainment Scaling (GAS) (Kiresuk et al, 1994; see Appendix, p. 292). The COPM and GAS are complementary approaches used to identify, articulate and measure goals (Lowe et al, 2006, Wallen et al, 2007). Although five goals were identified, the therapist, Sally and Travis made a collaborative decision to focus intensively on practising a single goal: putting on a top. Travis' participation in the goal setting and prioritization process was crucial for both ownership of the goal and motivation to engage in practice. Travis was videotaped attempting to dress his upper body to establish his baseline performance and to provide visual feedback and motivation to Travis and Sally during the intervention period (Table 8.5).

Participation
Sally had identified potential participation restrictions associated with Travis going to school next year. Her focus was for him to gain skills to maximize his future participation potential. As Sally did not identify current participation restrictions at home or in the community no formal measure of participation was used. The *Assessment of Preschool Children's Participation* (Petrenchik et al, 2006) would be appropriate if required.

Table 8.4 Assessment findings for the Canadian Occupational Performance Measure

Occupational Performance Area	Importance (1–10)	Performance (1–10)	Satisfaction (1–10)
(1) Dress upper body	9	3	2
(2) Use scissors to cut paper	7	2	2
(3) Pull up trousers	7	3	2
(4) Throw a ball with two hands	6	4	2
(5) Turn pages of a book	5	5	3

Table 8.5 Assessment findings for Goal Attainment Scaling; putting on a top

Attainment level	Score	Eating
Baseline	−2	Travis does not attempt the task of putting on his T-shirt and jumper. His parents provide full assistance with putting on a T-shirt and jumper 100% of the time
Less than expected outcome	−1	Within 2 weeks, Travis will place his right and left arms into sleeves with verbal prompts. His parents will provide physical assistance for all other components of the task
Expected outcome	0	Within 2 weeks, Travis will place both arms into the sleeves of a T-shirt and pull his top over-head with verbal prompts. Minimal physical assistance will be required to adjust the back of the top
Greater than expected outcome	+1	Within 2 weeks, Travis will place both arms into the sleeves and pull his T-shirt over-head without prompts. Minimal physical assistance will be required to adjust the back of the top
Much greater than expected outcome	+2	Within 2 weeks, Travis will put his T-shirt on independently 100% of the time. No assistance will be required.

Stage 5: contextual factors: environmental and personal

Environmental

Travis was enrolled to go to a mainstream school next year with his age peers. Unlike preschool, he was expected to access all areas of the curriculum independently as he was not eligible for integration aide assistance or school-based therapy funding.

Although supportive and aware of his needs, Travis' family found it difficult to implement a home programme as both parents worked. The grandparents were willing to assist in any home-based therapy but lacked confidence. Time constraints in the mornings also meant Travis' parents dressed him on workdays.

Personal
Travis did not have any identified cognitive, language or learning difficulties. He was a determined and active 4-year-old boy who enjoyed a challenge. He was very motivated to participate in the goal-setting process.

Stage 6: management plan

Summary of assessment findings
Despite full passive range of movement, Travis had a high level of spasticity in his affected elbow flexors, forearm pronators, long finger flexors and thumb adductors (Table 8.2). These finding were consistent with observation of abnormal posturing during the AHA. Overactivity in adductor pollicis and opponens pollicis resulted in a 'thumb-in-palm' deformity and difficulty grasping, holding and releasing objects.

Travis exhibited slight but unsustained repetitive mirror movements in both hands during the finger alternation task. This is normal for a child of Travis' age and is unlikely to influence bimanual performance. Similarly, the Pick-up Test did not indicate significant impairment of tactile sensibility.

The COPM enabled Sally to prioritize dressing of the upper body as the most important issue for Travis and the GAS allowed the specific elements of goal achievement to be measured. Analysis of Travis' baseline performance provided critical information on the specific variables limiting Travis' ability to put on a top independently related to person, task and environment factors. Environmental factors included his parents tending to perform the task for him, and the resultant limited learning opportunities. The task was more or less easy depending on the style of top Travis needed to don. Travis' difficulties planning the sequence of movements and limited range of movement in his impaired hand and spasticity led to poor initiation of grasp of the top with his impaired hand. In the assessment session Travis was able to remember simple sequences of movement when shown.

Understanding the contextual factors allowed the therapist and family to plan the timing of intervention. For Travis, an intensive period of intervention needed to coincide with preschool holidays and his parents' annual leave.

Stage 7: implement plan

Botulinum toxin A injections
Before starting therapy, Travis received injection of BoNT-A into brachialis, brachio-radialis, flexor digitorum superficialis, pronator teres, pronator quadratus, adductor pollicis and opponens pollicis of his right upper limb. The injections occurred 1 month prior to starting therapy. Therapy coincided with Sally's annual leave and Travis' holidays. The 1-month period also allowed for resolution of any excessive grip weakness as a result of injection to the fingers and thumb. The role of BoNT-A was to reduce

spasticity and theoretically improve Travis' ability to learn to execute the required movement for the task (i.e. grasp and hold).

Splinting
In the week following his injections, Travis was fitted with a customized overnight resting splint to provide a sustained stretch to his right wrist flexors, long finger flexors and thumb adductors/flexors. Travis wore his splint for a minimum of 6 hours per night when sleeping (Tardieu et al, 1988) and Sally was advised that Travis would need the splint indefinitely while he was growing. Because of the muscles selected for injection, the commonly used 'functional position' (Figure 8.2) was inadequate to provide stretch to the injected muscles. Therefore, the therapist made a 'ball' splint (Figure 8.3) to stretch to the long finger flexors and adductor pollicis and opponens pollicis. No day splints (i.e. neoprene, Lycra, functional thermoplastic) were recommended as positioning a joint passively during active movement limits the ability to strengthen antagonistic muscles and reduces sensory feedback.

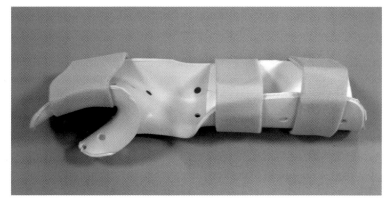

Figure 8.2
Resting splint in
'functional position'.

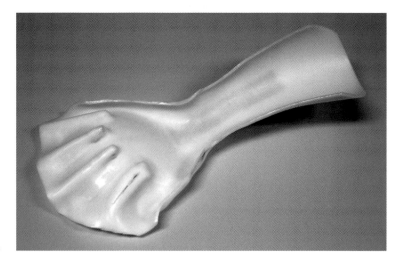

Figure 8.3
Resting 'Ball' splint.

Goal-directed training

One month following injections of BoNT-A, Travis commenced a 2-week goal-directed training programme (see Chapter 4). The programme involved three outpatient sessions per week and a home programme involving task practice for 20 minutes in the morning and 20 minutes in the afternoon, 7 days a week. Goal-directed training involves the following four stages (Mastos et al, 2007).

(1) Eliciting a purposeful goal that takes into consideration the client's age and level of cognitive impairment.
(2) Analysing the task performance with careful attention to the contributions of the environmental and task factors that help or hinder performance, as well as the person's skills and abilities.
(3) Planning the intervention, including the use of structured practice and effective feedback.
(4) Evaluating outcomes using validated tools.

The first two stages of goal-directed training occurred during the initial assessment and the COPM and GAS provided baseline measures of performance against which to evaluate outcomes in stage four. Stage three, the intervention plan, was developed based on Travis' stage of motor learning, with the aim of finding creative opportunities for repeated practice and ways of providing feedback on performance.

Session one

Because Travis had never put on his own top before, he still needed to learn the specific steps and movement sequences required. Travis was at the verbal–cognitive stage of motor learning (Fitts and Posner, 1967). He began with a loose fitting short-sleeved shirt to simplify the task. Involving Travis in solving the problem of how to don the top enabled him to be an active learner and problem-solver. Engaging Travis in this way enhanced the cognitive effort required, which is known to be an important component of skill acquisition and retention (Sherwood and Lee, 2003). Together, the therapist and Travis analysed the task and broke it into small steps with simple key words (verbal cues) developed to describe the actions (Box 8.2).

Box 8.2 Steps for dressing upper body

(1) Find front and bottom of top.
(2) Place top on lap.
(3) Find hole for right arm.
(4) Pull top over right arm with left hand.
(5) Lift top and put head through.
(6) Push left arm through hole.
(7) Pull front of top down with two hands.
(8) Pull back of top down with left hand.

Before attempting any steps, Travis verbalized the steps using the key words. In addition, the therapist demonstrated what was required. Self-talk and watching demonstrations are two strategies that assist with the acquisition of motor skills.

Travis practised the first step. He was asked to identify what went wrong when he was unsuccessful and helped to find ways to improve his performance. If required, the therapist provided physical assistance and verbal feedback to assist in the guiding and planning of movements and the sequencing of the step. The step was practised repetitively with graded physical and/or verbal assistance until he was able to use the simple key words consistently and perform the step successfully. At the conclusion of the first session, Travis was able to perform the first four steps successfully. Sally and Travis continued with the practice of the first four steps at home and used a logbook to record their practice. Because of Travis' high level of cognitive ability, he was able to engage actively in the problem-solving process. Children with cognitive impairments may need more structured assistance and significantly more time to learn a task. Children with specific difficulties with memory may benefit from memory aides such as pictures or photos of task sequences or strategies they are learning. In some cases, children may not achieve independent performance of high-level tasks.

SESSION TWO
Travis was able to remember and successfully demonstrate the first four steps. Progressive repetitive practice of the next steps was undertaken. At the conclusion of the session, Travis was able to perform the task independently. Success was inconsistent and verbal cues required at times. This indicated that Travis had reached the motor stage of learning where repeated practice is most important. Sally and Travis continued practice of the full task at home.

SESSION THREE
Travis was independent with the task of donning a T-shirt. The clothing was changed to a winter long-sleeved sweater and he practised this more challenging task repetitively. At the conclusion of the session, Travis successfully performed the task with assistance for steps 5, 6 and 7. Sally and Travis continued practice with the sweater at home with Sally progressively reducing the amount of physical assistance provided. Because Travis reached a greater than expected level of outcome following three sessions, the therapist introduced the second prioritized goal of cutting paper with scissors. Travis integrated practice of donning a top into his daily routine to consolidate his learning and to work towards the autonomous stage of motor learning while establishing a formal practice regimen of cutting with scissors.

SESSION FOUR
Travis was able to don a winter long-sleeved sweater independently. On occasions, minor assistance was required to assist with steps 7 and 8. Travis had improved greatly but he was not yet at the autonomous stage of motor learning where task performance was smooth, flexible and transferable to varying contexts. Travis was videotaped performing the task and shown the before and after video. He was very proud of himself and Sally said Travis was more motivated to perform a variety of other tasks independently.

SESSION FIVE AND SIX

The remaining sessions of the 6-week programme addressed the goal of cutting paper with scissors using the same principles of goal-directed training.

Stage 8: evaluate outcomes

Travis achieved his goal more rapidly than initially expected. Following four outpatient sessions and 4.5 hours of home practice he achieved +1 on the GAS. As a result, a second goal was introduced. Assessment using the modified Tardieu scale demonstrated reduced spasticity in the muscles injected with BoNT-A. The elbow R1/R2 difference was reduced by 50° and pronators by 20°. The complementary effects of the BoNT-A in the upper limb allowed Travis to use his hand more effectively during task practice, particularly when he needed to grasp the top. The AHA will be administered 3 months post-injection, prior to his review in the cerebral palsy clinic.

Following the six sessions, Sally reported she felt confident continuing with a home-based programme. By participating in the goal-directed training, Sally felt she had gained a better understanding of Travis' difficulty with daily tasks and had noted a change in both her and her husband's behaviour at home. Despite the pace of life at home, both parents were very aware of the need to allow Travis to practise difficult tasks while feeling supported and to assist in problem-solving when difficulties occurred. Travis was extremely proud of his achievements and Sally reported observing continued motivation to attempt tasks that he had previously avoided. Although Sally now felt more confident about Travis' transition to school, she and the therapist agreed to arrange a school-based meeting prior to the end of the year to ensure appropriate planning occurred and to maximize the success of the transition process.

Box 8.3 Key clinical messages

- Goal-directed training aims to facilitate acquisition of skills through active problem-solving and the formulation, practice and repetition of successful strategies.
- The COPM and GAS are complementary approaches used to identify performance issues and articulate and measure goals.

References

Boyd RN & Graham HK (1999) Objective measurement of clinical finding in the use of botulinum toxin type A for the management of children with cerebral palsy. *Eur J Neurol*, 6 (suppl 4), S23–35.

Canadian Association of Occupational Therapists (CAOT) (2002) *Enabling Occupation: An Occupational Therapy Perspective.* Ottawa: Canadian Association of Occupational Therapists.

Carlsson M, Hagberg G & Olsson I (2003) Clinical and aetiological aspects of epilepsy in children with cerebral palsy. *Dev Med Child Neurol*, 45, 371–6.

Carlsson M, Olsson I, Hagberg G & Beckung E (2008) Behaviour in children with cerebral palsy with and without epilepsy. *Dev Med Child Neurol*, 50, 784–9.

Cech DJ & Martin S (2002). *Functional Movement Development across the Life Span*. Philadelphia, PA: WB Saunders.

Duff SV & Gordon AM (2006) Activity limitation in hemiplegic cerebral palsy: evidence for disorders in motor planning. *Dev Med Child Neurol*, 48, 780–3.

Eliasson AC (2005) Improving the use of hands in daily activities: aspects of the treatment of children with cerebral palsy. *Phys Occup Ther Pediatr*, 23, 37–60.

Eliasson AC, Krumlinde-Sundholm L, Rösblad B, Beckung E, Arner M, Öhrvall A & Rosenbaum PL (2006) The Manual Ability Classification System (MACS) for children with cerebral palsy: scale development and evidence of validity and reliability. *Dev Med Child Neurol*, 48, 549–54.

Fitts PM & Posner MI (1967) *Human Performance*. Pacific Grove, CA: Brooks Cole Publishing.

Guzetta A, Bonanni P, Biagi L, Tosetti M, Montanaro D, Guerrini R & Cioni G (2007) Reorganisation of the somatosensory system after early brain damage. *Clin Neurophysiol*, 118, 1110–21.

Himmelmann K, Beckung E, Hagberg G & Uvebrant P (2006) Gross and fine motor function and accompanying impairments in cerebral palsy. *Dev Med Child Neurol*, 48, 417–23.

Hoare BJ & Imms C (2004) Upper-limb injections of botulinum toxin-A in children with cerebral palsy: a critical review of the literature and clinical implications for occupational therapists. *Am J Occup Ther*, 58, 389–97.

Jenks KM, de Moor J, van Lieshout EC, Maathuis KG, Keus I & Görter JW (2007) The effect of cerebral palsy on arithmetic accuracy is mediated by working memory, intelligence, early numeracy, and instruction time. *Dev Neuropsychol*, 32, 861–79.

Kantak SS, Sullivan KJ & Burtner P (2008) Motor learning in children with cerebral palsy: Implications for rehabilitation. In: Eliasson AC & Burtner P (eds) *Improving Hand Function in Children with Cerebral Palsy: Theory, Evidence and Intervention*. London: Mac Keith Press.

Kiresuk TJ, Smith JE & Cardillo JE (1994) *Goal Attainment Scaling: Applications, Theory and Measurement*. Hillsdale, Lawrence Erlbaum Associates.

Krumlinde-Sundholm L, Eliasson A-C & Forssberg H (1988) Obstetric brachial plexus injuries: assessment protocol ad functional outcome at the age 5 years. *Dev Med Child Neurol*, 40, 4–11.

Krumlinde-Sundholm L & Eliasson AC (2002) Comparing tests of tactile sensibility: aspects relevant to testing children with spastic hemiplegia. *Dev Med Child Neurol*, 44, 604–12.

Kuhtz-Buschbeck JP, Krumlinde-Sundholm L, Eliasson A-C & Forssberg H (2000) Quantitative assessment of mirror movements in children and adolescents with hemiplegic cerebral palsy. *Dev Med Child Neurol*, 42, 728–36.

Law M, Baptiste S, Carswell A, McColl MA, Polatajko H & Pollock N (2005) *The Canadian Occupational Performance Measure*, 4th edn. Toronto: Canadian Association of Occupational Therapists.

Lesny I, Nachtmann M, Stehlik A, Tomankova A & Zajidkova J (1990) Disorders of memory of motor sequences in cerebral palsied children. *Brain Dev*, 12, 339–41.

Lowe K, Novak I & Cusick A (2006) Low-dose/high concentration localised Botulinum toxin A improves upper limb movement and function in children with hemiplegic cerebral palsy. *Dev Med Child Neurol*, 48, 170–5.

Mastos M, Miller K, Eliasson A-C & Imms C (2007) Goal directed training: linking theories of treatment to clinical practice for improved functional activities in daily life. *Clin Rehabil*, 21, 47–55.

Palisano RJ, Rosenbaum PL, Bartlett D & Livingston MH (2008) Content validity of the expanded and revised gross motor function classification system. *Dev Med Child Neurol*, 50, 744–50.

Petrenchik T, Law M, King G, Hurley P, Forhan M and Kertoy, M (2006) *Assessment of Preschool Children's Participation*. Hamilton, ON: CanChild Centre for Childhood Disability Research.

Richards LG, Oloson B & Palmiter-Thomas P (1996) How forearm position affects grip strength. *Am J Occup Ther*, 50, 133–8.

Sanger TD, Chen D, Delgado MR, Gaebler-Spira D, Hallett M & Mink JW (2006) Definition and classification of negative motor signs in childhood. *Pediatr*, 118, 2159–67.

Sherwood DE & Lee TD (2003) Schema theory: critical review and implications for the role of cognition in a new theory of motor learning. *Res Q Exerc Sport*, 74, 376.

Steenbeek D, Ketelaar M, Galama K & Görter JW (2007) Goal attainment scaling in paediatric rehabilitation: a critical review of the literature. *Dev Med Child Neurol*, 49, 550–6.

Steenbergen B & Gordon AM (2006) Activity limitation in hemiplegic cerebral palsy: evidence for disorders in motor planning. *Dev Med Child Neurol*, 48, 780–3.

Steenbergen B, Verrel J & Gordon AM (2007) Motor planning in congenital hemiplegia. *Disabil Rehabil*, 29, 13–23.

Stiers P, Vanderkelen R, Vanneste G, Coene S, De Rammelaere M & Vandenbussche E (2002) Visual-perceptual impairment in a random sample of children with cerebral palsy. *Dev Med Child Neurol*, 44, 370–82.

Tardieu C, Lespargot A, Tabary C & Bret MD (1988) For how long must the soleus muscle be stretched each day to prevent contracture? *Dev Med Child Neurol*, 30, 3–10.

Thickbroom GW, Byrnes ML, Archer SA, Nagarajan L & Mastaglia MD (2001) Differences in sensory and motor cortical organization following brain injury early in life. *Ann Neurol*, 49, 320–7.

Valvano J (2004) Activity-focused motor interventions for children with neurological conditions. *Phy Occup Ther Pediatr*, 24, 79–107.

Vaz DV, Mancini MC, Fonesca ST, Veira DSR & de Melo Pertence AE (2006) Muscle stiffness and strength and their relaiton to hand function in children with hemiplegic cerebral palsy. *Dev Med Child Neurol*, 48, 728–33.

Wallen M, O'Flaherty SJ & Waugh MA (2007) Functional outcomes of intramuscular Botulinum Toxin type A and occupational therapy in the upper limbs of children with cerebral palsy: A randomised controlled trial. *Arch Phys Med Rehabil*, 88, 1–10.

Woods BT & Teuber HL (1978) Mirror movements after childhood hemiparesis. *Neurology*, 28, 1152–7.

Chapter 9

The role of botulinum toxin A injections in the lower extremity

Pam Thomason and Kerr Graham

Case study: Hamish

Hamish is a 5-year 5-month-old boy with spastic diplegic cerebral palsy, classified at Gross Motor Function Classification System (GMFCS; Palisano et al, 2008) level II. He will start school next year. A physiotherapist working in the community first referred Hamish to a tertiary centre when he was aged 2 years and 5 months for hip surveillance and for spasticity management, specifically inquiring about his suitability for injections of botulinum toxin A (BoNT-A). The steps involved in the clinical reasoning process used in this chapter are summarized in Figure 9.1 and described in Chapter 1.

Stage 1: initial data collection

Hamish was born at 25 weeks' gestation (birthweight 742 grams) as a result of maternal cervical incompetence. Hamish had a ventricular septal defect that closed spontaneously and had an uncomplicated postnatal period. He has had no seizures and is not taking any medications. Hamish showed delay in gaining motor milestones. He did not sit unaided until 11 months. He was diagnosed with spastic diplegic cerebral palsy by his neonatologist at the age of 2 years and magnetic resonance imaging (MRI) showed bilateral periventricular leukomalacia. He walked independently at 3 years 6 months of age. Hamish lives at home with both parents and a younger brother. He attends a local daycare centre 2 days per week. He has had a home-based physiotherapy programme and sees his physiotherapist every 2 weeks. See Box 9.1 for the GMFCS snapshot for level II.

Stage 2: identify and prioritize concerns

At age 3 years 2 months Hamish attended the out patient clinic for routine follow-up (Figure 9.2). Hamish's parents reported that he was crawling, pulling up to stand and walking short distances with the support of one person. He was keen to walk and

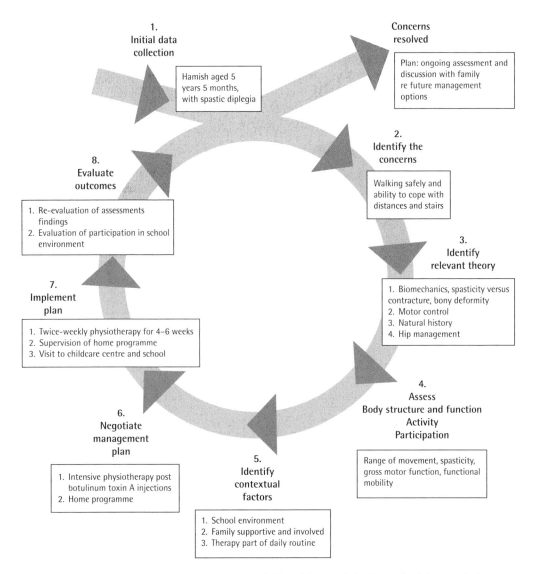

Figure 9.1 The intervention process used with Hamish: model adapted with permission from the Canadian Occupational Performance Process Model (CAOT, 2002).

energetically tried to step when held and tried to use a posterior walker. However, he felt 'tight' throughout his lower limbs and crossed his legs as he stepped and caught one foot on the other. He was unable to get his feet flat and could not stand still or walk on his own. It was getting hard for him to sit on the floor unless he 'W' sat and he could not sit with his legs out in front. He had to lie down to be dressed and it was difficult to get pants and particularly shoes and ankle–foot orthoses (AFOs) on, and Hamish disliked wearing AFOs for long periods.

His community physiotherapist reported that Hamish was consistently exhibiting spastic scissoring and equinus when standing and attempting to walk. It was becoming increasingly difficult for Hamish to dissociate his leg movements and this was directly hindering the progression of his walking ability. He had reduced range of passive abduction and his physiotherapist had concerns regarding his hip status.

Box 9.1 GMFCS level II snapshot[1]

Proportion of people with cerebral palsy classified as GMFCS II: 18–30%

Proportion of people classified as GMFCS level II who

- have a severe intellectual disability (IQ <50): about 20%;
- have a severe visual impairment: about 13%;
- have epilepsy: about 25%;
- have behavioural problems: less than 5%;
- have hip displacement requiring surgery: about 10%;
- walk alone at home by age 2–3 years: 24%;
- walk alone at home by age 4–12 years: 89%.

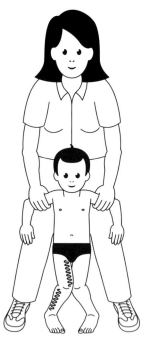

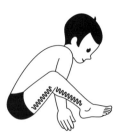

Figure 9.2 Drawing of Hamish (at age 3 years and 2 months) sitting and standing showing his difficulty with ability to stand with extended knees and feet flat which impaired his balance, thus requiring support. Difficulties with long sitting meant Hamish had difficulty freeing his hands for play and other activities in this position.

1   See Chapter 2: p. 17 for details of the sources used to derive these data.

At this time, Hamish was examined under anaesthesia to separate the degree of contracture from the degree of spasticity in all lower limb muscle groups. Surgery undertaken was bilateral hip adductor lengthening (to regain a good range of hip abduction) combined with phenolization of the obturator nerve and injections of BoNT-A to the hamstrings and calf muscles bilaterally. Open hip adductor release in combination with phenolization of the anterior branch of the obturator nerve is used to manage early hip displacement in children with cerebral palsy (Khot et al, 2008). This significantly reduces adductor spasticity and improves range of movement of hip abduction allowing better congruity of the hip joint and hip development. This management is used when the hips are at risk of further displacement. The advantage of phenol is that it reduces spasticity for up to 24 months and it can be directly placed on to the anterior branch of the obturator nerve under visual observation at the time of surgery. Since then, Hamish's management has included several episodes of care involving injection of BoNT-A to multiple lower limb muscles.

Hamish is now 5 years and 5 months, GMFCS level II and will start school next year. He uses a posterior walker to walk longer distances outside and wears bilateral hinged AFOs. Presenting issues are that Hamish is walking independently but with precarious balance. He is having frequent falls. His parents have noticed that Hamish seems to have difficulty stopping and turning and they think this might be contributing to his falls. They have also noticed that he seems to tire quickly when walking in the community. His community physiotherapist reports that his AFO tolerance has decreased and he is walking in equinus when not in his AFOs. He is wearing out a pair of shoes (at the anteromedial aspect of the toe) in 6 weeks and she is concerned about his safe mobility at school next year (Figure 9.3).

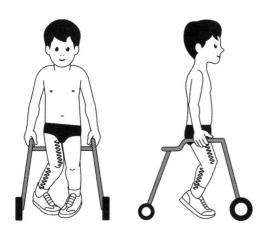

Figure 9.3 Drawing of Hamish's standing posture at age 5 years and 5 months. The continued effect of spasticity means it is difficult to stand with feet flat and hips and knees extended which limits his ability to balance, walk independently and achieve more complex motor skills such as climbing stairs and running.

Stage 3: identify relevant theory

Spasticity management options
A number of spasticity management options could be considered for Hamish including selective dorsal rhizotomy, multilevel injections of BoNT-A or intrathecal baclofen pump (see Chapter 4). At 3 years and 2 months, Hamish showed diffuse spasticity in his lower limb muscles. At this time he was not ambulant, and at GMFCS level II had a 10% risk of hip displacement that would require surgery (hip migration percentage of greater than 40%) (Hägglund et al, 2007). On assessment by a multidisciplinary team, it was felt that the overriding issue of hip displacement dictated management for Hamish. His antero-posterior pelvis radiograph results showed a migration percentage of 33% on the right and 46% on the left. Migration percentage is the measurement of the amount of the ossified femoral head that is lateral to the acetabular margin as measured on the antero-posterior pelvic radiograph: 10% or below is considered normal. Hamish's migration percentages were very significant and were likely to progress if untreated. Selective dorsal rhizotomy or intrathecal baclofen would address the issue of spasticity but not the issue of tight hip adductor muscles that was already present.

Ideally, the appropriate management option was a combination of measures to stabilize Hamish's hips, manage his lower limb spasticity and set a platform for a physiotherapy programme geared towards standing, independent walking and accelerated gross motor function. The most appropriate first-line management for Hamish was multilevel injections of BoNT-A combined with management of his hips. Recent studies (Crowner et al, 2007; Howell et al, 2007) suggesting severe adverse events from excessively high doses of BoNT-A have encouraged some practitioners to introduce 'Botox bearing protocols'. In this type of protocol, adductor spasticity is managed by a limited lengthening of the adductor longus and gracillis, phenolization of the obturator nerve in the groin, and BoNT-A injections to the hamstrings and calf muscles bilaterally.

Biomechanical considerations
Spastic diplegia often results in relatively symmetrical generalized lower limb spasticity in which the lower limbs are held in a posture of hip adduction, flexion and internal rotation, knee flexion and ankle plantar flexion. The result of this posture is an inability to achieve a base of support in standing, difficulties with long sitting and stepping and balance (Figures 9.2 and 9.3). Over time, persistent spasticity and abnormal biomechanical alignment lead to muscle and joint contracture and bony deformity that will require timely surgical intervention somewhere between the ages of 8 to 12 years (Bache et al, 2003).

Motor planning
Difficulties in isolating movements in the lower limbs may result from combinations of disordered motor control as well as the overriding effect of spastic co-contraction at multiple levels. The focus of spasticity management is to relieve the spastic co-contraction to enhance the opportunity for learning, practising and refining more normal motor patterns (Shepherd, 2003). However, disorders of motor planning go

beyond the execution of the motor task, which spasticity and other biomechanical factors impede. Children with cerebral palsy commonly have difficulty with anticipatory planning of motor actions (Steenbergen et al, 2006). This is evidenced in slow, inefficient execution of activities, poor anticipatory control and the tendency to plan and execute incremental components of a task rather than an integrated task with a clear and appropriate end-point (Steenbergen et al, 2007). Children with motor planning difficulties tend to acquire new skills at a slower rate than others. Motor planning relies on the ability to receive and utilize sensory information (proprioceptive, tactile and kinaesthetic), to develop and retrieve memories, including motor images of previous movement plans, to anticipate (predict and respond to) changing events and to execute the resulting motor plan (Cech and Martin, 2002; Steenbeek et al, 2007).

Hip surveillance
Hip surveillance is required for every child with cerebral palsy (Wynter et al, 2008). Hip surveillance is the process of monitoring and identifying the critical early indicators of progressive hip displacement. Early identification is an essential part of the strategy for prevention of hip displacement and its sequelae (see Chapter 2).

Stage 4: assessment of body structure and function, activity and participation
Following data collection and discussion of parental concerns and priorities, assessments were selected for Hamish. Priorities for Hamish were centred around his potential ability to access and function at a mainstream school next year. At the International Classification of Functioning, Disability and Health (ICF, World Health Organization, 2001) level of body structure and function, measurements of passive range of movement, muscle length and the modified Tardieu were evaluated. At the level of activity and participation the Gross Motor Function Measure (GMFM) and the Functional Mobility Scale (FMS) were completed (see Appendix for description of these assessments, pp. 292 and 294). A standardized two-dimensional video was recorded to evaluate Hamish's gait. Hamish's assessments are displayed in Table 9.1.

Table 9.1 Assessments for Hamish

Body structure and function	Activity	Participation
Range of movement, muscle length and spasticity Range of movement modified Tardieu	*Gross motor function* Gross Motor Function Measure Gait – visual gait analysis	Not formally tested
	Functional mobility Functional Mobility Scale	

Assessment findings for range of movement and spasticity are displayed in Table 9.2. At age 5 year and 5 months spasticity may be contributing less to Hamish's limitations of range of movement, and muscle contracture may be more apparent. Comparison with previous examinations showed that psoas, hamstrings and calves were tighter and his left knee had a fixed flexion deformity, and his rotational profile showed increasing internal rotation. An anterior-posterior pelvic radiograph showed a left hip migration percentage of 27% and a right of 19%, which was considered satisfactory, and an improvement on his hip migration results at 3 years of age.

His gross motor function and mobility scores are listed in Table 9.3. His FMS score of 5, 5, 2 confirms that he walks independently for short distances but uses his posterior

Table 9.2. Body structure and function assessment findings, Hamish aged 5 years 5 months[a]

Range of movement, muscle length and modified Tardieu	Left side	Right side
Thomas Test: psoas length	−15°	−10°
Popliteal angle hamstring length	70° (80°)	60° (70°)
Passive knee extension	−2°	0°
Soleus length	10°	15°
Gastrocnemius length	5° (−35°)	7° (−30°)
Hip abduction adductor length	20°	25°
Hip internal/external rotation	60°/30°	50°/35°
Femoral neck anteversion	32°	25°

a. Measures in parentheses indicate R1 spastic catch (Tardieu).

Table 9.3 Activity performance assessment findings, Hamish aged 5 years 5 months

Activity performance	
Gross motor function Gross Motor Function Measure	67.8
Functional mobility Functional Mobility Scale	
5 m	5 (independent)
50 m	5 (independent)
500 m	2 (use walker)

For details of scoring FMS – see Appendix, Figure A.4, p. 293.

walker when walking in the community over long distances. His GMFM–66 score of 67.8% indicates that he is functioning well for someone of GMFCS level II at that age (Rosenbaum et al, 2002). Visual gait analysis shows that when barefoot Hamish is able to walk easily and quickly but has trouble stopping to turn at the end of the walkway. His feet remain in equinus throughout stance, with a toe–toe pattern on the left and toe–heel on the right. The problems with foot clearance persist. In the coronal plane his hips are internally rotated, worse on the left, with pelvic retraction on the left. His foot progressions are internal bilaterally. In the sagittal plane his hips and left knee do not extend fully. He gets full knee extension on the right. Hamish shows spasticity with some degree of muscle contracture and worsening mal-alignment but his hip status is satisfactory.

Stage 5: contextual factors: environmental and personal

Environmental
Hamish is attending daycare 2 days a week. He will attend a mainstream school next year. At this stage, it is critical for Hamish to maintain functional and safe mobility for the transition to school next year. Strategies to maintain independent mobility at school and safety for Hamish in the playground need to be discussed both with the school and Hamish's family.

Personal
Although Hamish has some executive functioning difficulties related to poor motor planning, he does not have an intellectual impairment. He is keen to participate in all school activities and wants to be able to keep up with the other children at school next year. Hamish's parents work, Jane part time and Peter full time. They have no extended family living near by to help with Hamish.

Stage 6: management plan

Summary of assessment findings
Assessment confirmed that spasticity in combination with muscle contracture was contributing to Hamish's mobility problems with calf spasticity limiting his ability to stand with feet flat and maintain his balance (as seen by the significant dynamic catch (R1) of his calf muscles at around $-30°$, Table 9.2). Hamstring spasticity of $80°$ with fixed contracture at the left knee joint of $2°$ (Table 9.2) needs to be considered. Any degree of knee flexion contracture at this early age is significant as this tends to worsen with time and will lead to deterioration in gait and function over time. Hamish's need for speed and endurance to participate actively at school is also an important factor.

Following assessment and discussion with the family, the following goals were established for Hamish.

(1) Prevent and reduce muscle contracture.
(2) Improve standing balance and ability to start and stop.
(3) Improve endurance when walking.

These translated into the following functional goals:

- Hamish would be able to stand still on flat feet;
- Hamish would be able to walk and stop on request;
- Hamish would be able to stand still and count to ten slowly;
- Hamish would be able to walk with a walker outside on flat ground for 10 minutes.

To facilitate these goals Hamish required multilevel injections of BoNT-A to psoas hamstrings and calf. Tibialis posterior was also thought to be contributing to his internal foot progression so this was injected as well. Under general anaesthetic it was felt that muscle contracture was present in the gastrocnemius and Hamish had plaster of Paris below-knee casts applied as well. These remained on for 2 weeks followed by a return to wearing AFOs.

Stage 7: implement plan

Post botulinum toxin A

Fourteen days after the BoNT-A injections Hamish's community physiotherapist attended his home and implemented a programme. Frequency of physiotherapy was increased to twice weekly at this time and continued at this intensity for 6 weeks. Frequency of physiotherapy should increase after BoNT-A injections (Desloovere et al, 2007) to take advantage of the reduction of spasticity to improve range of movement and promote functional gains. Frequency should be determined on an individual basis and will be dependent on the child's age, functional level, compliance, family factors and therapist availability and funding. Hamish's physiotherapist instituted the following programme:

Goal 1: prevention and reduction of muscle contracture

HAMSTRINGS
Long sitting, including the use of a 3-point splint on the left knee, was initially undertaken for 15 minutes at a time and increased to 30 minutes. Care with positioning was explained to Hamish and his family to ensure good pelvic and lumbar spine posture during this time. This was done initially with the use of a wedge cushion to sit on. Hamish did this at the end of the day while he watched a favourite DVD to encourage him to stay in this position.

CALF
While casts were on Hamish was encouraged to stand with his heels down and knees straight. Initially he wore the 3-point splint on his left knee to maintain knee extension.

Various upper limb activities and games were used to maintain compliance and interest in this task. This was done weekly in his therapy session. When his casts were removed, stretching was undertaken in a standing lunge position both barefoot, and in shoes and AFOs. Each stretch was maintained for 1 to 2 minutes and Hamish had to do ten on each leg. These stretches were done in therapy sessions and also daily, as part of his home programme.

PSOAS
Hamish undertook prone lying for 15 minutes each day for the first 4 weeks post injections, at bedtime while stories were being read.

Goal 2: improve standing balance and ability to start and stop
Activities to improve standing balance were included as part of therapy sessions. Start and stop activities as well as fast and slow gross motor games were encouraged at home and at childcare. A visit to Hamish's childcare centre was carried out by his community physiotherapist 3 weeks after his injections to facilitate their use of the games and to help them understand and support Hamish's needs. Ways to manage Hamish's difficulties with motor planning and the effect of this on his ability to acquire and refine new motor skills were shared with parents and childcare workers. This included showing them how to assist Hamish to discover strategies that worked for him within games. Example strategies included slowing down his movements at appropriate moments and helping him to identify the key components of games that need his attention. In addition, the physiotherapist reinforced the importance of repetitive practice of motor activities; Hamish will need more practice than most children his age to acquire motor skills (Valvano, 2004; Eliasson, 2005).

Goal 3: improve endurance when walking
Walking and stair climbing were incorporated into therapy sessions by the use of treasure hunting for objects placed around the house and garden to encourage increased amounts of walking. The duration of this activity was increased at each session along with the difficulty of the terrain and distances covered until he could achieve 10 minutes without needing to rest. A structured walking programme both with and without the walker was followed on the weekends. A rewards chart helped Hamish achieve time targets.

The therapists visited his school so that issues regarding Hamish's mobility could be discussed with the school staff and a plan for using the walker outside during lunch breaks was put in place. Hamish's community physiotherapist provided reports and supporting documentation to assist the school with requests for funding for integration support for Hamish. It is important that this planning process is carried out by the community physiotherapists as they are the primary therapists responsible for Hamish's care. The role of the consultant physiotherapist from the tertiary centre is to advise the family and community physiotherapist about current and future management options for Hamish and how this may impact on his ability to participate at school and in the community.

Stage 8: evaluate outcomes

Six months post BoNT-A Hamish returned to the tertiary centre for assessment.

His parents reported that he had settled into school well and was coping well with the physical demands of school. His community physiotherapist reported that he was walking well at school with fewer falls. He was continuing to do his home stretches although calf stretching was becoming difficult again as a result of the return of calf spasticity. He was using his posterior walker outside at school for safety only and often left it behind on the sports ground at lunch times. At this stage, Hamish was walking well independently at home, at school and in the community. His FMS scores were 5, 5, 5, indicating that he could walk 500 metres without using his walker. His GMFM was 64.6%. Hamish's range of movement scores are presented in Table 9.4.

Gait evaluation from video assessment showed that when walking barefoot Hamish had a feet flat pattern with early heel rise more on the left than the right. He still had some difficulty with foot clearance in swing and reduced knee flexion in swing. In the coronal plane pelvic retraction persisted on the left and there were bilateral internally rotated hips and foot progressions worse on the left. In the sagittal plane his hips and knees did not extend fully with the pelvis in anterior tilt. In AFOs his gait was unchanged other than for increased internal foot progression. Hamish was now able to stop and turn around.

Physical examination and gait observation revealed that Hamish was developing bony torsion abnormality and increasing mal-alignment. There was increasing hip internal rotation bilaterally with decreased external rotation and increasing femoral neck anteversion. Gross motor function had also decreased slightly. This is part of the natural history of cerebral palsy (Bell et al; 2002; Gough et al, 2004).

At this time BoNT-A may now have limited further application in Hamish's case. Hamish is now 6 years old and starting to get muscle contracture as noted by his

Table 9.4. Assessment findings, 6 months post BoNT–A, Hamish aged 6 years[a]

Range of movement, muscle length and modified Tardieu	Left side	Right side
Thomas Test: psoas length	–5°	0°
Popliteal angle hamstring length	55° (60°)	45° (55°)
Passive knee extension	0°	0°
Soleus length	5°	10°
Gastrocnemius length	–10° (–35°)	–5° (–20°)
Hip abduction adductor length	15°	20°
Hip internal/external rotation	70°/20°	60°/30°
Femoral neck anteversion	40°	30°

a. Measures in parentheses indicate R1 spastic catch (Tardieu).

reducing range of dorsiflexion at the ankle and reduced abduction range at the hip despite BoNT-A and a continuing stretching programme. Botulinum toxin A acts to reduce spasticity but cannot affect fixed contractures. For many children there comes a time where BoNT-A is no longer useful but orthopaedic surgery may not be indicated as yet. At this age Hamish is not ready for single event multilevel surgery (SEMLS) (see Chapters 4 and 10) because as he continues to grow muscle contractures and bony deformity (femoral anteversion, tibial torsion) may progress significantly or remain fairly static, so it is too early to make a definitive decision about surgical prescription. Future surgery may include psoas and gastrocnemius lengthening, medial hamstring lengthening or transfer and varus derotation osteotomies of both femurs. It is important to discuss surgery and its timing with the family, including the necessity of waiting and that BoNT-A is no longer required at this stage. The consultant physiotherapist and orthopaedic surgeon will be involved in discussing these issues along with the community physiotherapist. It is important that the community physiotherapist has ongoing contact with the child's orthopaedic surgeon at this time. Figure 9.1 illustrates the cycle of clinical reasoning for Hamish.

Box 9.2 Key clinical messages

- Combined interventions aimed at stabilizing hips and managing lower limb spasticity set a platform for standing, independent walking and development of function.

- Botulinum toxin A can reduce spasticity but cannot affect contractures and is most useful in managing spasticity in young children with cerebral palsy.

- Goal-directed physiotherapy is important after BoNT-A injections to take advantage of the reduction of spasticity to improve range of movement and promote functional gains.

References

Bache CE, Selber P & Graham HK (2003) Mini-Symposium. Cerebral Palsy: the management of spastic diplegia. *Curr Orthop*, 17, 88–104.

Bell KJ, Ounpuu S, DeLuca PA & Romness MJ (2002) Natural progression of gait in children with cerebral palsy. *J Pediatr Orthop*, 22, 677–82.

Canadian Association of Occupational Therapists (CAOT) (2002) *Enabling Occupation: An Occupational Therapy Perspective.* Ottawa: Canadian Association of Occupational Therapists.

Cech DJ & Martin S (2002) *Functional Movement Development across the Life Span.* Philadelphia, PA: WB Saunders.

Crowner BE, Brunstrom JE & Racette BA (2007) Iatrogenic botulism due to therapeutic botulinum toxin a injection in a pediatric patient. *Clin Neuropharmacol*, 30, 310–13.

Desloovere K, Molenaers G, De Cat J, Pauwels P, Campenhout AV, Ortibus E, Fabry G & De Cock P (2007) Motor function following multilevel botulinum toxin type A treatment in children with cerebral palsy. *Dev Med Child Neurol*, 49, 56–61.

Eliasson AC (2005) Improving the use of hands in daily activities: aspects of treatment of children with cerebral palsy. *Phys Occup Ther Pediatr*, 25, 37–60.

Gough M, Eve LC, Robinson RO, Shortland AP (2004) Short-term outcome of multilevel surgical intervention in spastic diplegic cerebral palsy compared with the natural history. *Dev Med Child Neurol*, 46, 91–7.

Hägglund G, Lauge-Pedersen H, Wagner P (2007) Charactersistics of children with hip displacement in cerebral palsy. *BMC Musculoskeletal Dis*, 8, 101.

Howell K, Selber P, Graham HK, Reddihough D (2007) Botulinum neurotoxin a: an unusual systemic effect. *J Paediatr Child Health*, 43, 499–501.

Khot A, Sloan S, Desai S, Harvey A, Wolfe R & Graham HK (2008). Adductor release and chemodenervation in children with cerebral palsy: a pilot study in 16 children. *J Child Orthop*, 2, 293–9.

Palisano RJ, Rosenbaum PL, Bartlett D & Livingston MH (2008) Content validity of the expanded and revised gross motor function classification system. *Dev Med Child Neurol*, 50, 744–50.

Rosenbaum PL, Walter SD, Hanna SE, Palisano RJ, Russell DJ, Raina P, Wood E, Bartlett DJ and Galuppi BE (2002) Prognosis for gross motor function in cerebral palsy: Creation of motor development curves. *JAMA*, 288, 1357–63.

Shepherd R (2003) Optimizing motor performance in infants and children with cerebral palsy. *Dev Med Child Neurol Suppl*, 45, 17–19.

Steenbeek D, Ketelaar M, Galama K & Görter JW (2007) Goal attainment scaling in paediatric rehabilitation: a critical review of the literature. *Dev Med Child Neurol*, 49, 550–6.

Steenbergen B & Gordon AM (2006) Activity limitation in hemiplegic cerebral palsy: evidence for disorders in motor planning. *Dev Med Child Neurol*, 48, 780–3.

Steenbergen B, Verrel J & Gordon AM (2007) Motor planning in congenital hemiplegia. *Disabil Rehabil*, 29, 13–23.

Valvano J (2004) Activity-focused motor interventions for children with neurological conditions. *Phys Occup Ther Pediatr*, 24, 79–107.

World Health Organization (2001) *International Classification of Functioning, Disability and Health. Short Version.* Geneva: WHO.

Wynter M, Gibson N, Kentish M, Love SC, Tomason P & Graham HK (2008) *Consensus Statement on Hip Surveillance for Children with Cerebral Palsy: Australian Standards of Care.* Victoria: CP Australia.

Chapter 10

Physiotherapy following single event multilevel surgery (SEMLS)

Adrienne Harvey

Case study: Ruby

Ruby (Figure 10.1) is an 8-year-old girl with spastic diplegic cerebral palsy referred for assessment by her orthopaedic surgeon because she was being considered for single event multilevel surgery (SEMLS). She was referred for preoperative assessment and management, postoperative rehabilitation and postoperative assessment to quantify the outcome of the surgery. The steps involved in the clinical reasoning process used in this chapter are summarized in Figure 10.2 and described in Chapter 1.

Stage 1: initial data collection

Ruby was born at 29 weeks' gestation weighing 848 grams. Her diagnosis of cerebral palsy was made by her paediatrician when she was 2 years of age and magnetic resonance imaging (MRI) performed at that time showed periventricular leukomalacia. She began commando crawling at 12 months of age, sitting at 15 months and reciprocal crawling at 18 months. She walked at approximately 32 months of age. She was classified at Gross Motor Function Classification System (GMFCS; Palisano et al, 2008) level II (Box 10.1).

Physiotherapy treatment and assessment with a community physiotherapist began for Ruby when she was 2 years old. She was given botulinum toxin A (BoNT-A) injections (eight times) between the ages of 3 and 8 years to manage her spasticity. The sites for injections included gastrocnemius, adductors and hamstrings.

Ruby began using hinged (articulated) ankle–foot orthoses (AFOs) from the age of 26 months. On referral, she was using three-point knee extension splints for 30 minutes every day while long sitting to stretch her hamstrings. She could ambulate without

Figure 10.1 Ruby before her operation.

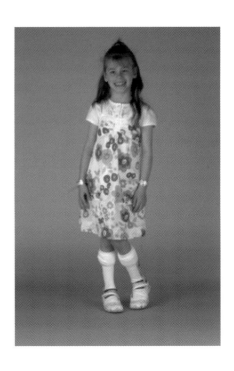

Box 10.1 GMFCS level II snapshot[1]

Proportion of people with cerebral palsy classified as GMFCS II: 18–30%

Proportion of people classified as GMFCS level II who

- have a severe intellectual disability (IQ <50): about 20%;
- have a severe visual impairment: about 13%;
- have epilepsy: about 25%;
- have behavioural problems: less than 5%;
- have hip displacement requiring surgery: about 10%;
- walk alone at home by age 2–3 years: 24%;
- walk alone at home by age 4–12 years: 89%.

assistive devices but used a wheelchair for longer distances, such as at the shopping centre or for family outings and school excursions. Ruby attended the local primary school and was in grade 2 at the time of assessment. She enjoyed playing with her friends at school. She lived at home with her parents and younger brother. Her father was an electrician and her mother worked as a part-time receptionist.

1   See Chapter 2: p. 17 for details of the sources used to derive these data.

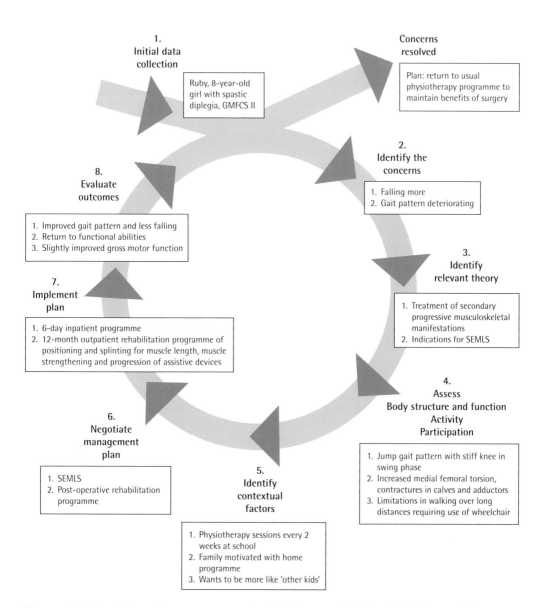

Figure 10.2 The intervention process used with Ruby: model adapted with permission from the Canadian Occupational Performance Process Model (CAOT, 2002). GMFCS, Gross Motor Function Classification System; SEMLS, single event multilevel surgery.

Stage 2: identify and prioritize the concerns

Ruby's parents were concerned that recently she was not responding to the BoNT-A injections. She was falling more (one to two falls per day). Her walking pattern was deteriorating with more 'turning in' of her legs and dragging her feet with her shoes wearing out at the toes very quickly. She was walking less and getting tired easily. Ruby reported that she was not able to do some of the activities her friends at school could do, like jumping. Her parents reported that Ruby had started noticing her limitations and verbalized these concerns at home.

A report from Ruby's community physiotherapist highlighted tightness in her calves causing difficulties with the fit of her orthoses. Her increasing hip internal rotation was interfering with her function and gait and, along with the dragging of her feet, was causing her to fall more. Overall, the main concerns were the deteriorating gait pattern with increased hip internal rotation, calf tightness and dragging of the feet, all affecting Ruby's function.

Stage 3: identify relevant theory

The primary underlying brain lesion in cerebral palsy is static; however, the musculoskeletal manifestations may be progressive (Bache et al, 2003). The secondary abnormalities seen in children with cerebral palsy, such as muscle contractures and bony deformities, are amenable to treatment however, the primary abnormalities resulting from the brain lesion are difficult to alter, with the exception of spasticity (Gage and Novacheck, 2001). One aim in the management of spasticity using modalities including BoNT-A injections is to prevent the development of fixed contractures (Graham and Selber, 2003). Botulinum toxin injections are indicated primarily in younger children aged between 2 and 6 years (Cosgrove et al, 1998; Graham et al, 2000). One aim of the injections is to defer the need for more extensive surgical correction, based on clinical, radiological and gait analysis assessment, until the child is at an optimal age to ensure the most benefits are obtained (Bache et al, 2003; Chapter 4).

Most children who have early spasticity management will still require orthopaedic surgery for the correction of fixed deformities due to the progressive nature of the musculoskeletal deformities (Graham and Selber, 2003). It is now generally accepted that the surgical correction of musculoskeletal deformities for the correction of gait deviations should be performed in one session (Browne and McManus, 1987; Nene et al, 1993; Abel et al, 1999, Fabry et al, 1999; Saraph et al, 2002; Bache et al, 2003; Graham and Selber, 2003). This ensures only one admission to hospital and one rehabilitation period, and can be denoted as single event multilevel surgery (SEMLS) (Bache et al, 2003; see Chapter 4). The frequently used procedures are muscle–tendon lengthenings, tendon transfers, rotational osteotomies and bony stabilization procedures (Bache et al, 2003).

Ruby's early management included BoNT-A injections for her spasticity. When she presented for assessment, the effect of the injections was wearing off. She was at a stage where her muscle and bony deformities were becoming worse and her gait and function were beginning to deteriorate. It was at this point that she was considered to be at an appropriate age and stage for surgical intervention. Determining the timing of gait correction surgery in children with cerebral palsy involves a balance between when enough growth has occurred to ensure the child will not require extensive surgery again at a later stage, yet not so much growth that the deformities are severe and are difficult to manage.

Stage 4: assessment of body structure and function, activity and participation

Ruby's activity limitation was classified according to the GMFCS (Palisano et al, 1997, 2008; see Chapter 2). She was classified as level II because she could walk indoors and outdoors and climb stairs holding onto a railing but experienced limitations walking on uneven surfaces (see Figure 2.1 in Chapter 2). A number of outcome measures were selected, centred on the International Classification of Functioning, Disability and Health (ICF, World Health Organization, 2001), to assess Ruby based on her age, the main concerns and the pending intervention. These are presented in Table 10.1.

Body functions and structures

THREE-DIMENSIONAL GAIT ANALYSIS (3DGA)
Ruby had a 3DGA as part of her presurgical assessment. Some clinicians believe that gait analysis is mandatory for the optimal treatment of problems relating to ambulation in cerebral palsy to assess dynamic gait problems accurately and allow more precise decision-making (Gage and Novacheck, 2001). A contrary view is that the variability seen in gait analyses questions their routine use (Wright, 2003). Gait analysis was considered important to understand Ruby's pathological gait pattern and to provide an objective outcome measure after surgery (Graham and Selber, 2003). The results of Ruby's gait analysis along with information from other measures of body structures and

Table 10.1 Assessments for Ruby

Body functions and structures	Activities and participation
Three dimensional gait analysis (3DGA)	Functional Mobility Scale (FMS)
Physical examination: spasticity, range of movement, muscle strength	Gillette Functional Assessment Questionnaire Walking Scale (FAQ)
Radiology	Gross Motor Function Measure (GMFM)
	Video assessment of gait

function and activity performance enabled an individualized surgical prescription to be implemented for her. The gait analysis also enabled her gait pattern to be classified according to the deformities in the sagittal plane. Based on the classification by Rodda et al (2004), Ruby had a jump gait pattern. Her gait analysis data showed a stiff knee gait pattern, equinus at the ankle and some flexion at the hip. Figure 10.3 illustrates the different sagittal gait patterns seen in children with spastic diplegia. In the transverse plane she also showed marked internal rotation of her hips with an internal foot progression angle.

PHYSICAL EXAMINATION: SPASTICITY, RANGE OF MOVEMENT AND MUSCLE STRENGTH

Spasticity was assessed using the modified Ashworth Scale (MAS) and the modified Tardieu scale. The MAS grades the degree of resistance to passive movement in relevant muscle groups (Bohannon and Smith, 1987). The modified Tardieu scale was used to assess the point in the joint range where a velocity dependent 'catch' was felt during a quick stretch of relevant muscles (Boyd and Graham, 1999, see Appendix, p. 289). Passive range of movement by goniometry was used to assess the relevant lower limb muscle lengths and joint range. Manual muscle testing to examine strength was assessed using the Medical Research Council (MRC) Scale (Medical Research Council, 1978). Table 10.2 summarizes the main physical examination measurement findings for Ruby preoperatively.

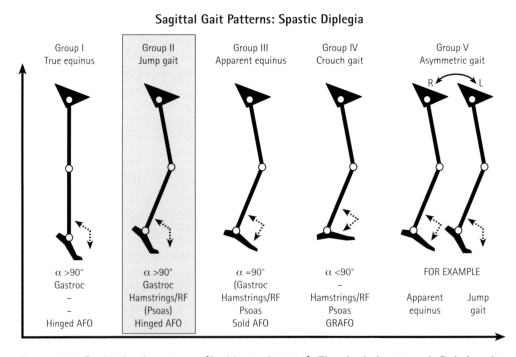

Sagittal Gait Patterns: Spastic Diplegia

Group I True equinus	Group II Jump gait	Group III Apparent equinus	Group IV Crouch gait	Group V Asymmetric gait	
$\alpha > 90°$	$\alpha > 90°$	$\alpha = 90°$	$\alpha < 90°$	FOR EXAMPLE	
Gastroc	Gastroc	(Gastroc	Hamstrings/RF		
–	Hamstrings/RF	Hamstrings/RF	Psoas	Apparent	Jump
–	(Psoas)	Psoas	GRAFO	equinus	gait
Hinged AFO	Hinged AFO	Sold AFO			

Figure 10.3 Sagittal gait patterns (Rodda et al, 2004). The shaded pattern is Ruby's gait pattern (jump gait).

Table 10.2. Main findings from Ruby's physical examination

	Right	Left
Range of movement		
Hip flexor length	8° extension	2° extension
Hamstrings (popliteal angle: hip and knee at 90°)	50°	53°
Knee joint extension	0°	2° fixed flexion
Calf length – knee flexed to 90°	11° dorsiflexion	0°
Calf length – knee extended	2° plantarflexion	14° plantarflexion
Adductor length	25° from midline	28° from midline
Hip internal rotation	72°	71°
Hip external rotation	22°	20°
Spasticity		
Hamstrings	Mild spasticity, catch at 65°	
Calves	Severe spasticity, catch at 20° (R) and 10° (L) plantarflexion	
Adductors	Moderate spasticity, catch at 15°	
Rectus femoris spasticity	Moderate	Moderate
Muscle strength (MRC)		
All hip muscles were weak and graded as 3 (able to move against gravity only)		
Quadriceps were slightly weak (Grade 4) and were able to work against some resistance but there was a quadriceps lag of 20° bilaterally		
Calves and ankle dorsiflexors were also weak (Grade 3)		

RADIOLOGY
Radiological examination of Ruby's hips and feet showed that she had mild hip displacement and mild planovalgus deformity of her feet. Figure 10.4 shows Ruby's pelvic radiograph before her operation.

Activities and participation

FUNCTIONAL MOBILITY SCALE (FMS)
The FMS was chosen to assess mobility preoperatively and to monitor mobility status over the postoperative rehabilitation period (see Appendix, p. 293). Preoperatively Ruby's FMS score was 5, 5, 1. She was able to walk independently at home and at school on level surfaces only (score 5) and required the use of a wheelchair for longer distances such as the shopping centre (score 1).

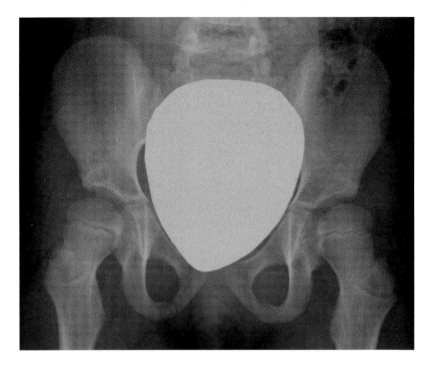

Figure 10.4 Ruby's pelvic radiograph showing some hip displacement.

GILLETTE FUNCTIONAL ASSESSMENT QUESTIONNAIRE (FAQ) WALKING SCALE
The FAQ is a 10-level categorical scale that assesses the walking ability of children with disabilities via parental report (Novacheck et al, 2000). Preoperatively Ruby's parents reported her as level 6 on the FAQ (walks more than 15–50 feet [4.5–15 metres] outside the house but usually uses a wheelchair or stroller for community distances or in congested areas).

GROSS MOTOR FUNCTION MEASURE (GMFM)
The GMFM was used to assesses change in Ruby's gross motor function over time (Russell et al, 2002; see Appendix, p. 294). Preoperatively Ruby's GMFM–66 score was 65.63% (95% CI 62.87–68.39).

VIDEO ASSESSMENT OF GAIT PATTERN
Visual assessment of Ruby's walking showed internal rotation of her hips bilaterally with a resulting internal foot progression angle. She showed incomplete knee extension in stance phase (left side worse than right) and a stiff knee pattern in swing phase. She displayed equinus at her ankles bilaterally and dragged her feet during swing phase, the left side worse than right.

The outcome measures selected in Ruby's case reflected her management needs at this time with the impending gait correction surgery. They focused around body functions and structures and activity limitation. There are other measures available for children with cerebral palsy. A systematic review of evaluative activity limitation measures used in children with cerebral palsy critically examined the psychometric properties and clinical utility of eight outcome measures (Harvey et al, 2008). The GMFM (Russell et al, 2002) and Activities Scale for Kids (ASK, Young et al, 2000) showed the most robust psychometric properties for cerebral palsy. Other useful measures that can be used for this age group of children include the Pediatric Evaluation of Disability Inventory (PEDI) (Haley et al, 1992) and the Functional Independence Measure for Children (WeeFIM) (Msall et al, 1994), which are described in the Appendix (pp. 292 and 295).

Stage 5: identify contextual factors

Ruby attended a mainstream school and received 10 hours per week of integration funding to assist her at school. Her community physiotherapist saw her every 2 weeks at school. She did not require assistive devices at school for mobility but would take her wheelchair on school outings. She sometimes lost her balance in the playground or when moving between classes if she was distracted or there were many other children moving around her.

Both of Ruby's parents worked and, with a younger brother at home, things were quite busy. Ruby was motivated to do her physiotherapy and stretching at home and her parents were diligent at carrying out her home programme, although time did not always permit long sessions. Ruby wanted 'to be able to do what the other kids could do' and often became frustrated with her abilities and her exercises. She attended swimming lessons every week and went to dance classes.

Stage 6: negotiate a management plan

Based on the assessment findings the surgical prescription for Ruby involved the following:

- bilateral femoral derotation osteotomies;
- bilateral Strayer's gastrocnemius recessions;
- bilateral percutaneous lengthening of adductor longus;
- bilateral transfer of rectus femoris to semitendinosus;
- botulinum toxin injections to calves, medial hamstrings and psoas muscles.

Botulinum toxin injections at the time of surgery were added as an adjunct for pain relief and for the prevention of spasms, thus ensuring comfortable and effective positioning postoperatively (Barwood et al, 2000). The surgery and the postoperative rehabilitation programme were discussed with Ruby and her family at a pre-admission clinic prior to her surgical admission. At this appointment the family met with all therapists and practitioners who would be involved in Ruby's care. Liaison between her community physiotherapist and the hospital physiotherapist began in the early preoperative stage to ensure a postoperative programme could be implemented effectively. The equipment requirements for the home setting were assessed by the occupational therapist to enable a smooth transition to home following her inpatient stay.

Stage 7: implement the plan

Described below is Ruby's rehabilitation programme following her SEMLS based on guidelines developed at The Royal Children's Hospital, Melbourne, Australia. The inpatient programme and postoperative monitoring are implemented by the hospital physiotherapists and the majority of the outpatient therapy occurs in the community with the child's usual physiotherapist. These guidelines are intended to be broad to ensure individual children have programmes tailored to them incorporating their type and severity of cerebral palsy, findings from assessment of body functions and structures, activities and participation, as well as personal and environmental factors.

Inpatient management

Ruby was admitted to hospital on the day of her surgery and returned to the orthopaedic ward with an epidural in situ for her early postoperative pain relief. She had below-knee plaster casts for support of her gastrocnemius lengthenings. Her femoral osteotomies were internally fixed with a plate and screws. Zimmer knee immobilizers were used to maintain knee extension. The femoral osteotomies necessitated a 3-week period of non-weight bearing following surgery. Other bony surgery would also generally have required a 3-week period of non-weight bearing; however, following surgery to soft tissues only (muscle lengthenings and transfers) the children can often commence standing and walking after 5–7 days.

Early physiotherapy consisted of positioning to maintain good alignment (Figure 10.5):

(1) symmetrical supine lying to ensure neutral rotation of her hips – Day 1;
(2) prone lying for 1–2 hours per day to maintain hip flexor length – Day 2;
(3) long-sitting for 3–4 hours per day to maintain hamstring length – Day 3.

Active-assisted and passive knee range of movement exercises commenced at Day 3 to ensure that Ruby's rectus femoris transfers did not become adhered to underlying muscle or subcutaneous tissue. This was performed three times daily with a repetition of 15–20. Ruby was discharged home on Day 6 using a wheelchair with leg extensions to maintain knee extension. She maintained a home programme of positioning and knee exercises as described above. She also performed non-weight bearing strengthening exercises for quadriceps (e.g. knee extension over a rolled towel progressing to over the edge of the bed), hip extensors (e.g. prone hip extension) and hip abductors (e.g. hip abduction in side lying). As per the rectus femoris transfer protocol, the goal for achievement of knee flexion range of movement was to reach 30° by discharge (week 1), 60° by the end of week 2 and 90° by the end of week 3.

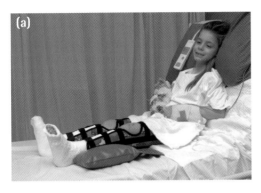
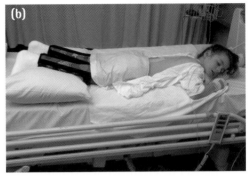

Figure 10.5 (a) long sitting and (b) prone lying postoperatively.

On discharge, the hospital physiotherapist communicated with Ruby's community physiotherapist and a letter was sent detailing the procedures that had been performed on Ruby, her non-weight bearing status, her status on discharge and explaining the aims of the programme for the coming few weeks. The community physiotherapist was now managing her programme in consultation with the hospital physiotherapist; hence good communication between the two was extremely important for Ruby's overall programme.

Within the first few weeks at home Ruby gradually returned to school, beginning with attending for three mornings a week and increasing the time as she was able. Ruby's community physiotherapist visited her at school and educated her teachers regarding her non weight-bearing status and her reduced mobility. Her physiotherapist also gave advice regarding transfers and the need for providing Ruby with extra assistance in the short term with her mobility around the school, for transfers and for going to the toilet. The physiotherapist explained to the school that as a result of the extensive nature of Ruby's surgery she would initially have reduced function and mobility and would require a wheelchair and later assistive devices for mobility, but that as she progressed through her rehabilitation she would eventually return to her previous functional level.

Outpatient management
Ruby returned to the outpatient clinic at 3 weeks and received the following interventions:

- plasters removed;
- radiology of her osteotomies;
- casting for her orthoses;
- application of fibreglass casts in preparation for weight bearing.

At 3 weeks she commenced weight bearing, initially standing in the parallel bars with her zimmer knee splints on. She progressed quickly with her physiotherapist to standing and walking using a posterior walker, initially with and then without the zimmer splints (Figure 10.6).

From 3–6 weeks postoperatively Ruby's programme consisted of the positioning and range of movement, weight bearing and walking and strengthening exercises (predominantly non-weight bearing strengthening). The zimmer knee splints that had been used throughout the day and night were now being used at night and for a period of long sitting each day. Her community physiotherapist saw her twice weekly at home and her parents did exercises with her daily.

At 6 weeks Ruby returned to the clinic. The report from her community physiotherapist was that she was progressing well and further guidance for the progression of her programme was required. Her casts were removed and she was fitted with her solid (non-articulated) AFOs. The 6–12 week stage of the postoperative programme is the critical stage for children when the most gains can be made. An effective strengthening programme is required to ensure an optimal outcome from the surgery. Ruby's strengthening programme was increased to include progressive resistive strength training and functional strengthening activities such as stair climbing, step-ups and sit-to-stand activities (see Figure 10.7).

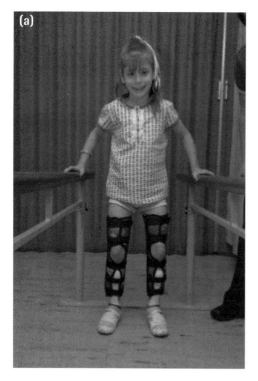

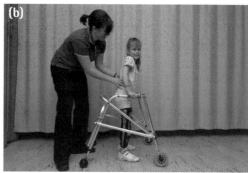

Figure 10.6 (a) Standing in parallel bars with zimmer splints on and (b) progressing to walker.

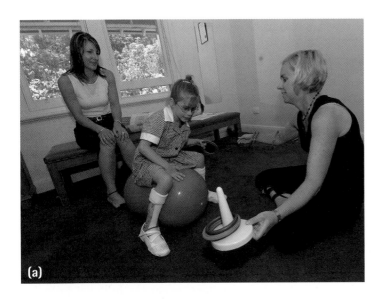

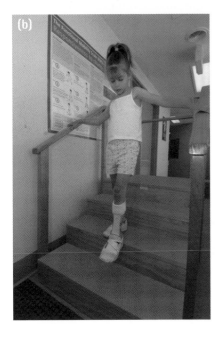

Figure 10.7 (a) and (b) strengthening exercises.

Hydrotherapy at this stage is an important part of the programme and Ruby began this weekly after cast removal. Hydrotherapy provides an environment where the child can move more easily with their body weight supported and aims to improve their strength, mobility and endurance. Ruby's physiotherapist was now seeing her three times weekly to ensure she was progressing at this critical stage. At 3 months the physiotherapist introduced crutches. She used her walker at school and was practising with crutches at home.

From 3–6 months postoperatively Ruby continued with her programme. The focus had shifted away from the muscle length and positioning, to increasing her strengthening programme. Recreational and fitness activities were also incorporated into her programme, including bicycle riding with her family and horse riding at the weekends. At 6 months she stopped using the walker and had progressed to independent walking at home and crutches at school. She still required a wheelchair for longer community distances.

From 6–12 months postoperatively Ruby returned to her usual physiotherapy sessions (every 1–2 weeks) and maintained a home strengthening programme with her parents. She resumed swimming weekly and riding her bicycle and returned to her dance classes at 9 months.

Orthotic prescription following SEMLS depends on the surgical procedures involved and the individual presentation of each child. Most children are initially prescribed solid AFOs. Progression depends on biomechanical alignment and strength and length of key muscles. Progression to hinged AFOs only occurs when and if there is adequate calf tension to ensure a competent plantar flexion–knee extension couple, full knee joint extension and adequate quadriceps strength to ensure the child maintains knee extension during stance phase of gait. A small group of children are prescribed ground reaction AFOs (GRAFOs) in the initial postoperative phase if they demonstrate crouch gait preoperatively with a small fixed flexion contracture at the knees. These are essentially used as a postoperative tool for 3–6 months and are then replaced with solid AFOs (Figure 10.8).

Stage 8: evaluate the outcomes

Children who undergo SEMLS require at least 12 months of rehabilitation and changes in mobility are seen up until 24 months (Harvey et al, 2007). In the clinical setting these children are monitored every 3 months for the first 12 months using two-dimensional video analysis and functional scales (Figure 10.9). Table 10.3 tracks Ruby's function and orthotic prescription over the 12-month rehabilitation period.

Following SEMLS a child's GMFCS level can change in the initial postoperative period (Harvey et al, 2007). This was demonstrated at 3 and 6 months postoperatively for Ruby and she functioned like a child in level III while recovering from surgery. It has also been demonstrated that following SEMLS children's mobility deteriorates initially and then improves over the 12-month rehabilitation period, as seen in Ruby's case (Harvey et al, 2007). Without gait correction surgery the child with cerebral palsy is at risk of function and gait deteriorating during their growing years. This is particularly pertinent during the adolescent years when rapid growth can lead to worsening deformities and impact on gait, thus making it difficult for the adolescent to remain ambulant (Johnson et al, 1997). Single event multilevel surgery aims to counteract this effect of natural history by preventing the deterioration, maintaining function and keeping the child ambulant. It is therefore expected that after SEMLS function will return to preoperative levels and perhaps some gains in function will be made. However, it is not expected that there will be substantial improvements in function.

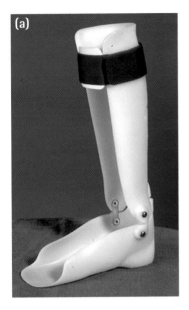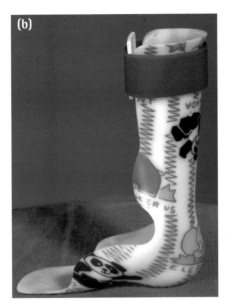

Figure 10.8 (a) Hinged ankle–foot orthosis (AFO) and (b) solid AFO. Braces fabricated by the Assistive Technology Department at Gillette Children's Specialty Healthcare, St. Paul, MN, USA. Reproduced with permission from Tom F. Novacheck, Gary J. Kroll, George Gent, Adam Rozumalski, Camilla Beattie and Michael H. Schwartz: Orthoses. In *The Identification and Treatment of Gait Problems in Cerebral Palsy* (2nd edn) edited by James R. Gage, Michael H. Schwartz, Steven E. Koop and Tom Novacheck. Clinics in Developmental Medicine no. 180–181. London: Mac Keith Press, 2009.

Table 10.3 Changes in functional measures and orthoses over the rehabilitation period

	GMFCS	FMS	FAQ	Orthoses
Before operation	II	5, 5, 1	6	Hinged AFOs
3 months after operation	III	3, 2, 1	5	Solid AFOs
6 months after operation	III	5, 3, 1	6	Solid AFOs
9 months after operation	II	5, 5, 1	6	Hinged AFOs
12 months after operation	II	5, 5, 1	6	Hinged AFOs

AFO, Ankle–foot orthosis; FAQ, Functional Activity Questionnaire; FMS, Functional Mobility Scale; GMFCS, Gross Motor Function Classification System.

A 3DGA and full clinical examination were performed at 12 months postoperatively to assess the outcome of the surgery. Ruby showed correction of the internal rotation at the hips and calf length was now restored to an adequate length. During gait she had an improved knee arc of motion in swing phase and better knee extension in stance phase (Figure 10.9). Her GMFM–66 score at 12 months postoperatively was 68.1% (95% CI 65.22–70.98) compared with 65.63% (95% CI 62.87–68.39) preoperatively. Although this difference is not statistically significant, it indicates that Ruby did improve on some items of the GMFM, such as stepping over an object, walking a straight line and jumping. Based on the motor growth curves, GMFM scores would normally be stable for a child her age; therefore, this difference can be considered clinically significant.

Ruby and her parents felt that the quality of her walking was improved with less turning in of her hips and, importantly, she was falling less. At 12 months after surgery her function had returned to preoperative levels; however, she was having some difficulties with higher-level activities such as jumping. The rehabilitation process had been a long one from the family's perspective, with functional gains appearing later than they had anticipated. However, they could see the improvements in her gait pattern.

At this stage Ruby was continuing to see her community physiotherapist once every 2 weeks to monitor her muscle strength and length, her gait pattern and her functional status. Every 6 months her community physiotherapist performed a full

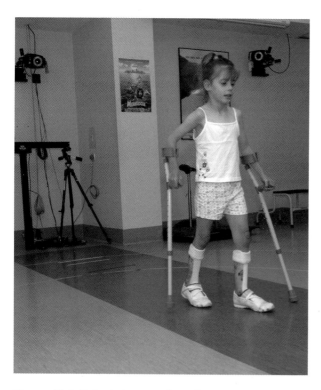

Figure 10.9 Ruby being monitored postoperatively using two-dimensional video in the gait laboratory.

assessment with physical examination, GMFM, video assessment of her gait and functional scales. After her 1-year post-surgical review the orthopaedic surgeon continued to monitor her every 6–12 months to ensure there was no deterioration or issues requiring addressing. Throughout her adolescent growth years, Ruby needs to be monitored carefully for any signs of recurrence of deformity and encouraged to remain fit and active.

Box 10.1 Key clinical messages

- Early management of spasticity includes botulinum toxin injections. The optimal age for multilevel orthopaedic surgery is when progressive gait deformities start to cause limitations in activities and participation.

- A comprehensive assessment using a number of tools is required to guide surgical decision-making and postoperative evaluation.

- Rehabilitation focuses on positioning, active-assisted exercises and strengthening as an inpatient followed by graduated strengthening programmes (progressive resistive strength training and functional strengthening), hydrotherapy and recreational and fitness activities on an outpatient basis.

- Careful orthotic and assistive device prescription is a key element of the postoperative programme.

References

Abel MF, Damiano DL, Pannunzio M & Bush J (1999) Muscle-tendon surgery in diplegic cerebral palsy: functional and mechanical changes. *J Pediatr Orthop*, 19, 366–75.

Bache CE, Selber P & Graham HK (2003) The management of spastic diplegia. *Curr Orthop*, 17, 88–104.

Barwood S, Baillieu C, Boyd R, Brereton K, Low J, Nattrass G & Graham HK (2000) Analgesic effects of botulinum toxin A: a randomized, placebo-controlled clinical trial. *Dev Med Child Neurol*, 42, 116–21.

Bohannon RW & Smith MB (1987) Interrater reliability of a modified Ashworth scale of muscle spasticity. *Phys Ther*, 67, 206–7.

Boyd R & Graham H (1999) Objective clinical measures in the use of Botulinum toxin A for the management of children with cerebral palsy. *Eur J Neurol*, 6, S23–35.

Browne AO & McManus F (1987) One-session surgery for bilateral correction of lower limb deformities in spastic diplegia. *J Pediatr Orthop*, 7, 259–61.

Canadian Association of Occupational Therapists (CAOT) (2002) *Enabling Occupation: An Occupational Therapy Perspective*. Ottawa: Canadian Association of Occupational Therapists.

Cosgrove AP, Corry IS & Graham HK (1998) Musculoskeletal modelling in determining the effect of botulinum toxin on the hamstrings of patients with crouch gait. *Dev Med Child Neurol*, 40, 622–5.

Fabry G, Liu XC & Molenaers G (1999) Gait pattern in patients with spastic diplegic cerebral palsy who underwent staged operations. *J Pediatr Orthop B*, 8, 33–8.

Gage JR & Novacheck TF (2001) An update on the treatment of gait problems in cerebral palsy. *J Pediatr Orthop B*, 10, 265–74.

Graham HK, Aoki KR, Autti-Ramo I, Boyd RN, Delgado MR, Gaebler-Spira DJ, Gormley ME, Guyer BM, Heinen F, Holton AF, Matthews D, Molenaers G, Motta F, Garcia Ruiz PJ & Wissel J (2000)

Recommendations for the use of botulinum toxin type A in the management of cerebral palsy. *Gait Posture*, 11, 67–79.

Graham HK & Selber P (2003) Musculoskeletal aspects of cerebral palsy. *J Bone Joint Surg*, 85, 157–66.

Graham HK, Harvey A, Rodda J, Nattrass GR & Pirpiris M (2004) The functional mobility scale. *J Pediatr Orthop*, 24, 514–20.

Haley SM, Coster WJ, Ludlow LH, Haltiwanger JT & Andrellos PJ (1992) *Pediatric Evaluation of Disability Inventory: Examiners Manual*. Boston, MA: New England Medical Centre.

Harvey A, Graham HK, Morris ME, Baker R & Wolfe R (2007) The Functional Mobility Scale: ability to detect change following single event multilevel surgery. *Dev Med Child Neurol*, 49, 603–7.

Harvey A, Robin J, Morris ME, Graham HK & Baker R (2008) A systematic review of measures of activity limitation for children with cerebral palsy. *Dev Med Child Neurol*, 50, 190–8.

Johnson DC, Damiano DL & Abel MF (1997) The evolution of gait in childhood and adolescent cerebral palsy. *J Pediatr Orthop*, 17: 392–6.

Medical Research Council of the United Kingdom (1978) *Aids to Examination of the Peripheral Nervous System: Memorandum No 45*. Palo Alto, CA: Pedragon House.

Msall ME, DiGaudio K, Rogers BT, LaForest S, Catanzaro NL, Campbell J, Wilczenski F & Duffy LC (1994) The Functional Independence Measure for Children (WeeFIM). Conceptual basis and pilot use in children with developmental disabilities. *Clin Pediatr*, 33, 421–30.

Nene AV, Evans GA & Patrick JH (1993) Simultaneous multiple operations for spastic diplegia. Outcome and functional assessment of walking in 18 patients. *J Bone Joint Surg Br*, 75, 488–94.

Novacheck TF, Stout J L & Tervo R (2000) Reliability and validity of the Gillette Functional Assessment Questionnaire as an outcome measure in children with walking disabilities. *J Pediatr Orthop*, 20, 75–81.

Palisano RJ, Rosenbaum PL, Walter S, Russell D, Wood E & Galuppi B (1997) Development and reliability of a system to classify gross motor function in children with cerebral palsy. *Dev Med Child Neurol*, 39, 214–23.

Palisano RJ, Rosenbaum PL, Bartlett D & Livingston MH (2008) Content validity of the expanded and revised gross motor function classification system. *Dev Med Child Neurol*, 50, 744–50.

Rodda JM, Graham HK, Carson L, Galea MP & Wolfe R (2004) Sagittal gait patterns in spastic diplegia. *J Bone Joint Surg Br*, 86, 251–8.

Russell D Rosenbaum PL, Avery L & Lane M (2002) *The Gross Motor Function Measure. GMFM-66 and GMFM-88 (Users' Manual). Clinics in Developmental Medicine No. 159*. Mac Keith Press: London.

Saraph V, Zwick E-B, Zwick G, Steinwender C, Steinwender G & Linhart W (2002) Multilevel surgery in spastic diplegia: evaluation by physical examination and gait analysis in 25 children. *J Pediatr Orthop*, 22, 150–7.

World Health Organization (2001) *International Classification of Functioning, Disability and Health, Short Version*. Geneva: WHO.

Wright JG (2003) Pro: interobserver variability of gait analysis. *J Pediatr Orthop* 23, 288–289.

Young NL, Williams JI, Yoshida KK, Bombardier C & Wright JG. (1996) The context of measuring disability: does it matter whether capability or performance is measured? *J Clin Epidemiol*, 49, 1097–101.

Chapter 11

Occupational therapy following upper extremity surgery

Josie Duncan

Case study: Adam

Adam was referred to a tertiary care facility for evaluation of his suitability for surgical management of his left upper limb. The steps involved in the clinical reasoning process used in this chapter are summarized in Figure 11.1 and described in Chapter 1.

Stage 1: initial data collection

Adam is a 10-year-old boy with left-sided spastic hemiplegia (asymmetrical cerebral palsy). He is ambulant (Gross Motor Function Classification System [GMFCS] level II; Palisano et al, 2008; see Box 11.1) and has some use of his left hand. He is classified at level II on the Manual Ability Classification System (MACS; Eliasson et al 2006; see Chapter 2). Two years previously, Adam received botulinum toxin A injections (BoNT-A) to pronator teres after which he had his usual therapy of one 30-minute session per fortnight. His parents reported that the positive benefits lasted for approximately 6 months.

Adam's family live in a large regional centre 2 hours' drive from the tertiary care hospital. He is in a grade appropriate to his age at the local school. His community occupational therapist has worked with him since he started school at 5 years of age. She has fabricated thermoplastic splints for him, worn at night, to prevent the development of secondary contractures in his wrist, fingers and thumb. Regular passive range of movement through forearm supination has also been encouraged to prevent pronation contracture. To address Adam's and his family's goals the community occupational therapist has also been engaging Adam in task-specific practice to optimize hand and upper limb skills for bimanual function.

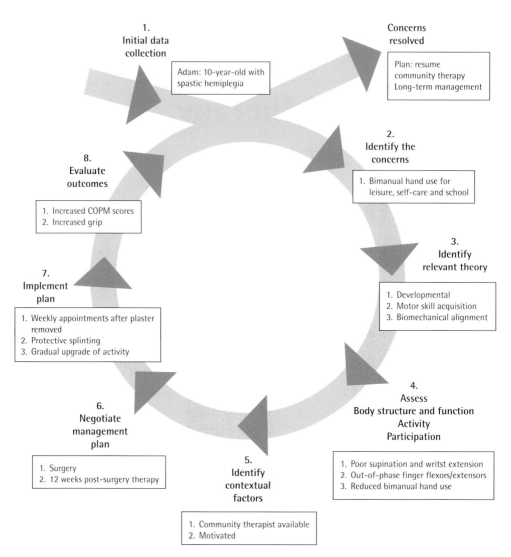

Figure 11.1 The intervention process used with Adam: model adapted with permission from the Canadian Occupational Performance Process Model (CAOT, 2002). COPM, Canadian Occupational Performance Measure.

Stage 2: identify and prioritize the concerns

Information about treatment priorities was sought from Adam, his parents and community therapist. Adam had expressed frustration with his difficulty handling a basketball when playing with his peers. He had a strong desire to handle the ball more competently using two hands. At home, he wanted to use his left hand more effectively to stabilize the PlayStation game control. At school, when cutting paper with scissors, Adam wanted to be able to hold and orient the paper better with his left hand. His

> **Box 11.1 GMFCS level II snapshot[1]**
>
> Proportion of people with cerebral palsy classified as GMFCS II: 18–30%
>
> Proportion of people classified as GMFCS level II who
>
> - have a severe intellectual disability (IQ <50): about 20%;
> - have a severe visual impairment: about 13%;
> - have epilepsy: about 25%;
> - have behavioural problems: less than 5%;
> - have hip displacement requiring surgery: about 10%;
> - walk alone at home by age 2–3 years: 24%;
> - walk alone at home by age 4–12 years: 89%.

parents were focused on encouraging independence and were keen for Adam to cut his own food at mealtimes. His community occupational therapist reported progressive pronation contracture despite inclusion of daily supination stretches in his home programme. His weak wrist extension also compromised his grip strength and thus limited his hand function. Adam had become increasingly uncooperative with therapy and educational interventions.

Stage 3: identify relevant theory

Developmental tasks of middle childhood
The ability to take part in age-appropriate daily activities related to caring for oneself, learning and recreation are key concerns in childhood. The child that is unable to participate in typical childhood occupations can become marginalized and socially isolated (Mandich and Rodger, 2006).

LEISURE
In middle childhood, play and leisure pursuits are increasingly undertaken with a peer group, but because of physical impairments children with cerebral palsy may be gradually excluded from group activities such as team sports, dance and other physical pursuits. At the same time, they become more aware of the impact and significance of their impairment, and peer interactions and friendships, physical well-being and self-esteem can be negatively affected (Cronin and Mandich, 2005). At this age, some children are choosing to self-exclude from physical activities (Imms, 2008).

---

1 See Chapter 2: p. 17 for details of the sources used to derive these data.

Self-care

The acquisition of self-care skills in childhood is intricately linked with the development of motor skills (Henderson, 2006). Self-management of personal care needs is important for the development of autonomy, self-efficacy, self-awareness and life satisfaction (Barnes and Case-Smith, 2004). Because of their atypical motor skill development children with cerebral palsy have an extended dependency on carers for self-care. This places additional stresses on family as well as the child.

School and classroom participation

Complex hand and upper limb movements are required for many tasks in the school environment including carrying large, small, heavy and fragile objects; opening doors, containers, and taking lids off pens; using scissors and ruling a line. Most activities are bimanual and as children progress through the school years, become increasingly complex with the expectation that they will be performed quickly and smoothly. Although Adam will not use his hemiplegic hand for tasks like handwriting, there is evidence that children with hemiplegia have increased difficulty achieving high-level tasks because of the impact of associated physical difficulties with posture and endurance as well as perceptual difficulties (DuBois et al, 2004).

Motor skill acquisition

In middle childhood, children without impairment experience a dramatic increase in the ability to calibrate movements precisely to the demands of a task. They develop more mature bilateral coordination skills, and increased dexterity and in-hand manipulation skills (Cronin and Mandich, 2005). In children with cerebral palsy, the combination of positive features such as spasticity and negative features such as weakness can result in muscle imbalance affecting the complex blend of stability and mobility necessary for coordinated movement (Eliasson, 1995; Brown and Walsh, 1999).

Biomechanical alignment and surgery

Atypical patterns of movement and immobilization in positions with mal-alignment can, over time, also lead to secondary structural changes to muscles, joints and surrounding soft tissues in the upper limb (Copley and Kuipers, 1999). Fixed contractures can be reduced by muscle–tendon lengthening or release (Chin et al, 2005). Tendon transfers can improve hand function by adjusting muscle imbalance. Static procedures such as joint stabilization, arthrodesis and tenodesis are sometimes performed where there is instability or dystonia, although children with dystonia can respond unpredictably to surgery. Some surgical procedures are deferred until after skeletal maturity to reduce the risk of recurrence of deformity with further growth (Chin et al, 2005). Not all children with cerebral palsy are candidates for upper limb surgery: careful assessment and patient selection is necessary. The efficacy of surgery for selected children is supported in several studies (Eliasson et al, 1998; Van Heest et al, 1999; Smeulders et al, 2005; see Chapter 4).

Stage 4: assessment of body structure and function, activity and/or participation

The problems identified by Adam and his parents were related to his difficulty participating in occupations appropriate for his age because of the impairment in his left upper limb. To determine Adam's suitability for surgery and develop a surgical plan, his upper limb assessment was videotaped. This enabled the surgeon to view the recording and formulate a surgical proposal. Specific assessments were completed of Adam's performance, and satisfaction with performance, of preferred activities and his upper limb motor skills and quality of movement.

Assessment of activity and participation

The Canadian Occupational Performance Measure (COPM, Law et al, 2005) was used as an assessment of activity limitation (see Appendix, p. 291). Adam and his parents were interviewed. Adam identified leisure activities (e.g. playing basketball) and his parents identified self-care and productivity/school activities (e.g. cutting food) as areas of priority. Clinical observation provided an additional opportunity to observe how Adam used his left hand in age-appropriate bimanual activities such as opening containers, ruling a line, cutting with scissors, using a knife and fork, doing up buttons, tying shoelaces and catching a ball, and to record the impact of Adam's impairments on his activity performance.

Assessment of body structure and function

Both passive and active range of movement (ROM) available in Adam's left arm and hand were measured using a goniometer and his grip strength was measured with a dynamometer. Quality of movement was measured using the Melbourne Assessment of Unilateral Upper Limb Function (Randall et al, 1999; see Appendix, p. 286).

Clinical observation of quality of movement and selective motor control in the hand while performing bimanual tasks revealed that Adam could actively extend his fingers and thumb when the wrist was stabilized in neutral. Palpation of the flexor carpi ulnaris tendon while Adam was moving his fingers revealed that it was contracting 'out of phase' with finger flexors. This resulted in wrist flexion and ulnar deviation when fingers flexed for grasp. This contributed to his very weak grasp. The results of Adam's assessments are presented in Table 11.1.

Stage 5: identify contextual factors: environmental and personal

Environmental factors

Adam attended a mainstream school where the community occupational therapist was funded by the state government to provide services for a total of 9 hours in the school year. Communication between the community occupational therapist and the tertiary care occupational therapist and surgeon was established to ensure appropriate exchange of information regarding Adam's treatment. The community occupational therapist was able to negotiate to 'stockpile' several of the year's sessions for treatment of Adam to reduce the number of trips the family would be required to make to the tertiary care

Table 11.1 Adam's pre-surgery scores on each measure

Assessment	Pre-surgery scores	
Canadian Occupational Performance Measure[a]		
Performance	3.25	
Satisfaction	3.25	
Passive range of movement		
Elbow	extension	−10°
	flexion	150° (full range)
Forearm[b]	supination	10°
	pronation	90° (full range)
Wrist[c]	extension	50°
	flexion	80° (full range)
Active range of movement		
Elbow	extension	−20°
	flexion	150° (full range)
Forearm[b]	supination	−90°
	pronation	90° (full range)
Wrist[c]	extension	−40°
	flexion	80° (full range)
Melbourne Assessment[d]	66%	
Grip strength		
Left	2 kg	
Right	15 kg	

a. Scores range from 1–10 with higher scores indicating better performance and satisfaction.

b. The zero starting position for measuring forearm movement is in the 'thumbs up' position, mid-way between pronation and supination.

c. The zero position for measuring wrist movement is neutral between flexion and extension.

d. Scores of 100% indicate unimpaired quality of movement.

centre for treatment postoperatively. Adam's family were very committed to optimizing any opportunity for improvement.

Personal factors
Adam was increasingly aware of his physical impairment and limitations. This was presenting as poor cooperation with therapy and educational interventions. His agreement and cooperation for the surgery and postoperative therapy was important and was secured because it was clearly linked to his goals around his leisure pursuits of basketball and PlayStation.

Stage 6: management plan

Summary of assessment findings
Measures of impairment suggested that poor active forearm supination and wrist extension were contributing to Adam's activity limitations. Evaluation of flexor carpi ulnaris revealed that it would contract appropriately if transferred to augment wrist extension. There was adequate passive wrist extension range for this procedure to be considered. Evaluation of finger extensors indicated that they had enough strength to extend the fingers if wrist flexion was limited after transfer of flexor carpi ulnaris to extensor carpi radialis brevis. While his pronation contracture had been progressively increasing, pronator teres had enough excursion to support transferring it to supplement his negligible active supination within the available range. Therefore tendon transfers were offered as a surgical option to Adam and his family as a way of increasing his ability to use his left hand actively in bilateral tasks.

Negotiated management plan
As the occupational performance issues Adam identified using the COPM involved his preferred leisure activities, he was motivated to accept the prospect of surgery and the associated therapy. It was important, however, that Adam and his family understood that surgery could not restore normal hand function. Following extensive discussion with the surgeon and tertiary care occupational therapist and consultation with the community occupational therapist, Adam and his family decided to proceed with the surgery. His community occupational therapist rescheduled seven 30-minute treatment sessions to occur in weeks 6 to 12 after surgery to support the treatment programme established with the tertiary care centre. Adam would also be seen at the tertiary care centre at weeks 4, 8 and 12 after surgery.

Based on the assessment findings, the surgical proposal for Adam was as follows:

(1) rerouting of pronator teres deep to the radius and reattachment on the dorso-radial side to act as a supinator; and

(2) transfer of flexor carpi ulnaris to extensor carpi radialis brevis, which releases the deforming wrist flexor (and ulnar deviator) and augments wrist extension and radial alignment. By virtue of the dorso-ulnar course of the transferred tendon, flexor carpi ulnaris also becomes a secondary supinator.

A period of 3 months therapy following surgery was specified as necessary for an optimal outcome.

The procedures identified as suitable for Adam are among a large number of possible procedures that are performed by hand surgeons for the range of musculoskeletal and biomechanical problems seen in children with cerebral palsy (Chin et al, 2005). Children of differing ages with differing presentations of involvement and severity can benefit from surgical intervention for a variety of reasons. Those with spastic hemiplegia who are quite functional (MACS levels I and II), with few contractures and some functional use of their hemiplegic upper limb, like Adam, are most likely to be offered surgery in the middle years of childhood. The goal is to improve the available but limited function, and will often have the added benefit of improving the appearance of the limb because of the rebalancing of deforming forces of hypertonic muscles. These children will generally have fewer procedures that are most often tendon transfers rather than releases.

Children with more functionally limiting spastic hemiplegia and quadriplegia, with minimal functional upper limb use (MACS levels IV and V), multiple contractures and/or a high risk of an increase in contracture, are more likely to be offered surgery as teenagers. The goal of surgery in those children is to reduce the dysfunction (e.g. reduce pain, and improve the ability of the child or carers to dress and clean the arm or hand), to reduce the extent of contracture (where splinting and maintaining range is not feasible) and to improve appearance. These children will often have multiple level corrections including muscle lengthening and releases. Botulinum toxin A and serial splinting can also be used to lengthen some shortened musculotendinous units, before surgery for a better outcome.

Stage 7: implement the plan

After surgery, Adam spent one night in hospital (tertiary care centre) and 4 weeks with his left hand immobilized in a plaster cast with wrist, finger and thumb in extension and forearm in supination. Four weeks postoperatively the plaster cast was removed at the hospital and the healed wounds were checked by the plastic surgeon. The occupational therapist at the hospital immediately fitted Adam with a low temperature thermoplastic splint to protect the transferred flexor carpi ulnaris tendon while still healing (Figure 11.2). The fingers and thumb were included in the splint to ensure maintenance of length in the extrinsic flexors and other soft tissues. The post-surgical splinting protocol involved a gradual reduction of wearing time (Table 11.2). The fit of the splint may require adjustment at week 5, as during the week after the cast is removed there is a gradual return of the hypertonicity that was inhibited during the post-surgical casting. The forearm did not require protective splinting but passive pronation was to be avoided to prevent damage to the transferred tendon.

In concert with the reduced splint wearing times there is a gradual increase in activation of transferred tendons where feasible. Guidelines for activation and re-education of the transferred pronator teres and flexor carpi ulnaris tendons included graded exercises and

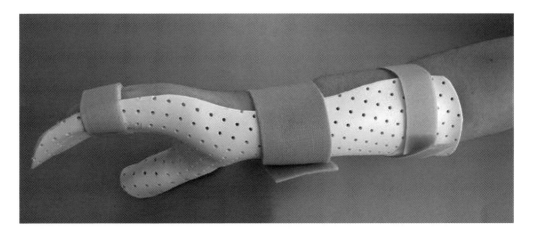

Figure 11.2: Post–surgical splint.

use of the hand in functional tasks. Weekly treatment and a home programme of daily exercises and activities were integral to achieving the best outcome for Adam (Figure 11.3). Optimal outcomes were ensured through regular liaison and collaboration between the community and tertiary care therapists. This was facilitated through use of TeleHealth systems providing a video link between centres. Using this technology reduced the number of occasions Adam and his family travelled to the tertiary hospital for review because Adam could demonstrate changes in movement and activity performance and the family and therapists in both centres could discuss progress and ongoing intervention via video.

Stage 8: evaluate the outcomes
Adam's performance and satisfaction with performance of his COPM goals and change on the upper limb measures at 6 and 12 months after surgery are shown in Table 11.3. Although the Melbourne Assessment showed only modest overall improvement of 4%, there was a positive change in reach, target accuracy, supination, hand-to-hand transfer and hand-to-mouth. Adam's grip was markedly stronger with increased active wrist extension with finger flexion. Using the COPM, clinically significant gains were perceived to have been made in all activities except the use of a knife and fork for cutting food. With improved grasp strength and a reduction in the severity of forearm pronation, Adam reported that he was able to hold the PlayStation control more securely and with better orientation. He was also more satisfied with his ability to hold a basketball using two hands because of reduced forearm pronation. Figure 11.4 shows his ability to extend the fingers with wrist extension and improved finger flexion with wrist extension. Figure 11.5 shows before and after positioning of the forearm, wrist and fingers.

Adam will require ongoing management of his spasticity. In addition, there is a potential for secondary contracture with growth that may require further surgery. Splints

Table 11.2: Post-surgical treatment protocol

Timing	Intervention focus
0 to 4 weeks	Plaster cast with wrist, finger & thumb extension and forearm supination
4 weeks	Plaster off; splint fitted for wrist, finger and thumb extension Remove splint for showers only Passive supination stretch initiated with splint on (Figure 11.3); avoid passive pronation
5 weeks	Splint off 2 hours daily. Splint may require adjustment to ensure a continued good fit Initiate low risk active grasp and release of light objects, which are of a size and texture that are easily grasped and held, to activate the flexor carpi ulnaris transfer for wrist extension with finger flexion Initiate active supination exercises (Figure 11.3) and activities to activate pronator teres transfer
6 to 12 weeks	Each week reduce splint wearing by another 2 hours daily until splint is off all day by 12 weeks Activity is gradually upgraded for wrist extension with finger flexion and forearm supination. Progressively more challenging grasp demands can be incorporated into functional bimanual tasks such as holding a bottle while opening it with the right hand, stabilizing the PlayStation control No basketball until 3 months post-surgery Scar management techniques including massage and silicone products (for example silicon gel sheet) are used as required to minimize hypertrophy
3–6 months	Monthly review for splint maintenance and fit, and integration of changed movement patterns into daily tasks
Beyond 6 months	Ongoing night splinting to maintain wrist, finger and thumb posture as needed

should be a feature of his long-term contracture management. As Adam matures, he can be encouraged to take a greater role in managing his own long-term health and well-being. This includes learning how to minimize contracture development and seek increased therapeutic input at strategic times to help him meet his goals and address occupational performance concerns.

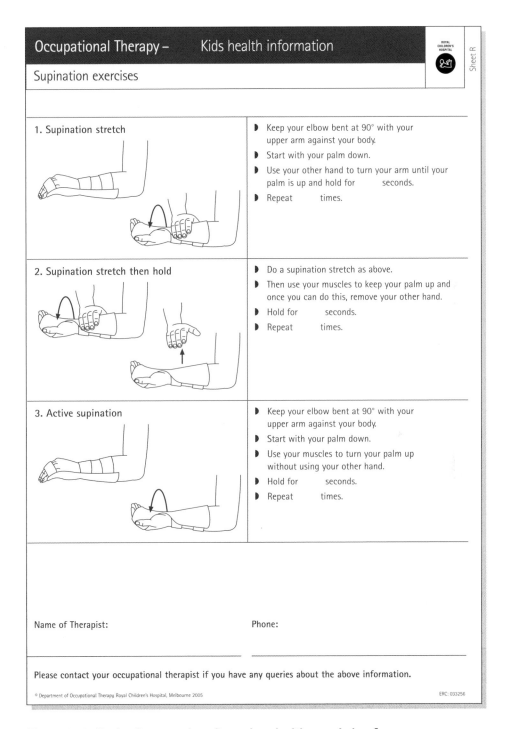

Figure 11.3. Supination exercises. Reproduced with permission from http://www.rch.org.au/emplibrary/ot/InfoSheet_R.pdf

Table 11.3. Evaluation of outcomes for Adam after surgery

	Pre-surgery	6 months post-surgery	12 months post-surgery	Change
Canadian Occupational Performance Measure				
Performance score	3.25	6.5	6.75	3.5[a]
Satisfaction score	3.25	8.0	6.25	3.0[a]
Melbourne Assessment	66%	70%	70%	4%
Grip strength	2 kg	9 kg	11 kg	9 kg[a]

a. A clinically important increase in score occurred either between pre- and post-assessments or where a change has been maintained at 12 months post-surgery.

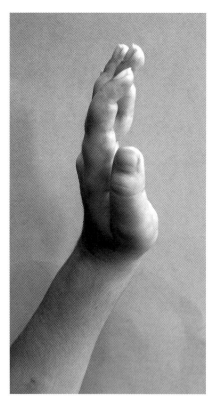 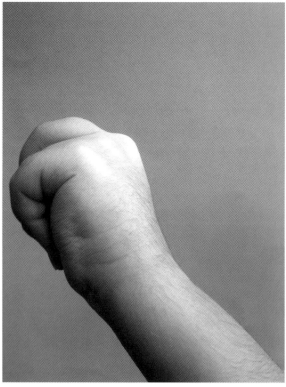

Figure 11.4 Post-surgery finger extension (a) and flexion (b) with wrist extension.

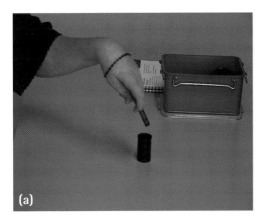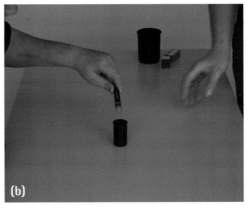

Figure 11.5 Video stills from the Melbourne Assessment: forearm, wrist and finger position before (a) and after (b) surgery.

Box 11.2 Key clinical messages

● Tendon transfer surgery can improve function and appearance of the upper limb in children classified at level II and III on the MACS by rebalancing the forces of hypertonic muscles.

● Comprehensive assessment is required for surgical planning. A videotaped assessment allows careful analysis of movement imbalance in the performance of functional tasks.

● Postoperative therapy must be timely to maximize surgery outcomes.

References

Barnes KJ & Case-Smith J (2004) Adaptive strategies for children with developmental disabilities. In: Christiansen CH & Matuska KL (eds) *Ways of Living: Adaptive Strategies for Special Needs*. Bethesda, MD: AOTA Press.

Brown JK & Walsh EG (1999) Neurology of the upper limb. In: Neville B & Goodman, R (eds) *Congenital Hemiplegia. Clinics in Developmental Medicine No. 150*. London: Mac Keith Press.

Canadian Association of Occupational Therapists (CAOT) (2002) *Enabling Occupation: An Occupational Therapy Perspective*. Ottawa: Canadian Association of Occupational Therapists.

Chin TYP, Duncan JA, Johnstone BR & Graham HK (2005) Management of the upper limb in cerebral palsy. *J Pediatr Orthop B*, 14, 389–404.

Copley J & Kuipers K (1999) *Management of Upper Limb Hypertonicity*. San Antonio, TX: Therapy Skill Builders.

Cronin A & Mandich MB (2005) *Human Development and Performance throughout the Lifespan*. New York, NY: Thomson, Delmar Learning.

DuBois L, Klemm A, Murchland S & Ozols A (2004) Handwriting of children who have hemiplegia: A profile of abilities in children aged 8–13 years from a parent and teacher survey. *Aust Occup Ther J*, 51, 89–98.

Eliasson AC (1995) Sensorimotor integration of normal and impaired development of precision movement of the hand. In: Henderson N A & Pehoski C (eds) *Hand Function in the Child: Foundations for Remediation.* St Louis, MO: Mosby.

Eliasson AC, Ekholm C & Carlstedt T (1998) Hand function in children with cerebral palsy after upper-limb tendon transfer and muscle release. *Dev Med Child Neurol*, 40, 612–21.

Eliasson AC, Krumlinde-Sundholm L, Rösblad B, Beckung E, Arner M, Öhrvall A & Rosenbaum PL (2006) The Manual Ability Classification System (MACS) for children with cerebral palsy: scale development and evidence of validity and reliability. *Dev Med Child Neurol*, 48, 549–54.

Henderson A (2006) Self-care and hand skill. In: Henderson A & Pehoski C (eds) *Hand Function in the Child: Foundations for Remediation*, 2nd edn. St Louis, MO; Mosby Elsevier.

Imms C (2008) *Participation of Australian Children who have Cerebral Palsy: The Middle Years.* Melbourne: School of Physiotherapy, Faculty of Health Sciences, La Trobe University.

Law M, Baptiste S, Carswell A, McColl M, Polatajko H & Pollock N (2005) *Canadian Occupational Performance Measure.* Ottawa, ON: CAOT Publications ACE.

Mandich AD & Rodger S (2006) Doing, being and becoming: their importance for children. In: Rodger S & Ziviani J (eds) *Occupational Therapy with Children: Understanding Children's Occupations and Enabling Participation.* Carlton, Victoria: Blackwell Publishing.

Palisano RJ, Rosenbaum PL, Bartlett D & Livingston MH (2008) Content validity of the expanded and revised gross motor function classification system. *Dev Med Child Neurol*, 50, 744–50.

Randall M, Johnson L & Reddihough D (1999) *The Melbourne Assessment of Unilateral Upper Limb Function: Test Administration Manual.* Melbourne: The Royal Children's Hospital.

Smeulders M, Coester A & Kreulen M (2005) Surgical treatment for the thumb-in-palm deformity in patients with cerebral palsy. *The Cochrane Database of Systematic Reviews*, Issue 4. Art. No.: CD004093. DOI: 10.1002/14651858.CD004093.pub2

Van Heest AE, House JH & Cariello C (1999) Upper extremity surgical treatment of cerebral palsy. *J Hand Surg Am*, 24, 323–30.

Chapter 12

Navigating school-based needs and technological supports for secondary schools

Margaret Mayston

Case study: Lucy

Lucy is a 12-year-old girl with above average intelligence who is about to progress from primary to secondary school. She enjoys mathematics and science, and wants to be a physicist. Lucy has been classified as level V on the Gross Motor Function Classification System scale (GMFCS; Palisano et al, 1997, 2008; see Box 12.1) and level IV on the Manual Ability Classification Scale (MACS; Eliasson et al, 2006, 2007; see Chapter 2). She has used a powered wheelchair for 2 years, but requires assistance for transfers and personal care. Lucy has some verbal communication but mostly uses an assistive communication device and has a lap-top computer for written work. The steps involved in the clinical reasoning process used in this chapter are summarized in Figure 12.1 and described in Chapter 1.

Box 12.1 GMFCS level V snapshot[1]

Proportion of people with cerebral palsy classified as GMFCS level V: 13–16%

Proportion of people classified as GMFCS level V who

- have a severe intellectual disability (IQ <50): about 85%;
- have a severe visual impairment: about 60%;
- have epilepsy: about 80%;
- have behavioural problems: about 10%;
- have hip displacement requiring surgery: about 65%;
- use a feeding tube: 42%;
- walk alone or with support at home by age 4–12 years: 0%.

---

1   See Chapter 2: p. 17 for details of the sources used to derive these data.

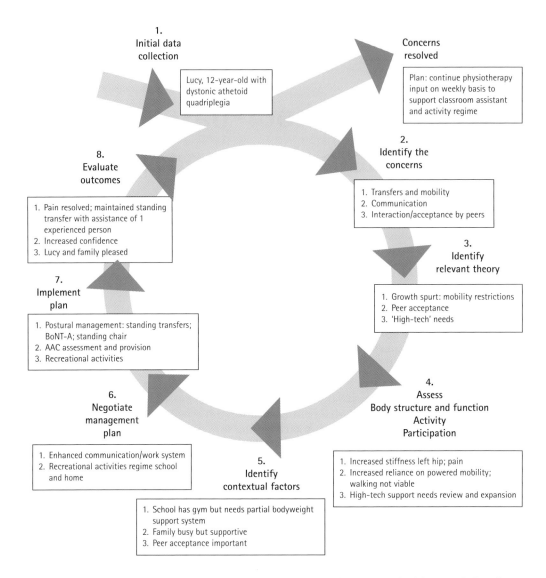

Figure 12.1 The intervention process used with Lucy: model adapted with permission from the Canadian Occupational Performance Process Model (CAOT, 2002). AAC, augmentative and alternative communication; BoNT-A, botulinum toxin A.

Stage 1: initial data collection

Lucy attends mainstream school and the community health care teams (for junior and senior school) wish to determine what input will be needed to assist Lucy to achieve optimally in secondary school and realize her goal of going to university. Transition plans began when Lucy was in year 5, when she was almost 11 years old. The purpose of this meeting was to review recent assessments and to finalize the transition plan.

Lucy was born at full term after an uneventful pregnancy, but there were complications during the initial forceps delivery. The cord prolapsed causing asphyxia and an emergency caesarean was performed. The diagnosis of dystonic athetoid quadriplegia with spasticity was confirmed when she was 2 years old. She has had multidisciplinary therapy input since she was 10 months old. More recently therapy has been provided at school in sports sessions, but she has had regular individual physiotherapy, occupational therapy and speech and language therapy after school. In addition she goes horse riding once a fortnight during a school sport session and goes swimming with the family at weekends. The family also goes bike riding and she uses an adapted tricycle, although she is slow and cannot keep pace. Her mother does Pilates exercises with her several times a week; thus her social and recreational activity has predominantly revolved around the family.

Lucy has a younger sister (aged 8 years) and her parents are her main carers. Her father has a printing business and her mother, although at home full time, works when she can: she is an artist.

Stage 2: identify and prioritize concerns

Lucy's concerns
Lucy is most concerned about how she will integrate into her new school and how she will carry her lap-top computer and books when moving between classrooms. She is also concerned about how she will negotiate the school to get to classes in different locations, as well as the time taken to do this. She has also highlighted the need for privacy while toileting, especially as her periods have started, and she is particularly anxious about how she will make and maintain friendships and socialize with her peers. She recognizes that her communication skills need assessment and revision to enable her to interact successfully with her peers.

Parental concerns
Lucy's parents share her concerns but also want to ensure that Lucy maintains her standing transfers and muscle length as she has now entered a phase of rapid growth and will experience less variety of postural positions during the day. They have already observed that Lucy has seemed stiffer in the last few months and that she has some pain in her left hip. They wonder if this is because Lucy has been walking less, and has not regularly used her Bronco walker (Bronco Gait Trainer, Snug seat/R82 A/S Denmark, similar to the Arrow walker, Triaid Inc, USA or Theraplay Ltd, UK) since she was 8 years old (Figure 12.2).

All, including Lucy, have agreed that assisted walking will no longer be a significant form of mobility for her. Appropriately, this decision had been made earlier in Lucy's development when it was realized that walking would not be maintained into the future, although her parents still find it difficult to perceive a future without Lucy using some kind of assisted walking, at least at home. Lucy has had a variety of

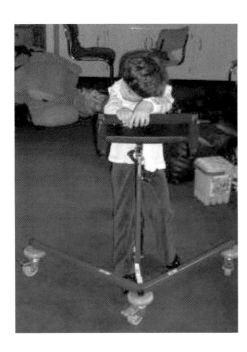

Figure 12.2 Eight-year-old Lucy using Bronco gait trainer.

orthoses for her lower limbs. She has had hinged and fixed ankle–foot orthoses (AFOs) to support her feet and provide good alignment, but has found them uncomfortable because of the constant movement from her involuntary spasms associated with the dystonia. Lucy has a Lycra body suit that she likes as it makes her feel more stable and more able to access her switch-operated communication device and lap-top computer. Although she has used a powered chair for the last 2 years she has also used a walking frame under the supervision of her physiotherapist. She needs assistance via a gaiter to keep her left arm forwards onto the grip of the walker; her lower limbs do not move fluently; and she has difficulty taking weight on her left leg as a result of the hip/knee flexion.

The most important issues identified by Lucy and her parents included the following:

- concern about reduced opportunities for standing and danger of increasing hip/knee flexion contracture and pain;
- the need to review mobility and assisted transfers;
- the increased need for more sophisticated technological aids for school work and communication;
- to enable Lucy to negotiate the transition to adolescence with its challenges of independence, socialization, recreation and formulation of future career aspirations to work towards optimal satisfying participation in adult life. This will include management of the balance of family and peer relationships.

Stage 3: identify relevant theory

Transition stage from childhood to teenager/adolescent
This is a challenging stage even if children do not have a motor disability. It is a time of changing demands educationally, socially and in terms of personal independence as children enter the transition from childhood to adolescence and adulthood.

It has already been decided that walking will no longer be prioritized for Lucy but that an emphasis on standing and stepping for transfers will be relevant for her. This is difficult for Lucy's parents to accept but they are beginning to appreciate the effort it takes for Lucy to walk with assistance, and that the powered chair will give her more opportunities for future independence. It is well accepted, although not well documented, that the pubertal growth spurt is a time when walking ability may need to be reviewed, and also a time when maintenance of muscle length is a particular challenge, especially for children who lack selective movement control (O'Dwyer et al, 1989; Gormley et al, 2004; Voormann et al, 2007;). At all times it is important to monitor hip location and spinal integrity as hip dislocation or spinal asymmetry can interfere with the ability to sit and function, and could impede Lucy's ability to continue to negotiate assisted standing transfers. Lucy has had regular hip and spine radiographs since she was 2, and so far her musculoskeletal integrity has not necessitated surgical intervention.

This stage is also one when the young person needs to begin to separate from the family and develop friendships and become more independent socially. Experience of working with and discussing this issue with children in GMFCS levels IV and V suggests they seem to have particular challenges in making and keeping genuine friends. It may also be that consideration needs to be given to changing the attitudes of other children and professionals in the mainstream school.

Participation

SOCIAL/RECREATIONAL
This is Lucy's main area of concern. It has been shown that socialization and participation are significant challenges for children with disability and areas in which they usually score lower than their peers (Maher et al, 2008). Recreational activities and general exercise are important for the health of all the population but also provide an opportunity for socialization and participation, and development of these activities could enable Lucy to integrate more with her peers and to provide a gradual separation from the family as she enters adolescence.

Mobility and transfers
Lucy's parents particularly identified the potential problems of increased flexor contractures associated with the expected period of rapid growth, reduced options for mobility in secondary school, and recent reduced walking practice, in addition to their dissatisfaction with Lucy's orthotic provision.

It has been decided that Lucy will focus on her wheelchair skills and only practise walking under supervision of the physiotherapist, with the aim of maintaining standing/stepping transfers. Following a lifespan view of management for children with cerebral palsy enables decisions about walking potential to be made before a child loses that ability, and it has been shown that early provision of powered mobility is beneficial (Bottos et al, 2001). Studies have also shown that a period of treadmill training with partial bodyweight support can be useful to maintain standing transfers (Schindl et al, 2000). In their study (Schindl et al, 2000), six of the ten children who participated were aged between 6 and 18 years and non-ambulant. Four of the six were shown to have improved transfer abilities following the 12-week training period, indicating that treadmill training may have advantages other than improvement of gait. Impairments that contribute to Lucy's increased stiffness, especially of her left hip and knee, are spastic hypertonia, dystonic spasms, reduced range of movement and impaired balance.

Another important aspect of assistance in transfers is the ability to take weight with the arms if possible. Lucy has limited upper limb use, especially on the left, but practices weight bearing using a gaiter on her left arm. She practises bilateral and unilateral grasp and release, but release is particularly difficult on the left. Since she has had the Lycra suit her arm use for switching has been easier because of the stability afforded by the suit, and her speech has shown some slight improvement in intelligibility. Developmental studies have shown that trunk stability is significantly influenced by sitting posture, which provides the postural background for upper limb skills (Hadders-Algra et al, 1999). There are several manufacturers of Lycra garments, and Lucy uses one which has no boning or solid supports. This is more comfortable for her, but still gives adequate trunk support via the Lycra panel reinforcement built into the suit. Some studies have shown Lycra suits can improve sitting balance and upper limb function, but result are conflicting because earlier suit designs used in these studies were not easy to put on and take off (Nicholson et al, 2001; Knox, 2003).

Lucy does not like the AFOs and prefers to wear well-fitting boots with ankle support and insoles. There is no good evidence to support the use of orthoses, although they are widely used (Morris, 2002).

As the increased tone with flexor spasms mostly affect her left hip and knee flexors, and is therefore focal, it is thought that botulinum toxin type A (BoNT-A) could be useful. It has been found that injection of BoNT-A can be useful in reducing painful muscle spasms (Barwood et al, 2000). Injection of BoNT-A has also been shown to reduce tone and enable easier practice of activities, and therefore can minimize the development of contractures (see reviews by Lannin et al, 2006; Ward, 2008).

Equipment needs
It is thought that standing practice can minimize the development of contractures and assist physiological functioning, e.g. digestion and bone mineral density, although there is limited evidence to support this (Tremblay et al, 1990; Stuberg 1992; Kecskemethy et al, 2008). The new school cannot support the use of a standing frame because of the

different class locations and space. Lucy is also not keen to pursue the standing frame in class as this will make her appear different from her peers.

It has been agreed that Lucy will be provided with a standing wheelchair at the start of the term in the new school, and she is looking forward to this (e.g. Balder Finesse, by Permobil represented worldwide; or the SIT, from Innovative Products Inc). New designs mean that these are more stable and robust to withstand the wear and tear of adolescent life.

Communication and class work
Lucy has limited upper limb skills. She is unable to use a pen or keyboard with either hand and operates her current powered chair via a joystick. She has the ability to operate switches and has reliable and consistent use of these. The use of assistive technology enables the user to participate in activities up to their cognitive potential, and fills the gap between the physical difficulties and their cognitive abilities.

The introduction of 'high-tech' systems has revolutionized the lives of people with severe motor impairments, so that even the most impaired person can access devices using head switches, infra-red technology and a variety of hand and other switch devices. Much still needs to be done, however, to enable the users to interact effectively with their peers to facilitate a lively mutual interaction, as the literature suggests that most interactions occur between child and adult (Clarke and Wilkinson, 2007, 2008).

Lucy has been using an augmented communication system for 3 years and although she can communicate verbally, she can only be understood for approximately 40% of the time by people who do not know her. She is confident in the use of her Mercury communicator when she is required to have complex verbal interactions. She has good keyboard skills and although she uses the mouse effectively with her right hand, she prefers to use a joystick control for the keyboard. She needs to grasp onto a grip on the wheelchair with her left hand to prevent her arm flying and causing postural instability while using the control on the right. Lucy will gradually be introduced to a more complex system with environmental controls that will allow her to become more independent.

School work will also be facilitated by a more sophisticated computer system that will enable Lucy independently to produce written work and access curricula and carry out topic work via the internet.

Stage 4: assessment of body structure and function, activity and participation restrictions

Based on the initial discussion with Lucy and her family, and consideration of relevant theory a list of assessments of body function, activity and participation was developed (Figure 12.3).

Body structure and function	Activity	Participation
Spastic hypertonia and range of movement (ROM) Tardieu test ROM (goniometry)	*Gross motor ability* Gross Motor Functional Measure-66	*School* School Function Assessment (SFA) (at start of the last term at primary school). The Functional Independence Measure (FIM) will be used when she starts at secondary school and is too old for the SFA
Pain Visual Analogue Scale (VAS; 1–5)	*Mobility and transfers* Functional Ambulation Capacity Clinical observation	*Social* Children's Assessment of Participation and Enjoyment (CAPE) and Preferences for Activities of Children (PAC)
Sitting balance Chailey Levels of Ability: sitting Clinical observation: support needed while reaching as used for SACND (Reid, 1995)	*Hand use* Clinical observation; possible use of Melbourne Assessment	
	Communication Assessment at specialized centre (e.g. ACE Centre Advisory Trust, Oxford, UK)	

Personal factors	Environmental factors
Self-perception profile for children if needed, but considered that CAPE/PAC were sufficient at this stage	Ramps and lift in place at school; check space between desks for manoeuvre of powered chair. Check school changing facilities etc

Figure 12.3 Assessments for Lucy. SACND, Sitting Assessment for Children with Neuromotor Dysfunction.

Participation
Her therapy team at primary school carried out the School Function Assessment (SFA, Coster et al, 1998; see Appendix, p. 298) and as expected this highlighted the area of participation, particularly as it was a significant goal area for Lucy and her family. The SFA criterion score for participation was 43 (raw score 15, Table 12.1), well below the cut-off score of 100 for children in classes 4–6. This was in contrast to her activity and performance score in the cognitive and behavioural tasks that were all at or above the criterion cut-off score, except for personal awareness; which was below the cut-off score because of her limited motor capacity. This was reinforced by the score from the Children's Assessment of Participation and Enjoyment (CAPE, King et al, 2004; see Appendix, p. 297) and the Preferences for Activities of Children (PAC), measures that are appropriate for children and adolescents aged 6–21. Table 12.2 shows Lucy's scores on the CAPE and as expected Lucy's diversity of social participation was low as social and recreational activities revolved mainly around the family.

Activity limitations

OBSERVATION OF ASSISTED MOBILITY, ASSISTED WALKING AND TRANSFERS
Lucy was classified at level V using the GMFCS (Palisano et al, 2008, see Chapter 2). She could transfer with the assistance of one person, and had been using a Bronco walker but had difficulty in using her left hand to hold on (Figure 12.2). She has mostly been using a powered wheelchair at school operated by a joystick and has used the manual chair for outings, pushed by a family member or carer.

- *Transfers:* Lucy has reliable use of her right arm for support but not the left, takes weight moderately well, and can take a few small steps to turn around when given

Table 12.1 Assessment findings from the School Function Assessment

School Function Assessment (SFA)		
	Criterion score	Criterion cut-off (4–6)
Part I Participation Regular classroom +5 settings	43	100
Part III Activity Performance: some of the physical tasks & cognitive behavioural tasks Recreational movement	0	100
Using materials	0	100
Functional communication task	100	100
Task behaviour/completion	100	81
Personal care awareness	43	100

Table 12.2 Assessment findings from the societal participation test

Children's Assessment of Participation and Enjoyment (CAPE)	
	Lucy's score (score range)
Overall	15 (0–55)
Domain Formal Informal	 1 (0–15) 14 (0–40)
Activities Recreational Active physical Social Skill-based Self-improvement	 5 (0–12) 3 (0–13) 4 (0–10) 2 (0–10) 1 (0–10)

'Diversity' scores are presented indicating number of activities in which Lucy participated in the past 4 months.

support at her trunk. Her score on the Functional Ambulation Category was 1 (FAC, Holden et al, 1984), that is, she needs constant help from one therapist for weight support and balance. With less experienced assistants than her mother and one-to-one carer, this ability would be scored at level 2; in these cases she needs to be hoisted.

- *Observation of wheelchair skills:* Lucy is proficient in her powered chair, can anticipate and negotiate obstacles and manoeuvre between rows of desks if there is sufficient space. She can travel at speed safely and is able to get between classrooms in good time, although she needs a little extra time to get settled and ready for the class.

GROSS MOTOR ABILITY
This was assessed using the Gross Motor Functional Measure (GMFM–66; Russell et al, 2002, see Appendix, p. 294) The GMFM–66 total score of 28 indicated that Lucy is significantly limited physically, particularly in higher-level activities such as standing and walking.

UPPER LIMB FUNCTION AND SITTING BALANCE
Lucy has been classified using the MACS (level IV; see Chapter 2) and hand skills have been assessed using The Melbourne Assessment of Unilateral Upper Limb Function (Randall et al, 1999; see Appendix, p. 286). The low score on the Melbourne Assessment is expected given that Lucy is fully dependent for all of her personal care activities. This

was particularly highlighted in the SFA, for which she scored well below the criterion cut-off score for her age in all areas of physical task performance in Part III (activity performance), e.g. criterion score of 30 for eating and drinking (criterion cut-off score 100). Lucy relies on her computer for all of her school work activities, and has limited use of the left hand for any activities.

COMMUNICATION AND SCHOOL WORK

Lucy has poor breath control and articulation that affect the quality of her speech, and lacks coordination of breathing and swallowing. Her communication has been assessed by the speech pathologist from the new community team who concluded that it would be helpful if Lucy was also assessed at a centre that specializes in 'high tech' communication aids and computerized access to the curriculum. Following this assessment it was considered that Lucy would benefit from an integrated system so that she can access various devices from one controller (e.g. Mini-Merc, Tobii ATI, USA; VS (Viking) Communicator 3 Pro Spectronics Inclusive Learning Technologies, Australia), and she will gradually be introduced to a system with increased complexity. This system will also enable her to send SMS (short message service) text messages to a mobile phone, which will increase her independence and will also help her family to cope with Lucy's increasing separation from them as they will be able to be in contact with each other if needed.

The assessment also produced recommendations related to her computer needs for production of school work. Lucy cannot use the keyboard directly but uses the joystick to access the software programmes. However, her access is highly dependent on precise positioning of the equipment. The lap-top computer will need to be mounted on a custom-made tray and easily folded away for ease of transportation between classrooms, and she will have access to a desk-top computer with all the peripherals such as CD-Rom/DVD, scanner and printer. She (and her classroom assistant and family) will require ongoing training with review of her technological needs at least every 2 years.

Body structure and function

MUSCLE TONE AND EXTENSIBILITY

Lucy has dystonic athetoid quadriplegia with spasticity. As there are no good measures of dystonia in children, the dystonic component of her diagnosis could not be directly measured. The spastic hypertonia element of her diagnosis was assessed using the Tardieu scale (see Appendix, p. 289), and muscle length of her hip flexors and hamstrings were assessed using goniometry. The findings were considered in conjunction with pain measures.

Goniometry revealed that her hip abduction is limited to 25° on the left, and 30° on the right, and that her hip flexors are also restricted. She has a slight fixed flexor contracture of her left knee (15°). It is important that knee flexors contractures do not progress, as a requirement of the standing wheelchair is that she has no greater than 25° fixed knee flexion. Lucy has had her hips monitored with regular radiographs since she was diagnosed at the age of 2 years, and to date there are no significant concerns that would warrant surgical intervention. Now that she is entering adolescence it is also important to monitor her spine as she will be spending more time in sitting, and her hip flexor spasms could affect her pelvic position and thus her spinal alignment. Both her hip location and spinal alignment are important factors in her continued ability to assist in standing transfers and for upper limb functioning.

SITTING BALANCE
There are few standardized tests available to measure sitting balance in children like Lucy. For example, the Sitting Assessment for Children with Neuromotor Dysfunction (SACND, Reid, 1995) is only valid for children up to the age of 10 years (see Appendix, p. 295). The Paediatric Reach Test (Bartlett and Birmingham, 2003) can be used (see Appendix, p. 295), but is difficult for children at GMFCS level V to perform. Clinical observations were that Lucy could sit when placed but that her balance was unreliable and she could not effectively, use her arms to prevent herself from falling. Functional tests of balance have not been studied extensively, particularly for children at GMFCS level V (Gan et al, 2008). It was therefore decided to make specific clinical observations about how long Lucy could sit without assistance, how much assistance was required for reliable sitting and what she could do with her upper limbs while sitting out of the chair with and without external support, and with and without the Lycra suit.

PAIN
A visual analogue scale (VAS) of 1–5 (where 1 is mild and 5 is excruciating, based on the McGill Pain Questionnaire, Melzack, 1975), was used for Lucy and she indicated that the pain in her left hip scored at 3 (distressing). Thus it was considered that this warranted some kind of intervention. This will be discussed at her regular orthopaedic appointment which is due at the end of her last term at primary school.

Stage 5: contextual factors: environmental and personal

Environmental factors
The new school has ramp access and also has a lift so that Lucy can get to the first floor classrooms. The school has a pool on site, but they need to have a hoist fitted so Lucy can get in and out of the pool. It has been decided that she will not attend all the physical education classes and sports lessons and will pursue other activities such as treadmill training during these lessons. The school gymnasium has a treadmill and will also get a bodyweight support system so that Lucy can participate in this activity while her peers are doing their physical education activities.

Personal factors

SELF-CONCEPT
It was decided not to test this specifically because the team felt that there were sufficient tests in place without adding another one at this stage. However, given peer acceptance and social isolation can be an issue for adolescents with disability, it was decided that

her assistant, family and team members would monitor Lucy's interactions and feelings during her first year at secondary school.

The family is very supportive, but her parents appreciate that they need to allow Lucy to socialize more with her friends and will facilitate her participation in after school clubs and social outings. Lucy would like to pursue her Pilates exercises in a class with other children and her mother has agreed to try and find a suitable venue for this. Lucy realises that she needs to keep up her weekly therapy sessions to enable her to get through the growth spurt and at the same time to maintain her current physical level.

Stage 6: management plan

Summary of assessment findings
Lucy is concerned about socialization and participation issues, which is reflected in the results of the outcome measures, particularly the SFA. The GMFM and SFA also indicate goal areas related to reducing her dependence in transfers and mobility. The GMFM, goniometry and VAS indicate that care needs to be taken to minimize flexor contractures of the left hip and knee, and to prevent pain from becoming a problem. Lucy currently indicates that her pain in the left hip is 3 on the VAS. Overall, Lucy is managing well and the team are confident that they can maintain her current activity/participation level despite the growth spurt and the psychological and social demands of the new school.

Negotiated treatment plan, including equipment review and provision
- Botulinum toxin injections to left psoas, adductors and hamstrings to reduce the spasticity and associated pain. Lucy will also need additional physiotherapy at this time to maximize the effects of the injections. The injection is planned to take place in the long holidays before the move to secondary school.
- Review of orthotic provision.
- Training and support to the full-time classroom assistant and liaison with school staff.
- Assisted transfers will be practised as part of her routine school and hygiene activities.
- Provision of powered wheelchair with standing capacity: training in its use as part of the therapy programme, including assisted transfer and hand switch practice.
- Participation in school swimming programme and after school club, plus inclusion in a Pilates class at school in physical education sessions. The introduction of the Pilates class is an innovation for the school, but one which is very much in keeping with the changes in physical activity classes of the general population. Lucy will also participate in the book club, which is held at lunchtimes once a fortnight, in addition to school outings.

- Lucy will give her class a presentation using her new Mini-Mercury communicator within the first month of the first term so that the class can get to know her and learn about her interests, aspirations and capabilities.
- It has been suggested that a buddy system might work to enable Lucy to receive support from her peers for some of the class and leisure activities. Her classroom assistant will also problem solve with Lucy and her peers ways to enhance her social integration.

The family will continue with their recreational activities of cycling and swimming at weekends, but will see if Lucy can join a swimming club with children of her own age. Lucy will be provided with a tricycle that has dual person capacity and can be adapted as the person grows (e.g. Draisin TWISTER, Quest 88 Limited), so that she can keep up with the family and experience successful participation. It is also a way the family can continue leisure activities together. Lucy's mother will continue the Pilates exercises with Lucy at home until school starts and then may reduce her input, although it is an activity which they enjoy together.

Stage 7: implement plan

Support in secondary school
The new wheelchair has been ordered for the start of the school year and the new therapy team will undertake training with Lucy to enable her to adapt to the new controls. Lucy will have a new classroom assistant and she is nervous about this. Her teaching assistant will be crucial to Lucy as she begins to bridge the gap between dependence and optimal independence, and will be an important element in Lucy's support as she develops her interaction with her peers (Hemmingson and Borell 2002; Schenker et al, 2005). It is therefore critical that this person clearly understands her role and can help Lucy and her peers to problem solve ways to access activities and increase her socialization.

Mobility and transfers
Lucy's orthoses have been reviewed and she will continue use of the Lycra suit. The AFOs that were causing discomfort have been discarded and she has a well-fitting pair of hiking boots with insoles. These can give support to her feet to maintain their integrity but unlike the AFOs do not restrict the ankle movement associated with her involuntary movements that caused the rubbing and discomfort.

It has been agreed that a course of BoNT-A will be considered. Her hips are located although both acetabula are shallow, and her range of abduction is sufficient (30° on the right and 25° on the left). However, it is hoped that the considerable pain she is experiencing may be alleviated by the BoNT-A injection to psoas, hamstrings and adductors. This will be done in the long vacation, a month before she starts secondary school, so that she can have extra physiotherapy input to maximize the effect of the injection and to enable her to start school pain free. Although the role of therapy in association with BoNT-A injection is not clearly defined, it is accepted that increased therapy is desirable in the period immediately following injection for about 4 weeks. Lucy will have therapy input three times a week for the first 2 weeks, reducing to once a week thereafter. When she is back at school her classroom assistant will carry out some of the required therapy activities during her physical education and sports classes to minimize time lost from school, but as soon as possible, it is expected that her physical education activities, the standing wheelchair and practice of transfers should be sufficient to maintain the effect of the injection. However, she will be regularly reviewed by the physiotherapist and her orthopaedic consultant.

The standing wheelchair will be used in school so that Lucy can regularly practice standing herself during lessons and at other times (it has been suggested that she does this four times per day for half an hour during appropriate sessions like art and domestic science). It is unclear for how long muscles need to be stretched to maintain length, but the use of the standing wheelchair and participation in swimming sessions should also contribute to maintenance of muscle length, strength and pain management.

Training for transfers will take place during regular school activities for personal hygiene and changing for pool and physical education activities, and similarly upper limb and sitting balance activities will be incorporated into school activities and physical education classes, especially the Pilates sessions.

Technology for communication and learning
The specialist centre assessing her communication needs suggested that a mini-computerized version of her Mercury system would ultimately enable Lucy to send text messages and prepare school presentation work more efficiently. Thus she is also learning to use her new Mini-Merc. With this device she has delivered a presentation to the class about herself and her interests and aspirations, and she very successfully contributes to class discussions. Lucy's joystick skills are limited and she can become tired taking notes using the on-screen keyboard and word prediction software, so her classroom assistant was asked to scribe for her using a wireless keyboard. This means that Lucy can make corrections if needed (see Figure 12.4 which shows an older teenager using the same device). As long as she has time to prepare in advance she is learning to manage these tasks well, and looking forward to being able to progress to using the instant messaging and texting features on her computer next term.

For a therapy programme to be successful it is important that the young person be positive and Lucy has agreed that she will regularly participate in the physical education classes, after school activities and therapy activities.

Stage 8: evaluate outcomes (end of term 1)

Qualitative outcomes
Lucy seems to be managing her new school well and making a contribution to her class and peer activities, however, integration into social and peer-based activities is a challenge. Her peers find it difficult to accept Lucy into all their activities because of her

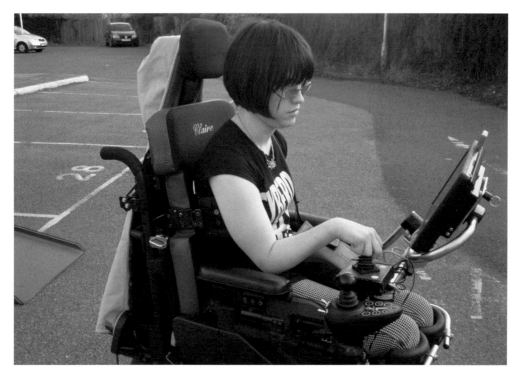

Figure 12.4 An adolescent using the Mini-Merc communicator.

limitations and the team will review ways that this can be addressed. Sitting balance and upper limb function have been maintained, and she transfers reasonably well with her classroom assistant. Lucy likes her very much, and it is considered that she has been a key contributor to the success of the transition so far. Lucy has cooperated well and has worked hard on integration with her peers.

Quantitative outcomes
Lucy has maintained her performance despite her growth spurt of 5 centimetres. Although growth tends to be less than that of typically developing peers for the child with severe impairment (Stevenson et al, 2006), clinical observation suggests that children with athetosis tend to grow normally, possibly because of their constant movements. She now reports only occasional pain of her left hip (VAS score of 1), and it seems that the BoNT-A injection and therapy followed by the recreational and standing activities has been effective. The classroom assistant is confident in carrying out her programme including standing transfers and will continue this under supervision of the physiotherapist. However, transfers carried out by people unfamiliar with Lucy will be done with the use of a hoist.

The physiotherapist will see her on a weekly basis during the school holidays to ensure that progress is maintained. Regular team reviews will take place, and she will continue regular appointments with the paediatrician and orthopaedic team to monitor her functioning and musculoskeletal status, particularly the latter as she enters a significant growth spurt and an altered regime of postural management. It is thought that Lucy will be able to maintain her current functional levels with the programme that has now been put in place, with bursts of physiotherapy input as needed. Lucy's family are adapting to the changed emphasis of peer versus family recreational activities and so far everyone is happy with the progress made in this challenging transition phase.

Box 12.2 Key clinical messages

- Transition into adolescence involves increasing educational, social and personal independence demands and working with families to plan for changes is important.

- Problem-solving equipment and technical solutions to physical, educational and social needs is critical to maximizing participation.

- Supporting young people to contribute actively to decision-making is a critical component of therapy.

- Physiotherapy at this stage also requires targeting of specific goals and monitoring of the musculoskeletal system, in this particular case, spine and hips.

References

Bartlett D & Birmingham T (2003) Validity and reliability of a pediatric reach test. *Pediatric Phys Ther,*15, 84–92.

Barwood S, Baillieu C, Boyd R, Brereton K, Low J, Nattrass G & Graham HK (2000) Analgesic effects of botulinum toxin A: a randomized, placebo-controlled clinical trial. *Dev Med Child Neurol*, 42, 116–21.

Bottos M, Feliciangeli A, Sciuto L, Gericke C & Vianello A (2001) Functional status of adults with cerebral palsy and implications for treatment of children. *Dev Med Child Neurol*, 43: 515–28.

Canadian Association of Occupational Therapists (CAOT) (2002) *Enabling Occupation: An Occupational Therapy Perspective*. Ottawa: Canadian Association of Occupational Therapists.

Clarke M & Wilkinson R (2008) Interaction between children with cerebral palsy and their peers 2: understanding initiated VOCA-mediated turns. *Augment Altern Commun*, 24, 3–15.

Clarke M & Wilkinson R (2007) Interaction between children with cerebral palsy and their peers 1: organizing and understanding VOCA use. *Augment Altern Commun*, 23, 336–48.

Coster W, Deeney TA, Haltiwanger JT & Haley SM (1998) *School Function Assessment*. San Antonio, TX: The Psychological Corporation.

Eliasson AC, Krumlinde-Sundholm L, Rösblad B, Beckung E, Arner M, Öhrvall AM & Rosenbaum P (2006) The Manual Ability Classification System (MACS) for children with cerebral palsy: scale development and evidence of validity and reliability. *Dev Med Child Neurol*, 48, 549–54.

Eliasson AC, Krumlinde-Sundholm L, Rösblad B, Beckung E, Arner M, Öhrvall AM & Rosenbaum P (2007) Using the MACS to facilitate communication about manual abilities of children with cerebral palsy. *Dev Med Child Neurol*, 49, 156–7.

Gan SM, Tung LC, Tang YH & Wang CH (2008) Psychometric properties of functional balance assessment in children with cerebral palsy. *Neurorehabil Neural Repair*, 22, 745–53.

Gormley ME, Krach LE & Murr S (2004) Non-operative treatment. In: Gage JR (ed.) *The Treatment of Gait Problems in Cerebral Palsy*: 250. London: Mac Keith Press.

Hadders-Algra M, van der Fits IB, Stremmelaar EF, Touwen BC (1999) Development of postural adjustments during reaching in infants with CP. *Dev Med Child Neurol*, 41: 766–76.

Hemmingson H & Borell L (2002) Environmental barriers in mainstream schools. *Child Care Health Dev*, 28, 57–63.

Holden MK, Gill KM, Magliozzi MR, Nathan J & Piehl-Baker L (1984) Clinical gait assessment in the neurologically impaired: reliability and meaningfulness. *Phys Ther*, 64, 35–40.

Kecskemethy HH, Herman DR, Paul K, Bachrach SJ & Henderson RC (2008) Quantifying weight bearing while in passive standers and a comparison of standers. *Dev Med Child Neurol*, 50, 520–3.

King GA, Law M, King S, Hurley P, Rosenbaum PL, Hanna S, Kertoy MK & Young N (2004) *Children's Assessment of Participation and Enjoyment and Preferences for Activities of Kids.* San Antonio, TX: The Psychological Corporation.

Knox V (2003) The use of lycra garments in children with cerebral palsy: a report of a descriptive clinical trial. *Br J Occup Ther*, 66, 71–7.

Lannin N, Scheinberg A & Clark K (2006) AACPDM systematic review of the effectiveness of therapy for children with cerebral palsy after botulinum toxin A injections. *Dev Med Child Neurol*, 48, 533–9.

Maher CA, Olds T, Williams MT & Lane AE (2008) Self-reported quality of life in adolescents with cerebral palsy. *Phys Occup Ther Pediatr*, 28, 41–57.

Melzack R (1975) The McGill Pain Questionnaire: major properties and scoring methods. *Pain*, 1, 277–99.

Morris C (2002) A review of the efficacy of lower-limb orthoses used for cerebral palsy. *Dev Med Child Neurol*, 44, 205–11.

Nicholson JH, Morton RE, Attfield S & Rennie D (2001) Assessment of upper-limb function and movement in children with cerebral palsy wearing lycra garments. *Dev Med Child Neurol*, 43, 384–91.

O'Dwyer N, Neilson P & Nash J (1989) Mechanism of muscle growth related to muscle contracture in cerebral palsy. *Dev Med Child Neurol*, 31, 543–47.

Palisano R, Rosenbaum P, Russell S, Walter D, Wood E & Galuppi B (1997) Development and reliability of a system to classify gross motor function in children with cerebral palsy. *Dev Med Child Neurol*, 39, 214–23.

Palisano RJ, Rosenbaum PL, Bartlett D & Livingston MH (2008) Content validity of the expanded and revised gross motor function classification system. *Dev Med Child Neurol*, 50, 744–50.

Randall MJ, Johnson LM & Reddihough DS (1999) *The Melbourne Assessment of Unilateral Upper limb Function: Test Administration Manual.* Melbourne: Royal Children's Hospital.

Reid D (1995) Development and preliminary validation of an instrument to assess quality of sitting in children with neuromotor dysfunction. *Phys Occup Ther Paediatr*, 15, 53–81.

Russell D, Rosenbaum PL, Avery L & Lane M (2002) *Gross Motor Function Measure (GMFM-66 & GMFM-88) User's Manual. Clinics in Developmental Medicine, No. 159.* London: Mac Keith Press Press.

Schenker R, Coster W & Parush S (2005) Participation and activity performance of students with cerebral palsy within the school environment. *Disabil Rehabil*, 27, 539–52.

Schindl MR, Forstner C, Kern H & Hesse S (2000) Treadmill training with partial body weight support in nonambulatory patients with cerebral palsy. *Arch Phys Med Rehabil*, 81, 301–6.

Stevenson RD, Conaway M, Chumlea WC, Rosenbaum PL, Fung EB, Henderson RC, Worley G, Liptak G, O'Donnell M, Samson-Fang L & Stallings VA (2006) Growth and Health in children with moderate to severe cerebral palsy. *Paediatrics*, 118, 1010–18.

Stuberg, W. (1992). Considerations related to weight bearing programs in children with developmental disabilities. *Phys Ther*, 72, 35–40.

Tremblay F (1990). Effects of prolonged muscle stretch on reflex and voluntary muscle activations in children with spastic cerebral palsy. *Scand J Rehabil Med*, 22, 171–80.

Voorman JM, Dallmeijer AJ, Knol DL, Lankhorst GJ & Becher JG (2007) Prospective longitudinal study of gross motor function in children with cerebral palsy. *Arch Phys Med Rehabil*, 88, 871–6.

Ward AB (2008) Spasticity treatment with botulinum toxins. *J Neural Transmission*, 115, 607–16.

Chapter 13

Strength training for adolescents

Nicholas F Taylor and Karen J Dodd

Case study: Tony

A physiotherapist working in a suburban community health service received a request to work with Tony, a sociable and verbally articulate 15-year-old boy with spastic diplegic cerebral palsy. Tony's mother initiated the referral and both parents attended the initial appointment. The steps involved in the clinical reasoning process used in this chapter are summarized in Figure 13.1 and described in Chapter 1.

Stage 1: initial data collection

Tony was born 15 weeks preterm. Tony was in the neonatal intensive care unit for 20 weeks during which he experienced a grade III periventricular haemorrhage and respiratory distress syndrome.

Eleven months after birth, Tony was referred to a developmental paediatrics programme where he received regular physiotherapy and occupational therapy until he began mainstream school at 6 years of age. He was classified as Gross Motor Function Classification System (GMFCS, Palisano et al, 2008; see Box 13.1) level II (see Chapter 2). He continued physiotherapy in intensive bursts during his school holidays, and his occupational therapist provided quarterly review consultations with the family. At 12 years of age he had single event multilevel surgery (SEMLS), which included bilateral tendo-achilles lengthening (see Chapter 4). Since then a physiotherapist had provided quarterly reviews to assess the suitability of his gait assistive devices and problem solve issues identified by his teachers.

Tony's parents currently work long hours in a local bakery they own. He is the youngest of three boys, all of whom live in the family home. Tony's oldest brother, who is 22 years old, works full time in the family business, and his other brother, who is 19 years old, is completing an apprenticeship as a pastry chef.

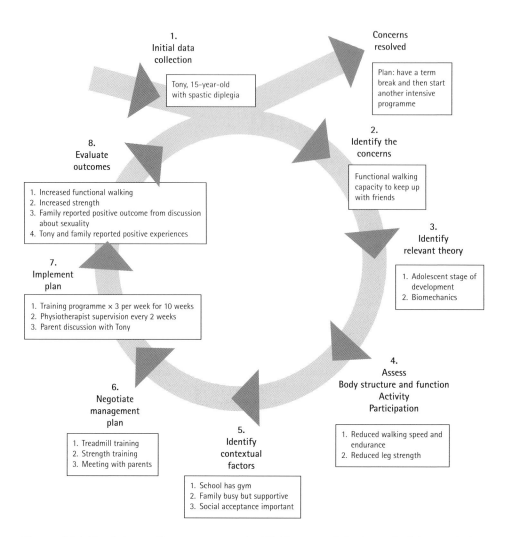

Figure 13.1 The intervention process used with Tony: model adapted with permission from the Canadian Occupational Performance Process Model (CAOT, 2002).

Box 13.1 GMFCS level II snapshot[1]

Proportion of people with cerebral palsy classified as GMFCS II: 18–30%

Proportion of people classified as GMFCS level II who

● have a severe intellectual disability (IQ<50): about 20%;
● have a severe visual impairment: about 13%;

1   See Chapter 2: p. 17 for details of the sources used to derive these data.

- have epilepsy: about 25%;
- have behavioural problems: less than 5%;
- have hip displacement requiring surgery: about 10%;
- walk alone at home by age 2–3 years: 24%;
- walk alone at home by age 4–12 years: 89%.

Stage 2: identify and prioritize concerns

Tony's parents were worried that Tony's walking had been deteriorating over the past year. They had noticed that he could not walk as far or as fast, that he had experienced a few falls at school, and that climbing up and down stairs took longer and he appeared less safe. His parents were unsure what to do because Tony didn't want to attend physiotherapy.

Tony was quiet through the interview but with prompting he agreed that his walking and stair climbing were worse (Figure 13.2). However, he said that he didn't care all that much except that he wanted to walk well enough to keep up with his friends at the weekends. He also said that physiotherapy was going to be useless because he wasn't a little kid any more.

Tony's and his parents' key concerns were as follows:

- his reduced walking distance and speed and wanting to be able to keeping up with friends;
- his increased risk of falls when walking;
- his reduced speed and safety in walking up and down stairs;

Stage 3: identify relevant theory

Adolescent stage of development

Adolescence is a period of transition that involves preparation for adult roles and independent living. It can be a difficult stage for adolescents with cerebral palsy (Hallum 1995; Palisano et al, 2007). The functional ability of young people with cerebral palsy can deteriorate during adolescence. For adolescents like Tony, classified as GMFCS level II, clinically significant declines in function during adolescence have been documented in the 66-item Gross Motor Function Measure (GMFM–66; Hanna et al, 2009). Adolescents with cerebral palsy walk less than they did as children (Johnson et al, 1997), and more than 50% of adults with cerebral palsy reported their gross motor function had deteriorated since they were children. There is evidence that activity limitations can negatively affect the social participation of adolescents with cerebral palsy (Schenker et al, 2005) therefore Tony's desire to walk well enough to keep up with his friends was significant.

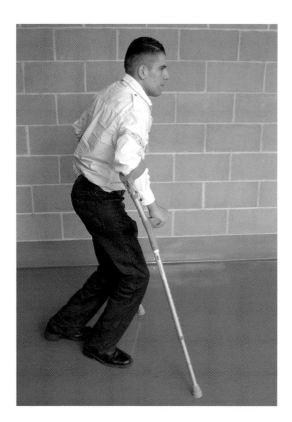

Figure 13.2 Tony walking with elbow crutches.

Adolescence is also important for developing social skills, being and feeling accepted and becoming interested in developing sexual relationships (Marn and Koch, 1999; King et al, 2000). One important aspect is the development of self-concept – how a person feels about themselves. Although research has shown that we should not assume that self-concept is impaired in young males with cerebral palsy, measurement of self-concept can be useful in determining what an individual considers important to how they feel about themselves as a person (Shields et al, 2006). Tony remained quiet during the interview and the few comments that he did make indicated that he did not want to be treated like a child. The physiotherapist decided that assessing self-concept might help with goal-setting and treatment planning because Tony had not clearly identified all of his concerns or the importance he placed on his performance in different areas.

Biomechanics
The main problem identified by Tony and his family was limitation of walking ability: in particular, walking speed, walking distance, going up and down stairs, and lack of safety when walking. A biomechanical approach to analysing problems identifies the impairments that contribute to limitations of walking, including muscle weakness, spasticity and reduced range of joint motion, impaired balance and lack of physical fitness.

MUSCLE WEAKNESS

Muscle weakness is common in people with cerebral palsy (Damiano et al, 1995; Wiley and Damiano, 1998), with strength deficits demonstrating a positive relationship with functional limitations for adolescents with cerebral palsy (Kramer and MacPhail, 1994). There is also evidence that increased muscle strength in young people with cerebral palsy can carry over into improved walking ability (Damiano and Abel, 1998; Eagleton et al, 2004), including improvements in crouch gait (Unger et al, 2006) and walking endurance (Andersson et al, 2003).

SPASTICITY AND REDUCED RANGE OF MOVEMENT

A relationship has been established between increased spasticity of leg muscles and knee angular velocity during walking in children with spastic diplegic cerebral palsy (Tuzson et al, 2003; Damiano et al, 2006). Also, younger children with cerebral palsy who received botulinum toxin to manage their spasticity and reduced range of movement demonstrated improvements in gait parameters such as increased knee extension during stance (Scholtes et al, 2007).

BALANCE

A significant correlation was found between poor standing balance and limitations in walking ability in young people with spastic diplegic cerebral palsy (Liao et al, 1997). Many factors can contribute to impaired balance including delayed responses in ankle muscles, inappropriate muscle sequencing, increased co-activation of agonists and antagonists, spasticity and muscle weakness (Woollacott and Shumway-Cook, 2005). Reactive balance training in children with cerebral palsy resulted in improved balance responses in standing (Woollacott and Shumway-Cook, 2005), although it is not known if these improvements carried over into improved postural control during walking.

CARDIORESPIRATORY FITNESS

A lack of cardiorespiratory fitness can also contribute to reduced walking endurance. Rimmer (2001) highlighted the impact of reduced physical fitness on long-term health for people with cerebral palsy which led to Damiano (2006) advocating for more intense physical training programmes (see Chapter 4). Children and adults with cerebral palsy demonstrate levels of cardiorespiratory fitness 21–61% lower than norm-referenced data (Lundberg 1978; Lundberg 1984; Fernandez et al, 1990). However, relatively few training programmes have been evaluated.

Stage 4: assessment of body structure and function, activity and participation

Based on the initial discussion with Tony and his family, and consideration of relevant theory a list for assessments of body structure and function, activity and participation was developed (Table 13.1).

Activity

Table 13.2 summarizes the assessment findings of the activity level assessments for Tony.

Table 13.1 Assessments for Tony

Body structure and function	Activity	Participation
Muscle strength 1RM leg press	*Walking speed* 10 m walk self-selected 10 m walk fast	Children's Assessment of Participation and Enjoyment (CAPE)
Muscle endurance Repetitions at 50% 1RM	*Walking endurance* 6-minute Walk Test	
Spasticity and Range of movement Tardieu test	Timed Stairs Test	
Balance Paediatric reach test	Gross Motor Function Measure – E	
Self-concept Self-perception profile for adolescents		

1RM, one-repetition maximum.

Table 13.2 Assessment findings for the activity limitation tests

Activity level	
Self-selected walking speed over 10 m	35 m/min
Fast walking speed over 10 m	43 m/min
6-minute walk test	183 m
Timed Stairs Test	22 s
Gross Motor Function Measure – E	47%

m, metres; min, minutes; s, seconds.

OBSERVATION OF WALKING

Tony's motor disability was classified at level II on the GMFCS (Palisano et al, 2008; see Chapter 2). He walked with a crouched gait (flat foot contact, ankle dorsiflexion, hips flexed, knees flexed around 25°, and pelvis neutral), and used bilateral ground reaction ankle–foot orthoses. The development of crouch gait with excessive ankle dorsiflexion has been associated with tendo-achilles lengthening procedures (Borton et al, 2001). Using two forearm crutches Tony could walk around the house and at his local school and for short distances outside. He used a self-propelled manual wheelchair for long distances or in less familiar and challenging environments such as the local shopping centre or over rough and variable terrain.

WALKING SPEED

Walking speed was tested by timing the middle 10 metres (m) of a 14 m walkway at both self-selected and fast walking speeds using Tony's normal assistive devices. Walking speed can be measured with high reliability in people with neurological impairments (Wade, 1992), and significant changes in walking speed have been found after interventions in young people with cerebral palsy (Dodd and Foley, 2007).

WALKING ENDURANCE

Walking endurance was tested by measuring how far Tony could walk in 6 minutes on a flat standardized course (see Appendix, p. 296). The test was completed twice, with the first trial regarded as practice.

TIMED STAIRS TEST

The Timed Stairs Test (Russell et al, 1993; see Appendix, p. 296) was used to measure Tony's ability to walk up and down stairs, a task that is commonly difficult for people with cerebral palsy, and an activity identified as becoming more difficult for Tony.

GROSS MOTOR FUNCTION MEASURE (GMFM, DIMENSION E)

Activity was assessed using dimension E of the GMFM (Russell et al, 2002) which measures walking, running, and jumping activities (see Appendix, p. 294). The GMFM dimension E was chosen because the items represented areas that Tony identified as being difficult.

Body structure and function

Table 13.3 summarizes the findings from assessments aimed at body structure and function for Tony.

MUSCLE STRENGTH

Muscle strength was measured using a one-repetition maximum (1RM) leg press (see Appendix, p. 288), that assessed the maximal weight he could control through his available range. The test was relevant because Tony used a crouch type gait, and the physiotherapist was concerned with improving the coordinated muscle action required for walking.

Table 13.3 Assessment findings for the tests of body structure and function

Body structure and function		
Muscle strength 1RM leg press	61 kg	
Muscle endurance Leg press repetitions at 50% 1RM	28	
Tardieu test	Knee R2–R1: 20° (X=2) Ankle R2–R1: 14° (X=1)	
Range of movement	Knee at V1: –5° extension Ankle at V1: +20° dorsi-flexion	
Standing balance Pediatric Reach Test	Total: 54 cm Forward: 22 cm Right: 12 cm Left: 14 cm	
Self-concept Self-perception Profile for Children[a]	Global self worth Scholastic Social Athletic Appearance Job skills Romantic appeal Behaviour Close friendship	2.9 2.6 1.9 2.0 1.7 2.2 1.6[b] 3.1 2.0

1RM, one-repetition maximum; R1, joint angle of muscle reaction (catch) at a V3 (as fast as possible) speed; R2, full passive range of movement (R2) at a V1(as slow as possible) speed; X, the intensity and duration of the muscle reaction (the resistance felt when muscle is passively stretched).
a. Scores range from 1–4. b. Most important to Tony.

MUSCLE ENDURANCE
Muscle endurance was measured by counting the number of seated leg press repetitions that could be completed using a weight equal to 50% of Tony's 1RM (see Appendix, p. 287).

SPASTICITY AND RANGE OF MOVEMENT
The Tardieu scale provided a clinical measure of spasticity (Boyd and Graham, 1999). For this assessment, the passive range of movement at the knee and ankle at slow

velocity provided a quick screening assessment to identify any gross impairments of leg range of movement (see Appendix, p. 289).

STANDING BALANCE

Tony's standing balance was assessed with the standing section of the Pediatric Reach Test (Bartlett and Birmingham, 2003). The test measured the distance Tony could reach forward and to each side without losing balance or taking a step (see Appendix, p. 295).

SELF-CONCEPT

Tony's self-concept was measured because there were indications in the initial interview that relationships with his friends were of concern to him. Self-concept was measured with the Self-Perception Profile for Adolescents (Harter, 1988; see Appendix, p. 299).

Participation

The Children's Assessment of Participation and Enjoyment (CAPE) provided an indication of Tony's level of societal participation (King et al, 2004; see Appendix, p. 297). Tony's intensity of participation was low, but he participated in at least one recreational activity each week. The social activities Tony identified tended to be done at home, with friends or family, although he had been to the movies twice in the last 4 months (Table 13.4).

Table 13.4 Assessment findings from the societal participation tests

Children's Assessment of Participation and Enjoyment (CAPE)	
	Tony's score (score range)
Overall (range)	23 (0–55)
Domain	
Formal	2 (0–15)
Informal	21 (0–40)
Activities	
Recreational	7 (0–12)
Active physical	2 (0–13)
Social	7 (0–10)
Skill-based	2 (0–10)
Self-improvement	5 (0–10)
'Diversity' scores presented indicating number of activities in which Tony participated in past 4 months.	

Stage 5: contextual factors: environmental and personal

Environmental factors
Tony attended a mainstream school in his neighbourhood. The school had a fully equipped gymnasium, including a wide range of weights machines, steppers and motorized treadmills with very slow minimum speeds of 0.1 kilometres per hour (kph) and the capacity to increase this in increments of 0.1 kph. The gymnasium was staffed by one of the physical education teachers at the school and was open until 5.00 pm Monday to Friday.

Personal factors
Tony's family was supportive but very busy. They ran a family business in which Tony's mother, father and eldest brother all worked long hours, including weekends. Tony was coping well with his school work and was doing better than the class average in mathematics and science.

Tony no longer wanted to participate in the type of individual therapy that he experienced throughout his childhood. Perhaps consistent with this, social acceptance with his peers had become increasingly important to him.

Stage 6: management plan

Summary of assessment findings
The assessment confirmed and documented the main problem identified by Tony and his family. His relatively slow self-selected and fast walking speeds, difficulty going up and down steps and lack of walking endurance all contribute to Tony finding it difficult to keep up with friends who had no physical impairment. His score of 47% in dimension E of the GMFM confirmed Tony's limitations in mobility.

The measures of body structure and function suggested that poor muscle performance could be contributing to Tony's walking limitations. He could leg press 61 kilograms (kg) through both legs, similar to the amount of weight that can be lifted by adults with cerebral palsy with high support needs (Taylor et al, 2004a), and much less than the average weight of more than 100 kg that can be lifted by able-bodied male adolescents (Christou et al, 2006). Tony could only do 28 repetitions when the weight was reduced to half, which is about 70% of what would be expected in people with other neurological disabilities (Taylor et al, 2006). These findings were also consistent with the observation of a crouch gait. Other possible contributing impairments, spasticity (Tardieu test) and range of movement, were considered minor, since there was a relatively small difference in knee joint angle of 20° between the fast and slow passive stretch (i.e. R2–R1) and he had close to full range available at his knee. The quick screening test of passive range of movement at slow speed at the ankle indicated increased range of dorsiflexion, again consistent with the observation of crouch gait.

Tony's global self-worth was generally positive, that is, he felt good about himself as a person. The three domains where he chose more negative rather than positive responses were romantic appeal (1.6), appearance (1.7), and social acceptance (1.9), and he nominated romantic appeal as the domain most important to him. On discussing these findings privately with Tony, he mentioned that he was interested in beginning to date one of the girls in his class. He hadn't dated before, although most of his friends had dated briefly. He had asked this girl to come to the movies with him, but she had laughed off the suggestion and had not spoken much to Tony since. Tony said he thought she didn't want to go out with him because he had a disability, and because he 'walked weirdly'. He was clearly upset and said 'I probably won't ever have a girlfriend'.

Tony's overall participation score of 23 was a bit lower than group averages of about 26.5 (interquartile range 10) reported for young people with cerebral palsy (Imms, 2008). Despite participating in a variety of activities, the intensity of Tony's participation was very low. The companion measure to the CAPE, the Preferences for Activity of Children (PAC), also revealed that social participation was very important to him, suggesting that interventions should aim to include a social component.

The contextual factors confirmed there were resources available at his school. The gymnasium at the school allowed the physiotherapist to plan an intervention that did not make too many demands on his busy family, and provided potential for social interaction with his peers.

Negotiated treatment plan
The following treatment plan was developed to improve Tony's functional walking capacity: an exercise programme at the school gymnasium to be completed three times a week for one school term (10 weeks). The two key elements of the treatment plan were:

- task specific treadmill training;
- a progressive resistance exercise programme for major leg muscles.

Following the discussion with Tony about the incident with the girl in his class and his generally negative view of his physical attributes (assessed in the self-concept tool) the therapist arranged a meeting with Tony's parents to talk about the issues he had raised.

Stage 7: implement plan

Treadmill training
Tony's treadmill training programme aimed to improve the speed and distance he could walk. Contemporary clinical practice suggests that task-specific repetitive practice of walking is required to improve walking performance. One of the main advantages of treadmill training is that it reduces the biomechanical constraints on walking and provides an environment for repetitive gait practice during which adolescents can maintain a more rhythmical and efficient walking pattern at higher speeds. A recent clinical controlled trial evaluating the effects of a school-based, partial bodyweight

support treadmill training programme, conducted twice a week for 6 weeks, for children with cerebral palsy, aged 5 to 14 years, found that treadmill training can improve the walking speed and might also improve walking endurance in some children (Dodd and Foley, 2007; see Chapter 4).

Young people who have very poor balance during walking or who cannot adequately maintain an upright standing posture without support can be fitted with a partial bodyweight support system. This comprises a harness fitted around the child's trunk and attached to an overhead support system, which is suspended over the treadmill. As Tony could walk relatively upright on a treadmill, he did not use a partial bodyweight support harness (See Figure 13.3).

The initial training intensity was set by Tony's physiotherapist. He trained on Monday, Wednesday and Friday for 10 consecutive weeks. At each session the treadmill was started at the lowest speed and this was gradually increased to a speed where Tony was able to step forward comfortably. Tony aimed to walk as upright as possible at a comfortable walking speed for up to 30 minutes. At the beginning he could only walk at a speed of 21.2 m/min for 6 minutes on the treadmill. This was very slow given that 8- to 16-year-old children without impairment walk at an average free speed of 110.5 m/min, when measured in the 6-minute walk test (Morinder et al, 2008). At each

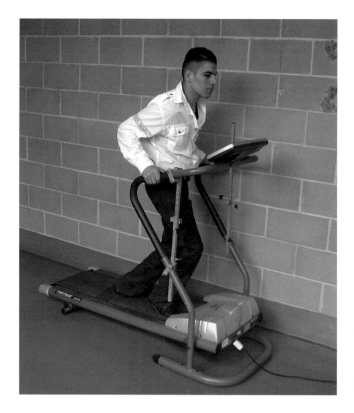

Figure 13.3 Tony walking on a motorized treadmill. The therapist encouraged correction of the crouch posture during treadmill training sessions.

session Tony attempted to walk faster and to increase the amount of time he walked for up to 30 minutes.

Tony's therapist attended the gymnasium every 2 weeks to check his progress. In week 4, she saw that he could comfortably walk at 25.4 m/min. This suggested that he was ready to progress and he was asked to walk an extra 10 minutes at each session.

Strength training

Tony also started a progressive resistance strength training programme in his school gymnasium to improve the ability of the major antigravity leg muscle groups to generate force. Progressive resistance exercise programmes can improve muscle strength in people with cerebral palsy with strong trends suggesting that the improved ability to generate force can carry over into an improved functional ability (Dodd et al, 2002, 2003; see Chapter 4). The major muscle groups targeted were the ankle plantar flexors, the knee extensors and the hip extensors. Because Tony had never done weight training before, he commenced with weight machines. Weight machines are safer for novices than exercising with free weights such as dumbbells because there is less chance of injury, such as having a weight fall on them. Tony's exercises are described in Table 13.5.

Completing the exercises with good form was emphasised. That is, Tony aimed to complete each exercise through his available range with control, both during the

Table 13.5 Summary of Tony's strength training programme

Strength exercises		
Exercise	Starting position	Description
Leg press	Seated, hips and knees flexed, feet placed flat on plate	Slowly push on the plate until knees are extended then return
Calf raise	Seated, both feet flat on floor, bar over distal thigh	Raise heels to come up onto toes so that the bar lifts up above the distal thigh, then return heels to floor
Knee extension	Seated, hips at about 90° and knees at about 110° bar placed over distal tibia	Push bar placed over distal tibia to extend the knee and then return
Hip extension	Standing, with both hands supported on rail. Cuff about ankle connected via pulley to weight stack	Maintain control with one leg, slowly extend leg with cuff about 20–30° . Repeat with each leg

concentric and eccentric phases of the exercise. Because Tony was particularly weak in the final 20° of knee extension as demonstrated by his crouch gait position, the therapist emphasized control of knee extension through the final 20° of extension of the leg press and knee extension exercises.

Exercise dosage was consistent with guidelines of the American College of Sports Medicine (2002). The initial training intensity was set at about 70% of Tony's 1RM. For example, the initial weight he lifted for the leg press was set at 40 kg (which is a bit less than 70% of the 1RM found at assessment). Tony aimed to complete three sets of 8 to 10 repetitions of each exercise, with a 2-minute rest period between each set.

His physiotherapist attended the first training session where he taught Tony his programme and liaised with his physical education teacher, who would be providing supervision while Tony trained during the week. The teacher was familiar with progressive resistance training principles so the physiotherapist had confidence that Tony would receive appropriate supervision. When Tony's therapist attended the gymnasium after 2 weeks the weights were evaluated and progressed to make sure that the training load continued at approximately 70% of 1RM. After 2 weeks Tony was doing three sets of 12 repetitions of his seated leg press at 40 kg and he was ready to progress. His leg press 1RM had increased to 75 kg, so his training load was increased to 52.5 kg. Tony should feel as though he worked 'hard' (at least five on the CR–10 rating of Perceived Exertion Scale [Foster et al, 2001]) at the end of each exercise session. The key principles of strength training are highlighted in Box 13.2.

Factors to promote programme adherence
A key factor in the success of any exercise programme is adherence; which can be enhanced by attending to the following factors (Taylor et al, 2004b).

- The therapist's key roles are to set up the programme, be knowledgeable about exercise modalities (treadmill training and strength training), be able to problem solve and progress the programme, and provide support and motivation. In Tony's case the therapist also provided information, support and contact details to the physical education teacher who was on duty in the gymnasium.
- Social support from family members and others is important when introducing a physical activity programme for a person with a physical disability. Although

---

Box 13.2 Key principles of strength training

(1) Relatively few repetitions (2 to 3 sets of 8 to 10 repetitions, 2 to 3 times per week).

(2) Relatively high load (only lift the amount of weight that can be lifted through full range with good form 8 to 10 times or 70% of one repetition maximum).

(3) Progress load (when able to complete 3 sets of 10 repetitions, increase the weight lifted).

Tony's family was very busy and could not attend the gymnasium with Tony, they attended the initial assessment session and endorsed the agreed programme. In addition, they bought him a new pair of runners with a popular brand name. Two friends who agreed to attend the gymnasium with him provided social support. Both friends were promising footballers who used the gymnasium to get fit for the coming season by completing a programme devised by their physical education teacher. This was a vital part of the programme for Tony, because social inclusion was important to him.

- Programme factors: a programme with a relatively small number of exercises is important for adherence. Tony's initial programme involved only four strengthening exercises and treadmill training. A log book where exercise repetitions and weights are recorded can also promote adherence (see Figure 13.4 for an example). Tony filled out his exercise log during each session and it became a source of pride and motivation to him and formed the basis of evaluating and upgrading the programme. The third important programme factor was the availability of accessible equipment. In this case, Tony could easily access his school's exercise equipment without cost.

- Autonomy, motivation and understanding were all important elements in Tony's programme. He needed to choose to participate. The therapist affirmed Tony's goals for treatment, they worked together to develop the programme and to problem solve how the programme would be implemented. In addition, the therapist developed a written agreement with Tony, which he signed to demonstrate his understanding and willingness to participate. Tony became enthusiastic about the programme because he saw it as a way of getting fit like his friends rather than as 'therapy'. Treadmill training and strength training both involve relatively intense training; therefore, it is important that the person chooses to participate. This is particularly important when working with adolescents who are capable of making informed choices.

Meeting with Tony's parents
With Tony's permission, the therapist described the incident between Tony and the girl at school. Tony's parents were unaware of his concerns but because Tony was quiet at home, they weren't surprised he hadn't told them. They weren't sure how to help him.

The therapist discussed how helping Tony to have a strong sense of self was one way to combat the negative effects of perceived discrimination, and that helping him participate socially with his peer group was important. This was hard for Tony's parents because he needed more assistance with transport to community facilities than other adolescents his age.

Tony's parents felt comfortable about talking to him about school, girlfriends and sexuality in general, but wondered how to find out about any particular issues he might have because of his disability. To assist them, the therapist looked for and provided information from the local family planning association who had numerous resources

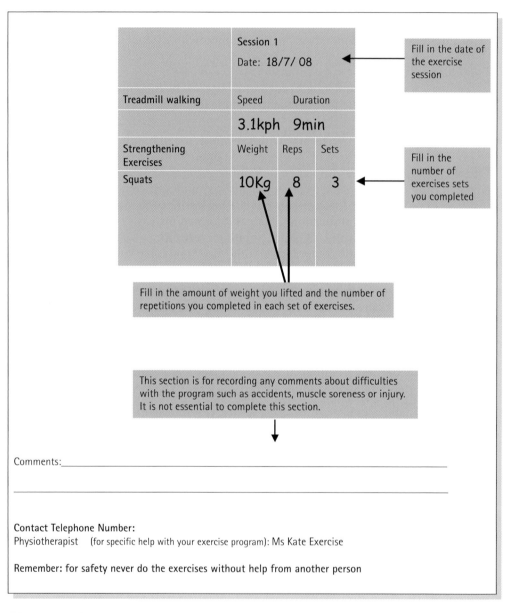

Figure 13.4 Exercise Log Book.

Exercise Record Week One

	Session 1 Date:			Session 2 Date:			Session 3 Date:		
Treadmill walking	Speed		Duration	Speed		Duration	Speed		Duration
Strengthening Exercises	Weight	Reps	Sets	Weight	Reps	Sets	Weight	Reps	Sets
Squats									
Heel raises									
Step ups									

Comments:_____

_____

Figure 13.4 continued

(books, pamphlets and a DVD) to assist parents to explain and discuss sexuality with adolescents with disabilities.

Stage 8: evaluate outcomes

After 10 weeks, each outcome measure was readministered to determine the programme's effectiveness. There were no changes in the Tardieu scale, joint range of movement, the self-concept scale or on the stair climbing test. Changes in the balance test scores were found, but these seemed small and unlikely to be clinically important. Large and clinically significant changes were seen in muscle strength as measured with the 1RM leg press (35% increase in weight lifted) and in muscle endurance using 50% 1RM leg press (13 more repetitions). Large changes were also detected in dimension E of the GMFM (an increase from 47 to 62%), walking endurance as measured with the 6-metre Walk Test (an increase of 95 m over 6 minutes) and in fast walking speed over 10 m (an increase from 43 m/min to 52 m/min). These outcomes showed the programme had been successful in addressing many of the concerns initially identified.

The qualitative assessment of the programme was very positive. Tony's mother said, 'Before he couldn't walk as far and he got very tired. Now he can walk 1 to 2 km, and he hasn't been falling.' However, the most significant improvement was the change in Tony's participation. Tony said, 'Last weekend I went to the movies with my friends and before I was using my wheelchair to get around and this was a real hassle because sometimes there are steps that make it hard to use the wheelchair, but now I can walk heaps more on my own. I love it.'

Tony's parents were pleased they had raised the issues of girlfriends and sexuality. Together with his older brothers, they had talked about how he might approach other girls, develop friendships and go out together with a group of friends. They discussed sexuality and answered all of the questions that Tony had about his body and what he could expect. His parents said they were glad this issue had been raised; because they tended to focus on his walking and general mobility they had just not realised how grown up he had become.

Tony and his parents were happy with his progress, but they all wanted to have a term break. There is evidence that improvements after a relatively short strengthening programme can be sustained in the absence of specific intervention for up to 12 weeks (Dodd et al, 2003). Therefore, the physiotherapist made a time to meet Tony and his parents again in 12 weeks' time. A summary of the clinical reasoning process can be reviewed in Figure 13.1.

> **Box 13.3 Key clinical messages**
>
> ● Adolescence is a difficult time of transition for individuals with cerebral palsy, because functional ability can deteriorate, and it is a time for developing social skills.
>
> ● Treadmill training reduces the biomechanical constraints on walking and provides an environment for repetitive practice to improve walking.
>
> ● Progressive resistance training can increase muscle strength that can carry over into an improved ability to do tasks and can be seen as a socially desirable form of exercise by adolescents with cerebral palsy.

References

American College of Sports Medicine (2002) Progression models in resistance training for healthy adults. *Med Sci Sports Exerc*, 34, 364–80.

Andersson C, Grooten W, Hellsten M, Kaping K, Mattsson E (2003) Adults with cerebral palsy: walking ability after progressive strength training. *Dev Med Child Neurol*, 45, 220–8.

Bartlett D, Birmingham T (2003) Validity and reliability of a pediatric reach test. *Pediatr Phys Ther*, 15, 84–92.

Borton DC, Walker K, Pirpiris M, Nattrass GR & Graham HK (2001) Isolated calf lengthening in cerebral palsy: Outcome analysis of risk factors. *J Bone Joint Surg Br*, 83, 364–70.

Boyd RN & Graham HK (1999) Objective measurement of clinical findings in the use of botulinum toxin type A for the management of children with cerebral palsy. *Eur J Neurol*, 6, S23–35.

Canadian Association of Occupational Therapists (CAOT) (2002) *Enabling Occupation: An Occupational Therapy Perspective.* Ottawa: Canadian Association of Occupational Therapists.

Christou M, Smilios I, Sotiropoulos K, Volaklis K, Pilianidis T & Tokmakidis SP (2006) Effects of resistance training on the physical capacities of adolescent soccer players. *J Strength Cond Res*, 20, 783–91.

Damiano DL (2006) Activity, activity, activity: rethinking our physical therapy approach to cerebral palsy. *Phys Ther*, 86, 1534–40.

Damiano DL & Abel MF (1998) Functional outcomes of strength training in spastic cerebral palsy. *Arch Phys Med Rehabil*, 79, 119–25.

Damiano DL, Vaughan CL & Abel MF (1995) Muscle response to heavy resistance exercise in children with spastic cerebral palsy. *Dev Med Child Neurol*, 37, 731–9.

Damiano DL, Laws E, Carmines DV & Abel MF (2006) Relationship of spasticity to knee angular velocity and motion during gait in cerebral palsy. *Gait Posture*, 23, 1–8.

Dodd KJ & Foley S (2007) Partial body-weight-supported treadmill training can improve walking in children with cerebral palsy: a clinical controlled trial. *Dev Med Child Neurol*, 49, 101–5.

Dodd KJ, Taylor NF, Damiano DL (2002) A systematic review of the effectiveness of strength-training programs for people with cerebral palsy. *Arch Phys Med Rehabil*, 83, 1157–64.

Dodd KJ, Taylor NF & Graham HK (2003) A randomized clinical trial of strength training in young people with cerebral palsy. *Dev Med Child Neurol*, 45, 652–7.

Eagleton M, Iams A, McDowell J, Morrison R & Evans CL (2004) The effects of strength training on gait in adolescents with cerebral palsy. *Pediatr Phys Ther*, 16, 22–30.

Foster C, Florhaug JA, Franklin J, Gottschall L, Hrovatin LA, Parker S, Doleshal P & Dodge C (2001) A new approach to monitoring exercise training. *J Strength Cond Res*, 15, 109–15.

Fernandez JE, Pitetti KH, Betzen MT. (1990) Physiological capacities of individuals with cerebral palsy. *Hum Factors*, 32, 457–66.

Hallum A (1995) Disability and the transition to adulthood: issues for the disabled child, the family and the paediatrician. *Curr Probl Pediatr*, 25, 12–50.

Hanna SE, Rosenbaum PL, Bartlett DJ, Palisano RJ, Walter SD, Avery L & Russell DJ (2009) Stability and decline in gross motor function among children and youth with cerebral palsy aged 2 to 21 years. *Dev Med Child Neurol*, 51, 295–302.

Harter S (1988) *The Manual for the Self-Perception Profile for Adolescents.* Denver, CO: University of Denver.

Imms C (2008) *Participation of Australian Children who have Cerebral Palsy: The Middle Years.* Melbourne, School of Physiotherapy, Faculty of Health Sciences, La Trobe University.

Johnson DC, Damiano DL & Abel MF (1997) The evolution of gait in childhood and adolescent cerebral palsy. *J Pediatr Orthop*, 17, 392–6.

King GA, Cathers T, Polgar JM, MacKinnon E & Havens L (2000) Success in life for older adolescents with cerebral palsy. *Qual Health Res*, 10, 734–49.

King GA, Law M, King S, Hurley P, Rosenbaum PL, Hanna S, Kertoy MK & Young N (2004) *Children's Assessment of Participation and Enjoyment and Preferences for Activities of Kids.* San Antonio, TX: PsychCorp.

Kramer JF & MacPhail HE (1994) Relationships among measures of walking efficiency, gross motor ability and isokinetic strength in adolescents with cerebral palsy. *Pediatr Phys Ther*, 6, 3–8.

Liao HF, Jeng SF, Lai JS, Cheng CK & Hu MH (1997) The relation between standing balance and walking function in children with spastic diplegic cerebral palsy. *Dev Med Child Neurol*, 39, 106–12.

Lundberg A (1978) Maximal aerobic capacity of young people with spastic cerebral palsy. *Dev Med Child Neurol*, 20, 205–10.

Lundberg A (1984) Longitudinal study of physical working capacity of young people with spastic cerebral palsy. *Dev Med Child Neurol*, 26, 328–34.

Marn LM & Koch LC (1999) The major tasks of adolescence: implications for transition planning with youths with cerebral palsy. *Work*, 13, 51–58.

Morinder G, Mattsson E, Sollander C, Marcus C & Larsson UE (2008) Six-minute walk test in obese children and adolescents: reproducibility and validity. *Physiother Res Int*, 14, 91–104.

Palisano RJ, Copeland WP & Galuppi BE (2007) Performance of physical activities by adolescents with cerebral plasy. *Phys Ther*, 87, 77–87.

Palisano RJ, Rosenbaum P, Bartlett D & Livingston MH (2008) Content validity of the expanded and revised Gross Motor Function Classification System. *Dev Med Child Neurol*, 50, 744–50.

Rimmer JH (2001) Physical fitness levels of persons with cerebral palsy. *Dev Med Child Neurol*, 43, 208–12.

Reiner AM, Bjarnason HK (199) Growing up with cerebral palsy: the effect of physical maturity on individuals with cerebral palsy. *Dev Med Child Neurol*, 41 (suppl 80), 11.

Russell D, Rosenbaum PL, Gowland C, Hardy S, Lane M, Plews N, McGavin H, Cadman DT & Jarvis S (1993) *Gross Motor Function Measure Manual.* Hamilton, ON: McMaster University.

Russell D, Rosenbaum PL, Avery L & Lane M (2002) *The Gross Motor Function Measure. GMFM–66 and GMFM–88 (Users' Manual). Clinics in Developmental Medicine No. 159.* London: Mac Keith Press.

Schenker R, Coster WJ, Parush S (2005) Neuroimpairments, activity performance, and participation in children with cerebral palsy mainstreamed in elementary schools. *Dev Med Child Neurol*, 47, 808–14.

Scholtes VA, Dallmeijer AJ, Knol DL, Speth LA, Maathuis CG, Jongerius PH & Becher JG (2007) Effect of multilevel botulinum toxin a and comprehensive rehabilitation on gait in cerebral palsy. *Pediatr Neurol*, 36, 30–9.

Shields N, Murdoch A, Loy Y, Dodd KJ & Taylor NF (2006) A systematic review of the self-concept of children with cerebral palsy compared with children without disability. *Dev Med Child Neurol*, 48, 151–7.

Taylor NF, Dodd KJ & Larkin H (2004a) Adults with cerebral palsy benefit from participating in a strength training programme at a community gymnasium. *Dis Rehab*, 26, 1128–34.

Taylor NF, Dodd KJ, McBurney H & Graham HK (2004b) Factors influencing adherence to a home-based strength-training programme for young people with cerebral palsy. *Physiotherapy*, 90, 57–63.

Taylor NF, Dodd KJ, Prasad D & Denisenko S (2006) Progressive resistance exercise for people with multiple sclerosis. *Disabil Rehabil*, 28, 1119–26.

Tuzson AE, Granata KP & Abel MF (2003) Spastic velocity threshold constrains functional performance in cerebral palsy. *Arch Phys Med Rehabil*, 84, 1363–8.

Unger M, Faure M, Frieg A (2006) Strength training in adolescent learners with cerebral palsy: a randomized controlled trial. *Clin Rehabil*, 20, 469–77.

Wade DT (1992) *Measurement in Neurological Rehabilitation*. Oxford: Oxford University Press.

Wiley ME & Damiano DL (1998) Lower-extremity strength profiles in spastic cerebral palsy. *Dev Med Child Neurol*, 40,100–7.

Woollacott MH & Shumway-Cook A (2005) Postural dysfunction during standing and walking in children with cerebral palsy: what are the underlying problems and what new therapies might improve balance? *Neural Plast*, 12, 211–9.

Chapter 14
Transitions to adulthood

Mary Law and Debra Stewart

Transition periods such as moving into the adult world are critical developmental stages. Youth need to develop readiness skills for this next life phase. Transitions present significantly more challenges for youth with disabilities, their families and communities. At transitions, systems and services tend to be uncoordinated or fragmented and people lack the information needed to navigate the transition successfully. Youth with disabilities wish to become fully productive members of adult society. The current generation of young people with disabilities have grown up in their own homes and communities and have experienced a more integrated childhood than children with disabilities did a generation ago. Their capabilities – and expectations for the future – are greater.

The purpose of this chapter is to discuss the role of therapy in developing goals and initiating interventions to develop participation in societal roles as young people become adults. This stage of development is a time when services for people with cerebral palsy are often drastically reduced.

Case study: Isabella

Isabella is a young woman of 17 who is preparing to make the transition from living at home to attending university and living away from home in 2 years. Isabella has spastic diplegic cerebral palsy and is classified at level III on the Gross Motor Function Classification System (GMFCS) (Palisano et al, 2008; see Chapter 2 and Box 14.1). The occupational therapist at the local children's rehabilitation centre will be working with Isabella and her parents over the next 2 years as she prepares for this new phase of her life.

Isabella had attended the local children's rehabilitation centre for services since she moved to this area when she was 5 years old. Isabella walks at home and school using

---

Box 14.1 GMFCS level III snapshot[1]

Proportion of people with cerebral palsy classified as GMFCS III: 8–12%

Proportion of people classified as GMFCS level III who

- have a severe intellectual disability (IQ <50): about 30%;
- have a severe visual impairment: about 20%;
- have epilepsy: about 25%;
- have behavioural problems: less than 5%;
- have hip displacement requiring surgery: about 18%;
- use a feeding tube: 4%;
- walk alone at home by age 4–12 years: about 10%;
- walk with support at home by age 4–12 years: 36%.

---

forearm crutches, and uses a motorized scooter for longer distances and community mobility. Over the past 5 years, she has seen the physiotherapist and occupational therapist once or twice each year for individual review sessions. Since she was 14, she had been involved in several group rehabilitation services to develop fitness and exercise routines, and life skills. She is also a member of the teen group through the centre and participates in social functions held by this group each month. Her parents had requested occupational therapy assessment and services related to her transition to university. The steps involved in the clinical reasoning process used in this chapter are summarized in Figure 14.1 and described in Chapter 1.

Stage 1: initial data collection

The occupational therapist working in the transition programme at the centre contacted Isabella and her parents to set up an initial time to meet with them. The therapist travelled to their home for this first meeting because she found this location made it easier to gather information about a young person's living context. Isabella and her family live in a one storey house in a new suburb. Isabella has two younger sisters, aged 14 and 12.

In school, Isabella is currently finishing grade 11, with one more year before she graduates. Her school grades are very good, particularly in English, history and social sciences. Isabella's plan is to apply to attend a university about 1 hour away from her home. She wants to live in residence at the university. Once at university, she will be eligible for some attendant care services to assist with more complex activities of daily living such as cleaning and laundry.

---

1   See Chapter 2: p. 17 for details of the sources used to derive these data.

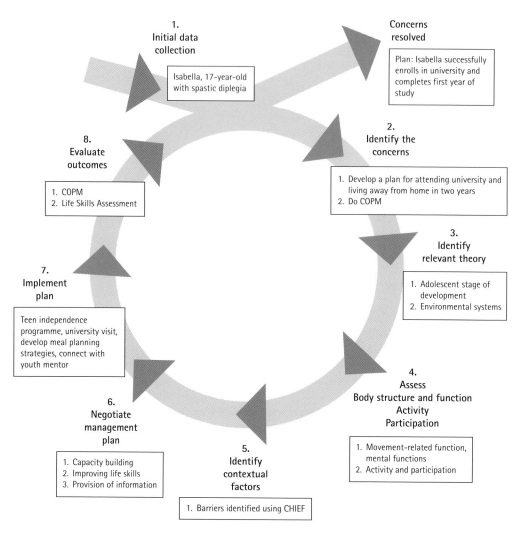

Figure 14.1 The intervention process used with Isabella: model adapted with permission from the Canadian Occupational Performance Process Model (CAOT, 2002). CHIEF, Craig Hospital Inventory of Environmental Factors; COPM, Canadian Occupational Performance Measure.

Stage 2: identify and prioritize concerns

During the meeting at Isabella's house, the occupational therapist explored the issues about transition to university with Isabella and her parents. The therapist used the Canadian Occupational Performance Measure (COPM) (Law et al, 2004) to help Isabella and her parents identify the issues about going to university that were concerning them. The COPM is an individualized measure designed to identify and detect change in a client's self-perception of occupational performance over time (see Appendix, p. 291). Using the COPM, the therapist asked Isabella and her parents to identify the daily occupations (self-care, work, school, leisure) that she might have difficulty performing while at university. The therapist stressed that these occupations also included any tasks/activities for which Isabella would direct her own care (e.g. working with attendant care services).

The issues identified by Isabella and her parents were as follows:

(1) making light meals/snacks;

(2) directing her attendant caregiver in performing instrumental activities of daily living (IADL) tasks (cleaning, laundry);

(3) organizing any necessary academic accommodations;

(4) doing things with friends;

(5) moving from class to class (particularly in the winter);

(6) managing money/budget while away at university;

(7) taking notes in lectures.

Isabella scored the importance of each issue using the COPM scale (her top five are 1–5 in the list above). Once these issues have been addressed, the remaining issues will be reviewed with Isabella and her parents. Table 14.1 outlines the COPM findings and initial scores for performance and satisfaction.

Table 14.1 Canadian Occupational Performance Measure results

Identified issues	Importance (range 1–10)	Performance (range 1–10)	Satisfaction (range 1–10)
Making light meals/snacks	9	4	6
Directing attendant caregiver in performing IADL tasks (cleaning, laundry)	8	3	2
Managing money/budget while away at university	6	5	9
Taking notes in lectures	7	7	8
Organizing any necessary academic accommodations	10	2	2
Do things with friends	10	6	3
Moving from class to class (particularly in the winter)	8	5	4

IADL, instrumental activities of daily living.

Stage 3: identify relevant theory and evidence

Developmental theories about adolescence and young adulthood
The transition from adolescence to adulthood has been described in the literature as a developmental process, with significant changes in social roles and expectations (Staff and Mortimer, 2003; Schulenberg et al, 2004). Recent literature takes a broad, life course perspective on transition, recognizing that all aspects of an individual's life should be considered (Stewart, 2006). This view fits with a new theoretical perspective called 'emerging adulthood' (Arnett, 2006). It acknowledges that young adults in their twenties, particularly in Westernized, developed countries, are delaying the attainment of key adult 'markers' such as moving away from the parents' home, marriage and having children. This perspective can serve as a guide to therapists, families and youth with disabilities in developing realistic expectations that fit with the current context.

The most appropriate theory to consider is the theory of developmental contextualism (Lerner, 1989; Lerner and Castellino, 2002). In developmental contextualism, Lerner emphasizes the integration of ideas about nature and nurture, with the influence of contextual factors on an individual's development. Lerner posits that an adolescent has the ability to change and these changes are dependent on the relative influences of their environment and their heredity (Lerner, 1989). Positive development occurs when there is a good fit between the adolescent and the context (family, society) in which they are developing.

The transition from adolescence to the adult world is an important stage in life. The most common domains for this transition for all youth are education, employment, living arrangements, community life, financial independence, social situations and leisure. Youth with disabilities go through the same transition processes as their peers without disabilities and face many of the same challenges. There are, however, unique issues and concerns related to having a disability. Several assumptions about transition are important to consider. First, transition is a dynamic complex process that involves all aspects of life. Second, youth with disabilities develop and change at different rates during any transition experience. Finally, disability is only one factor that will determine the success of a transition experience. Cerebral palsy remains an important factor as youth move into the adult world. Research indicates that youth with disabilities do not achieve similar outcomes to their peers in academic achievement, interpersonal relationships, community participation and employment (Cadman et al 1991; DePoy and Werrbach, 1996; Antle et al,1999; Wagner, 2005).

Person, environment and occupation
The theoretical model from occupational therapy that is used for this clinical situation is the Person–Environment–Occupation (PEO) model (Law et al, 1996). The PEO model depicts three inter-related components of occupational performance (person, environment and occupation). A child's performance is the outcome of the transactional relationship between the child, environment and occupation.

Although there are substantial personal challenges in transitions such as physical limitations and cognitive and communicative challenges, research to date has indicated that environmental barriers are the most significant challenges to youth as they move into the adult world (Stewart et al, 2001; National Center for Youth with Disabilities, 1996). Environmental barriers include physical inaccessibility, economic barriers to participation, misconceptions and stigma and social attitudes. Research indicates that social attitudes and social support, as an environmental strategy, facilitate a smooth transition into adult society (Beresford, 2004; Betz, 2004).

Part of transition to adulthood is the transfer of youth from children's rehabilitation services to adult services. Research indicates that these transitions involve both the person and environment in interaction (White, 2002). The multifaceted nature of the transition process requires researchers and service providers to use a comprehensive approach to planning and evaluating transition services (Luft, 1999). Multiple assessment strategies are recommended, including formal and informal methods, to address objective and subjective outcomes such as quality of life, activity performance, self-determination, use of supports, satisfaction and achievement of personal goals and dreams (Thoma and Held, 2002; Wehmeyer, 2002).

Research evidence
In a recent study on transition to adulthood for youth with physical and developmental disabilities, Stewart and colleagues (2007) developed best practice guidelines. Research and the grey literature were reviewed and summarized for an 'expert advisory panel' of youth, parents, community members, service providers, consultants and the research team. The group reviewed this evidence at a consensus conference and developed basic principles for transition services and supports, and best practice guidelines. The following principles for transition were stated from the consensus conference. All services and supports will

- apply a person-first, family-centred, culturally sensitive approach;
- employ a lifespan philosophy;
- be collaborative and interdependent;
- value citizenship and participation;
- have individualized choices and options;
- employ a programme orientation towards the future;
- focus on strengths and needs, not medical conditions (Stewart et al, 2007).

The best practice guidelines for policy, services, support and communities coming from this research are shown in Box 14.2.

Stage 4: assessment of body function and structure, activity and participation
Following identification of Isabella's goals for therapy through the COPM, the therapist, Isabella and her parents discussed a plan to gather more information

Box 14.2 Best practice guidelines

(1) Collaborative initiatives and policies for transition to adulthood are needed

- At the policy level, collaboration through an inter-ministerial team could develop policy around transition.
- At the service level, intersectoral collaboration and communication is essential. Plans for transfer between paediatric and adult service systems should start early and involve all services.
- At the community level, identify existing transition community networks, and if not there, create them. A coordinating body, such as social planning councils, could standardize this across regions.

(2) Building community capacity will enhance the transition process

- Community facilitators or 'navigators' should be created to support youth and families in planning for transition and navigating all of the systems and resources out there. They can also help to develop circles of support and networks. The position of a facilitator needs to be unencumbered, i.e. not affiliated with any service system, but rather be part of the community.
- At the community level, employers and other community members need to become aware of the capacity of youth with disabilities to contribute and participate. Families and youth also need support to advocate for inclusion, as it takes a great deal of time and energy.

(3) Information, resources and services need to be accessible and available to all

- A single point of access is needed for information, resources, networking and supports along the lifespan. The facilitators/navigators could work from this access point.
- At the policy level, access to a location that coordinates transition information (e.g. libraries – disability information service) is required.
- Governments and service systems should commit to disclosure about transition services in clear language and evidence of the benefits related to transition.
- At the service level, ensure a commitment to information exchange among professionals.
- At the community level, develop and hold annual transition workshops in different regions.

(4) Education and research is critical to successful development in this field

- Develop an educational strategy related to transition and educate people about the values, needs for supports, benefits of transition strategy and real life outcomes.
- Educate service providers, educators at all levels from elementary to post secondary and health professions students as well as the youth themselves, parents, community and employers about pathways to and strategies for successful transition.
- Develop educational materials for different audiences.

- Education of parents by parents is needed in communities.
- Develop continuing education courses to educate youth and parents to be navigators and peer mentors.
- In order for the peer-based initiatives to be successful, investment in infrastructure such as transportation, support for people participating in supporting others, is needed.
- Any new transition programme should have research and evaluation to demonstrate the benefits of these programmes, show how transition programmes can be effective, follow youth over time to learn what works and doesn't work, evaluate training or education models that are in place.
- Youth, parents, community, consumers should be included as part of the research team.
- Any transition project should focus on outcomes of participation, quality of life, opportunities, self-determination, self-advocacy, self-efficacy, as well as an overall cost benefit analysis (Stewart et al, 2007).

regarding her current activities and participation related to these goals. The COPM goals were as follows:

- make light meals/snacks;
- direct attendant caregiver in performing IADL tasks (cleaning, laundry);
- organize any necessary academic accommodations;
- do things with friends;
- move from class to class (particularly in the winter).

Further assessment and observation of Isabella performing these activities was used to identify factors that supported or limited her performance. This part of the assessment process was guided by the structure of the International Classification of Functioning, Disability and Health (ICF) (WHO, 2001).

Body function and structure

Neuromusculoskeletal and movement-related functions (e.g. range of movement; grasp and release; strength)
The goal of making a light meal or snacks (an ADL activity) required Isabella to have functional range of movement and strength in order to reach, grasp and manipulate objects. To assess these body functions, the therapist used a dynamic assessment approach (Elman, 2003; Thelen and Bates, 2003). Dynamic assessment is an approach to assessment and intervention that is based on research by Vygotsky (1978). The key characteristic of dynamic assessment is the use of 'assessment – intervention – reassessment' whereby a therapist observes performance, intervenes to support performance and then retests. With a dynamic assessment approach, body functions

and structures such as range of movement, strength and reach/grasp are not assessed independently but rather within the context of activity performance.

The therapist observed Isabella making lunch (sandwich, drink and apple) in her home. For Isabella, optimal functioning is achieved when she is sitting in a sturdy chair at a table. She has the necessary range of movement in both hands to grasp and release utensils (knife, fork, spoon), to slice and butter bread, to open and close packages and to assemble a sandwich. Range of movement in her upper extremities is limited to shoulder height when standing, and she is therefore not able to reach items in cupboards above this level. She also cannot bend down to reach items in cupboards below counter level. Her strength in her upper extremities is good against minimal to moderate resistance. She can lift a small pot, plate, bottle or can independently. She does not have the hand strength to open a new bottle or to use a manual can opener. Her sensory function in her upper extremity is adequate for function.

The results of the first part of this dynamic assessment process are reported here – the remaining process is detailed in the intervention implementation plan (Stage 7).

MENTAL FUNCTIONS (E.G. COGNITIVE, SELF-EFFICACY)
The therapist was able to review Isabella's school and psychoeducational reports to determine that cognitive functioning was an area of strength for her. Reports indicated that she demonstrates strong problem-solving and decision-making skills. Self-determination has emerged as an important area of functioning for young people in transition to adulthood. The therapist reviewed recent resources on self-determination that are available online (for example, see http://www.ncset.org/publications/ viewdesc.asp?id=962) and she then requested a meeting with Isabella, her teachers and her parents to identify current functioning and needs for support and development. The therapist chose to use an open-ended discussion in keeping with a dynamic assessment approach, as she wanted to ensure that all perspectives and needs were raised.

Activities

MAKE LIGHT MEALS/SNACKS
As described above, a dynamic assessment approach was used to conduct an observational assessment of Isabella's performance of this activity. Making a meal/snack is one example of the many life skills that young people have to develop in preparation for moving away from home. A number of assessment tools are available to assess a young person's current capacity and self-efficacy related to life skills. The therapist chose one measure to do with Isabella, to get an overall picture of her current capacities. The Ansell-Casey Life Skills Assessments are available online (www.caseylifeskills.org) and are relatively easy to complete.

Mobility (walking endurance and scooter use)
Isabella used forearm crutches to walk at home, in her high school and for very short distances in the community. For longer community trips, she used an electric scooter.

Walking endurance was tested using the 6-minute walk assessment procedure (see Appendix, p. 296). Such walking assessments are reliable and valid (Andersson et al, 2006). With Isabella, this assessment provided information for her to use to plan a strategy for mobility at university. Part of this strategy was to figure out in which situations she will walk using her forearm crutches and when she will use her electric scooter. Isabella was able to walk 90 metres (average of two test occasions) during this assessment.

Participation
The Life–H (Noreau et al, 2007) short version was used to provide an overall assessment of participation for Isabella (see Appendix, p. 298). Findings for the LIFE–H are recorded in Table 14.2.

Stage 5: contextual factors: environmental and personal

Environmental factors
Environmental factors were assessed using the Craig Hospital Inventory of Environmental Factors (CHIEF; see Appendix, p. 299). The CHIEF has been used to assess environmental factors affecting the participation of children and youth with physical disabilities (Law et al, 2007). Isabella's CHIEF scores are listed in Table 14.3.

Table 14.2 LIFE–H scores

LIFE–H scale	Isabella's score (range 0–9)[a]
Daily activities	
Communication	9.5
Personal care	7.4
Housing	5.6
Mobility	4.3
Nutrition	8.7
Fitness	3.5
Social roles	
Recreation	7.8
Responsibility	8.4
Education	7.5
Community life	6.9
Interpersonal relationships	8.3

a. Scores range from 0 (not able to do item) to 9 (able to participate without restriction).

Table 14.3 Mean perceived environmental barriers on Craig Hospital Inventory of Environmental Factors (CHIEF)

CHIEF subscale	Isabella's score[a]
Attitudes and social support	0.85
Institutional and government policies	1.98
Natural and built environment	2.20
School and work environment	2.35
Services and assistance	1.54

a. Score range 0–8; higher scores indicate more barriers.

Personal factors
Isabella is a highly motivated young woman who has done well in her academic grades in high school and is now keen to begin her university studies. Her family has saved funds over the years to enable her to attend university. She has a positive temperament and is very willing to try out potential solutions to issues that arise because of her disability. She is worried about meeting friends at university and wants to have fun as well as do well in her studies.

Stage 6: management plan

Summary of assessment findings
Using developmental contextualism theory, assessment findings focus primarily on the 'interactions' or 'relationships' between person and environment. In addition, occupational therapists focus on a person's occupations or the tasks and activities they participate in every day. For Isabella, there is a good fit between her and the context of her family who are supporting her, and her high school whose staff are encouraging her to develop independence. There is a good fit with her cognitive and affective function and the task of making a meal but there are some issues with current neurological functions and the task, which will require some environmental modification and skill development.

Negotiated treatment plan
The occupational therapist referred to the best practice guidelines to frame a treatment plan, which she then negotiated with Isabella and her family.

COLLABORATION
Any treatment plan for Isabella needs to focus on the importance of networking for everyone involved. This focus builds on the significant contribution of the environmental context to her successful planning and transition. This activity will include regular meetings with everyone involved, meetings between the high school and university and other 'adult' services. Also, mentoring from a young adult who has experienced this transition would fit in here (see under capacity building).

CAPACITY BUILDING

Capacity is a term that refers to the assets, abilities and strengths of people and communities. Isabella demonstrates many capacities already, particularly in her motivation and interests. Capacity building for many youth with disabilities relates to self-determination. Isabella would benefit from opportunities and experiences to realize her potential to determine and plan her own future and to learn how to direct another person, such as an attendant in the future, to complete tasks that are difficult or energy-consuming ones like shopping and cleaning.

Two specific plans relate to this area of focus for treatment.

(1) Youth KIT (Stewart et al, 2009) – provision of the Youth KIT, a resource about information, and developing skills in using information effectively have been identified as important supports for youth with disabilities in transition and their families. The Youth KIT can be used by Isabella to develop specific goals and interests for the transition ahead of her, and to help her identify the supports she will need.

(2) A second activity under this focus is identification of a 'navigator', a young adult who has 'graduated' from the treatment centre and is now at university and can help Isabella to navigate this system.

Capacity building also refers to the community, which is the context around a person. Isabella's parents need to develop the capacity to 'let go' and still support Isabella, and people at her high school need to develop the capacity to enable her self-determination. There is also a role for the occupational therapist to meet with people from the university community, to ensure that they have the capacity (the knowledge and skills) to support Isabella for a successful transition (Wynn et al, 2006).

INFORMATION AND EDUCATION

Because information and education are so important for a successful transition, it was decided to connect Isabella with relevant websites on transition to adulthood, and resources such as the student with disabilities websites (e.g. in Canada the National Educational Association of Disabled Students [NEADS]). Information can also be provided about local community websites that give important information about adult services and university websites. She will also need to be provided with educational materials (e.g. videos, booklets) to read and discuss with her parents and therapist. Attending a summer transition camp will also provide her with relevant information.

Stage 7: implement plan

The therapists reviewed all assessment information and recommendations, and discussed these findings with Isabella and parents. Together, they decided to implement the following actions:

● a referral to a summer teen independence programme with a focus on helping Isabella to develop self-efficacy and competence in the life skills needed for future independent living;

- therapist to meet with guidance counsellor and teacher regarding planning for the last year of high school and to discuss strategies to encourage self-determination. For example, Isabella will participate actively in writing her individualized education plan (IEP) and attend all school planning meetings about her;
- therapist to meet with Isabella and parents to design meal planning strategies and adaptations;
- therapist to provide Isabella and her parents with written resources on transition planning;
- therapist to accompany Isabella on a trip to the university. While there, she will connect with disability services and apply for attendant care and any other resources/supports she may need. She will also have a tour of the residence;
- seek a young adult mentor to meet with Isabella regularly, and to work through the Youth KIT with her.

Stage 8: evaluate outcomes

Evaluation of outcomes is completed through readministration of the COPM (see Table 14.4). This evaluation indicated that Isabella perceived important changes to her performance and satisfaction with performance for the activities of make light meals/snacks, direct attendant caregiver in performing IADL tasks (cleaning, laundry), organize necessary academic accommodations and move from class to class. Little change was perceived for the activity of doing things with friends.

Table 14.4 Canadian Occupational Performance Measure reassessment results

Identified issues	Baseline performance	Review performance	Baseline satisfaction	Review satisfaction
Making light meals/snacks	4	8	6	9
Directing attendant caregiver in performing IADL tasks (cleaning, laundry)	3	6	2	8
Organizing any necessary academic accommodations	2	7	2	6
Do things with friends	6	7	3	3
Moving from class to class (particularly in the winter)	5	8	4	9

Scores range from 1–10. Changes >2 points indicate clinically significant changes.

Box 14.3 Key clinical messages

- Transitions present significantly more challenges for youth with disabilities, their families and communities. At transitions, systems and services tend to be uncoordinated or fragmented and people lack the information needed to navigate the transition successfully.

- Environmental barriers present the most significant challenges to youth with disability as they transition (these include physical inaccessibility, economic barriers to participation, misconceptions and stigma, and social attitudes).

- Collaboration, communication and planning, as well as building community capacities enhance the transition process.

References

Andersson C, Asztalos L & Mattson E (2006) Six-minute walk test in adults with cerebral palsy: A study of reliability. *Clin Rehabil*, 20, 488–95.

Antle BJ, Frazee C, Contaxis G, Antle BJ, Frazee C, Contaxis G, Forma L, Nikou R, Self H, Tonack M &Yoshida K (1999) *Creating a Life of your Own: Experiences with Transition to Independence among Adults with Life-long Disabilities Final Report of Research Fellowship in Community Living.* Toronto, ON: West Park Hospital.

Arnett JJ (2006) Emerging adulthood: The Winding Road through the Late Teens through the Twenties. New York, NY: Oxford University Press.

Beresford B (2004) On the road to nowhere? Young disabled people and transition. *Child Care Health Dev*, 30, 581–7.

Betz B (2004) Transition of adolescents with special health care needs: review and analysis of the literature. *Issues Comprehen Pediatr Nurs*, 27, 179–241.

Cadman D, Rosenbaum P, Boyle M & Offord DR (1991) Children with chronic illness: Family and parent demographic characteristics and psychosocial adjustment. *Pediatr*, 87, 884–9.

Canadian Association of Occupational Therapists (CAOT) (2002) *Enabling Occupation: An Occupational Therapy Perspective.* Ottawa: Canadian Association of Occupational Therapists.

DePoy E, Werrbach G (1996) Successful living placement for adults with disabilities: Considerations for social work practice. *Soc Work Health Care*, 23, 21–34.

Elman J (2003) Development: It's about time. *Dev Science*, 6, 430–3.

Fougeyrollas P, Noreau L, Bergeron H, Cloutier R, Dion SA & St-Michel, G. (1998). Social consequences of long term impairments and disabilities: conceptual approach and assessment of handicap. *Int J Rehabil Res*, 21, 127–41.

Law M, Cooper B, Strong S, Stewart D, Rigby P & Letts L (1996) The person-environment-occupation model: a transactive approach to occupational performance. *Can J Occup Ther*, 63, 9–23.

Law M, Baptiste S, Carswell A, McColl MA, Polatajko, H & Pollock N (2004) *Canadian Occupational Performance Measure Manual*, 4th edn. Toronto, ON: CAOT Publications ACE.

Law M, Petrenchik T, King G & Hurley P (2007) Perceived barriers to recreational, community, and school participation for children and youth with physical disabilities. *Arch Phys Med Rehabil*, 88, 1636–42.

Lerner RM & Castellino DR (2002) Contemporary developmental theory and adolescence: developmental systems and applied developmental science. *J Adolesc Health*, 31, 122–35.

Lerner RM (1989). Developmental Contextualism and the life-span view of person-context interaction. In: Bornstein M & Bruner JS (eds) *Interaction in Human Development*: 217–39. Hillsdale, NJ: Erlbaum.

Luft P (1999) Assessment and collaboration: key elements in comprehensive and cohesive transition planning. *Work*, 13, 31–41.

National Center for Youth with Disabilities (1996). *Transition from Child to Adult Health Care Services: A National Survey*. Minneapolis, University of Minnesota.

Noreau L, Lepage C, Boissiere L, Picard R, Fougeyrollas P, Mathieu J, Desmarais G & Nadeau L (2007). Measuring participation in children with disabilities using the Assessment of Life Habits. *Dev Med Child Neurol*, 49, 666–71.

Palisano RJ, Rosenbaum PL, Bartlett D & Livingston MH (2008) Content validity of the expanded and revised gross motor function classification system. *Dev Med Child Neurol*, 50, 744–50.

Schulenberg J, Bryant A & O'Malley P (2004) Taking hold of some kind of life: how developmental tasks relate to trajectories of well-being during the transition to adulthood. *Dev Psychopathology*, 16, 1119–40.

Staff J & Mortimer JT (2003). Diverse transitions from school to work. *Work Occup*, 30, 361–9.

Stewart D (2006) Editorial: Evidence to Support a Positive Transition to Adulthood for Youth with Disabilities. *Phys Occup Ther Paediatr*, 26, 1–4.

Stewart D, Law M, Rosenbaum P & Willms D (2001) A qualitative study of the transition to adulthood for youth with physical disabilities. *Phys Occup Ther Pediatr*, 21, 3–21.

Stewart D, Antle B, Healy H, Law M & Young N (2007) *Best Practice Guidelines for Transition to Adulthood for Youth with Disabilities in Ontario: An Evidence-based Approach*. Hamilton, ON: CanChild Centre for Childhood Disability Research, McMaster University (http://transitions.canchild.ca/en/ltResources/transitionsummary.asp)

Stewart D, Freeman M, Burke-Gaffney J, Law M, Missiuna C, Shimmell L & Jaffer S (2009) *The KIT (Keeping It Together) for Youth, Research Version*. Hamilton, ON: McMaster University and Hamilton Family Network.

Thelen E & Bates E (2003) Connectionism and dynamic systems: are they really different? *Dev Science*, 6, 378–91.

Thoma CA & Held M (2002) Measuring what's important: using alternative assessments. In: Sax CL & Thoma CA (eds) *Transition Assessment. Wise Practices for Quality Lives*. Baltimore, MD: Paul Brookes Publishing Co.

Vygotsky LS (1978). *Mind and Society: The Development of Higher Psychological Processes*. Cambridge, MA: Harvard University Press.

Wagner M, Newman L, Cameto R, Levine P (2005) *National Longitudinal Transition Study2: Changes over Time in the Early Post-school Outcomes of Youth with Disabilities*. Menlo Park, CA: SRI International.

Wehmeyer ML (2002) Self-determined assessment. In: Sax CL & Thoma CA (eds) *Transition Assessment. Wise Practices for Quality Lives*. Baltimore, MD: Paul Brookes Publishing Co.

White PH (2002) Transition: a future promise for children and adolescents with special healthcare needs and disabilities. *Rheum Dis Clin North Am*, 28, 687–703.

World Health Organization (2001) *International Classification of Disability, Functioning and Health*. Geneva: WHO.

Wynn K, Stewart D, Law M, Burke-Gaffney J & Moning T (2006) Creating connections: A community capacity building project with parents and youth with disabilities in transition to adulthood. *Phys Occup Ther Paediatr*, 26, 89–103.

Chapter 15

The young adult with complex disability

Barbara Scoullar and Christine Imms

Case study: Simon

Simon is a 25-year-old man who has a diagnosis of severe bilateral spastic cerebral palsy (quadriplegia), Gross Motor Function Classification System (GMFCS, Palisano et al, 2008) level V and Manual Ability Classification System (MACS, Eliasson et al, 2006) level V (see Chapter 2). He receives his adult health care through the young adult complex disability service. This team includes a rehabilitation physician, a physiotherapist, an occupational therapist, a speech pathologists, a prosthetist/orthotist and a dietitian. Referrals can be made to other allied health, nursing, medical and surgical services as needed. The services Simon receives in one episode of care at the young adult complex disability service are described in this chapter (see Figure 15.1 and Chapter 1 for a description of the intervention model).

Stage 1: initial data collection

Simon attended the young adult complex disability service with Vivien, his single parent. There are no siblings and Simon has no contact with his father. On his first visit, Simon's history is reviewed with Vivien and their collective needs and priorities identified.

Previous services

After Simon was diagnosed at 6 months of age, he attended an early intervention programme where he received speech therapy, occupational therapy and physiotherapy. It was a conventional programme following a theoretical approach based on Bobath theory (Levitt, 1995, 2004; see Chapter 4). Although Simon had a significant physical disability and intellectual impairment he attended his local primary school. He had an aide who assisted him throughout the school day and he attended fortnightly physiotherapy, occupational therapy and speech therapy for 1 hour each. At this age Simon could walk with assistance using a K-walking frame for short distances and sat in

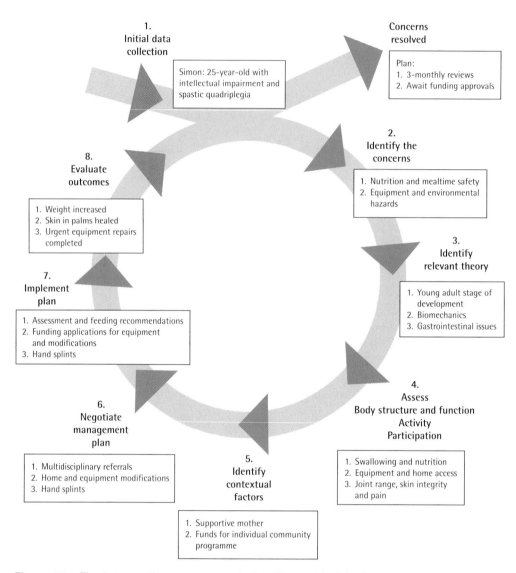

Figure 15.1 The intervention process used with Simon. Model adapted with permission from the Occupational Performance Process Model (CAOT, 2002).

a chair with additional supports. Until the age of about 12 years Simon would have been classified at GMFCS level IV. Other than a consistent yes/no response, he had no verbal communication but had some receptive language skills.

On reaching secondary school Vivien decided to send Simon to a special school for students with a physical disability that employed therapists as well as teachers. This school followed the principles of conductive education (Bourke-Taylor et al, 2007; see Chapter 2). By Grade 7, when Simon was 12, he could no longer walk with assistance and began mobilizing using an attendant manual wheelchair; his cognitive impairment precluded him from learning to use a motorized wheelchair. From age 12, Simon's gross motor performance was at GMFCS level V (see Box 15.1). This decline in his function is consistent with that shown in a longitudinal study of gross motor outcomes of children and adolescents with cerebral palsy (Hanna et al, 2008). Although Hanna et al show that children in GMFCS levels I and II tend to have stable gross motor skills through adolescence and into young adulthood, those in levels III to V show a trend for loss of gross motor function that appears to begin in middle childhood (Hanna et al, 2008). Of these three levels, the predicted loss in function of children in level IV was greatest at 7.8 points on the Gross Motor Function Measure (GMFM–66). This is a clinically important decline in function. In Simon's penultimate year at secondary school, when he was 17 years old, he was given an augmentative language device to try. He did not enjoy using it and Vivien found it cumbersome to use, and thought that he interacted well without it.

On leaving the secondary educational system a decision must be made as to what tertiary/vocational direction to follow. For those with a low cognitive ability there are three options: to attend a day placement for 1–5 days per week; to have a tailored individual programme; or to combine the first two options. The choice depends on family preference and what services are available locally. Simon has an individual support plan and associated funding that allows him to purchase support workers, occasional respite services and some equipment. Simon uses his support workers to take him to a tailored programme 5 days per week.

Medical history
Simon was born by emergency caesarean section following a normal pregnancy. His Apgar scores were 3 at 1 minute, 7 at 5 minutes and 8 at 10 minutes. His birth-weight was 2.65 kilograms (kg). He had apnoeic and cyanotic episodes requiring ventilation with generalized seizures. Delays in all areas of development were apparent from early life, along with poor growth and an increase in tone with poor selective control of movements. He has no hearing problems, has strabismus and wears glasses.

Simon had surgery to reduce saliva production when he was 12 years old. Vivien is concerned about this now as new evidence suggests there is an increase in decay through too little saliva washing over the teeth (Hallet et al, 2007). In the past Simon received dental services through the paediatric hospital as he usually required a general anaesthetic. Vivien has a referral to the public dental service where services are provided for people with a disability. However, the dental hospital does not have an intensive care unit which puts some clients at risk after procedures using an anaesthetic (Theroux and Akins, 2005).

Simon had a gastroscopy 4 years ago that found minor oesophagitis associated with reflux. He had a percutaneous endoscopic gastrostomy (PEG) 1 year later. Vivien only uses the PEG tube to deliver medication. As is common with people with severe cerebral palsy, Simon takes medication to enable regular bowel movements.

Simon has had a number of orthopaedic surgical procedures aimed at aligning joints and maintaining walking when he was younger. At 6 years of age Simon had adductor tenotomy and obturator neurectomy to correct imminent dislocation of the right hip, and 4 years later he required a Chiari osteotomy to reconstruct the hip. Simon then had several long admissions for investigation and management of pain that culminated in him having further hip surgery; a right girdle-Shanz excisional arthroplasty and valgus proximal femoral osteotomy with left excision of the femoral head, plus bilateral percutaneous hamstring releases. Following the final hip procedure, Simon developed an infected pressure sore on his right ischium. Two years later he had surgery to remove the plate from his right femur. Although Simon has a scoliosis, as is common in children with cerebral palsy (Graham, 2004), he did not have corrective surgery.

Box 15.1 GMFCS level V snapshot[1]

Proportion of people with cerebral palsy classified as GMFCS level V: 13–16%

Proportion of people classified as GMFCS level V who

- have a severe intellectual disability (IQ <50): about 85%;
- have a severe visual impairment: about 60%;
- have epilepsy: about 80%;
- have behavioural problems: about 10%;
- have hip displacement requiring surgery: about 65%;
- use a feeding tube: 42%;
- walk alone or with support at home by age 4–12 years: 0%.

Stage 2: identify and prioritize concerns
Vivien attended the clinic with a clear list of concerns that she wished to address with the team.

(1) Equipment needs: Vivien was concerned that some of Simon's equipment was in need of repair (e.g. the bath chair) or was too heavy for carers to use easily (e.g. the wheelchair) and would like all of Simon's equipment reviewed.

(2) Architectural concerns: Simon's support workers from the council recently indicated they were unhappy with the physical environment in the home and sent a list of complaints that they wanted addressed related to safe access to the front and back of the house, and in the bathroom.

---

1 See Chapter 2: p. 17 for details of the sources used to derive these data.

(3) Skin and joint integrity and pain: Simon's palms have become smelly and the skin is breaking down. His toes are painful and he has recently been refusing to wear shoes and socks.

(4) Eating and swallowing needs: Vivien has noticed that Simon coughs frequently during and after meals and she is concerned that he has been losing weight.

(5) Dental care: Vivien continues to find it difficult to manage Simon's routine dental care and she has become concerned about potential decay.

(6) Long-term care: as Vivian experiences increasing difficulty in managing Simon at home, she would like to talk to someone about long-term residential options for him.

Stage 3: identifying relevant theory

Young adult stage of development
The tasks of young adulthood in Western societies are typically defined in relation to taking responsibility, gaining employment, independently pursuing leisure interests, accommodation and relationships outside the immediate family (Gething et al, 1995; Donkervoort et al, 2007). To achieve these tasks, parental roles shift to allow increased autonomy in decision making. For the young person with severe and multiple disabilities however, many of these goals are unobtainable, thus the focus shifts to enabling community leisure participation, supporting social relationships, establishing long-term supported accommodation within or external to the family, and maintaining health and well-being through ongoing integrated health services. Parents or caregivers typically retain responsibility for many aspects of the young adult's life for many years, if not the rest of their lives.

Best practice guidelines for assisting young adults to transition from paediatric to adult services are described in Chapter 14. The clinic Simon transitioned into (the young adult complex disability service) was in an adult hospital that provided multidisciplinary clinical assessment and management, as well as appropriate referrals to hospital or community-based services, including mental health services. Managing the needs of a young adult with complex disabilities in an adult hospital system designed to provide services for older people and the sick, can present a number of challenges. For example, finding a suitable car park can be daunting and many families choose to travel by taxi, although this is expensive; there are no hoists for transferring or change tables in the toilets to manage continent care or even toilets large enough to enable assisted standing transfers; and usually there is no area where a client can be given their enteral feed while they wait.

Another key challenge for young adults is to identify and negotiate the services and resources they require to support their accommodation, equipment and leisure needs. Adult services present a new arena of funding sources and service providers, often with varying eligibility criteria and bureaucratic requirements. Young adults with severe and complex disabilities will continue to need an active advocate to attend medical appointments with them and to make decisions on their behalf. This requirement has legal ramifications, and family members need to negotiate relevant power of attorney requirements. Case managers and clinic therapists play an ongoing role in informing, educating and advocating for young adults with complex needs and their families.

Occupational performance coaching
Occupational performance coaching is a cognitive approach to therapy, initially described in relation to families of children with disability (Graham et al, 2009). Occupational performance coaching is grounded in family-centred care, is occupation based and focused on enabling participation in the community. Occupational performance coaching is intended for young people who do not have the capacity, because of age or impairment, to engage in cognitive interventions because they require moderate language and cognitive skills. Thus families or primary caregivers are engaged in a process of interactive problem-solving with the therapist. Therapy is goal focused and the emphasis is on detailed analysis of barriers to occupational performance. The therapist acts as a coach to the caregiver as solutions are sought that are congruent with the client's environmental context and participation goals. Parents are assisted to develop plans that they perceive are achievable, relevant and likely to work (Graham et al, 2009). Vivien had always been an advocate for Simon and this was particularly evident when devising his adult programme. The clinicians at the young adult complex disability service will continue to support Vivien in her planning by providing information, education and support as they work through Simon's and her issues and together select and guide the interventions that take place.

Biomechanical considerations
Musculoskeletal issues in individuals at GMFCS level V require lifelong management of joint position, skin integrity and pain. Pain is common in adults with severe physical disability (Houlihan et al, 2004), and at present Simon is refusing to wear shoes, and more recently socks, as a result of his painful toes. Simon has received therapy and orthopaedic management throughout his life aimed at managing his posture, preventing joint deformity and improving functional mobility and sitting. However, his long-standing hypertonicity, abnormal postures and impaired motor control have led to contractures in all four limbs and a worsening scoliosis.

Scoliosis is common in individuals with spastic quadriplegic cerebral palsy (McCarthy et al, 2006) and untreated scoliosis leads to significant problems with pain, seating, cardiorespiratory compromise and difficulties with caregiving. In adults with even relatively small spinal curves the scoliosis continues to progress after skeletal maturity and must be monitored (Graham, 2004). Because of the association between hip dislocation and development of scoliosis in children at GMFCS levels IV and V, postural management devices and programmes have been recommended through childhood. Postural management equipment includes supine or prone lying devices, standing frames and seating systems. Each of these is aimed at placing the child in good postural alignment for prolonged periods (greater than 6 hours per day is often recommended [Pountney et al 2009]). Although there is some low-level evidence of positive outcomes following postural management (Pountney et al, 2009) a recent review highlighted the lack of strong evidence in support of the postural management programmes to reduce hip deformity significantly and the significant impact that complying with such programmes can have on participation of the child and family, causing pain and disrupting sleep in the individual (Gough, 2009). Currently, Simon's equipment is aimed principally at supporting his participation, preventing skin breakdown and slowing further loss of range of movement.

Gastrointestinal considerations
Gastrointestinal disorders in individuals with cerebral palsy are common and are particularly prevalent in individuals in GMFCS level V (Sullivan et al, 2000; see Chapter 2 for further detail). Because of the risk of chronic lung disease associated with aspiration pneumonia, and the pain associated with reflux and constipation, careful review of Simon's weight, height, nutritional intake and oral feeding practices are important.

Carer health and well-being
Parents and caregivers of young people with severe physical disability are at significantly greater risk of a number of detrimental health outcomes including increased risk of emotional problems, back problems, migraine, intestinal ulcers, asthma, arthritis and pain (Brehaut et al, 2004). Assisting caregivers to locate appropriate health services for themselves and supporting their caregiving through timely prescription of appropriate equipment and respite are key components of providing an integrated health service to young people with severe and multiple disabilities.

Stage 4: assessment of participation, activity and body structure and function
Clinic personnel follow a multidisciplinary, family-centred approach to assessment and management. This means that preliminary interviews take place with Vivien, Simon and key members of the team so that Vivien does not need to provide the same information several times. The team uses an informal approach that aims to gather information about Simon's daily activities, as well as identify key concerns of the individual and family.

Activity and participation
Simon is dependent for all personal, domestic and community activities. Support workers visit each weekday to attend to his morning routine personal care needs and to accompany him on his outings and activities. Simon's community activities include trips to a music group, going to the football, ten-pin bowling, art classes and browsing in the shopping mall. Support workers come again at 8.00 pm each night to shower him and settle him into bed where he watches television. Vivien must turn Simon two or three times during the night and manage weekend care.

Simon's daily activities and participation are supported by a range of equipment (Table 15.1) and architectural modifications. The home has a ramp at the front entrance and a modified small bathroom. He has a single ceiling track hoist in his bedroom that

Table 15.1. Simon's history of equipment needs over the last 8 years

Equipment	Age prescribed, years	Needing now
Supported frame for sitting in a car	15	no
High/low electric bed with head and knee break	17	yes
Air flow mattress	17	yes
Gel wheelchair cushion and gel side support pads	18	yes
Ceiling hoist and slings	16	yes
Tilt in space wheelchair with leg raise and tray	18	yes
Mesh bath chair on castors	17	yes
Custom-made shoes	17	no

was once the lounge/dining room. A bath chair was provided following Simon's last surgery and is a large mesh shower seat on a mobile base. Simon has a high–low bed with head and knee break and an airflow mattress. The mattress was prescribed following his last hospital stay and the development of a pressure injury over his right ischial tuberosity.

Vivien owns a van with a rear entrance hoist and Simon mobilizes in an attendant carer wheelchair that was prescribed by his school therapists 4 years ago. The chair has tilt-in-space capability with back recline and elevating leg rests (Figure 15.2). Simon sits on an air cell cushion with foam back rest and chest pads. He is not reporting any pain and has no skin areas where pressure is a concern. Because of Simon's bony prominence at the elbows a padded surface backed by wood was attached to his Perspex wheelchair tray.

Body structures and function
During the clinic visit, Simon is hoisted onto a plinth and the doctor, occupational therapist and physiotherapist perform a physical examination. While Simon is hoisted he is weighed (46 kg) and when he is in supine his length is measured (161 centimetres). All clients are weighed at each clinic, initially to give a baseline and to determine their body mass index (BMI). If a client is under- or overweight it provides an alert for further investigation and management. Simon is underweight with a BMI of 17.7.

Simon cannot sit independently on the edge of the plinth and does not have any protective responses. He has a startle reflex. In supported sitting he has some head control in extension/flexion with a lateral pull to the left. Simon's ankles have 90° fixed contractures with his toes resting in various postures (Figure 15.3). Simon experiences pain when donning shoes and Vivien is reporting that donning socks is becoming painful. Simon is able to use the Pain Assessment Instrument for Cerebral Palsy (see Appendix, p. 288) to indicate that his level of toe pain when wearing shoes is a 6 (Boldingh et al, 2004).

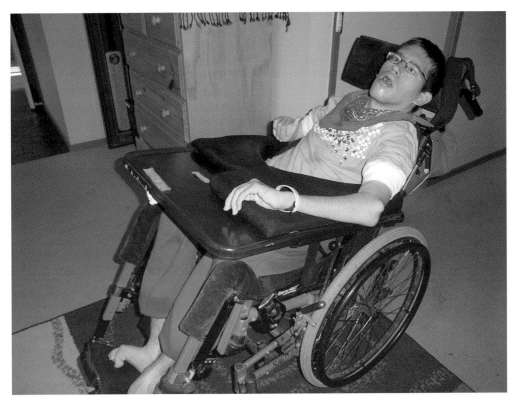

Figure 15.2 Simon's tilt-in-space wheelchair.

- Simon has increased tone most apparent in his right upper limb and left lower limb.
- Bilaterally his shoulders rest in abduction.
- He has fixed right elbow flexion contracture (90°) with dislocation of right and left ulna heads. He can extend his left elbow to 70°.
- Both forearms are pronated, the left more than 90°.
- His right wrist is held in 90° extension with no active flexion but it is possible to passively flex it to 45° extension.
- At rest, his right finger metacarpophalangeal joints are held in 55° flexion with no voluntary extension but near full passive range of extension.
- There is evidence of a low grade palmar infection of the right hand.
- Simon has a left concave scoliosis with right obliquity at the hip with the left hip mildly forward. Both knees have approximately 15° flexion contractures.

Simon is doubly incontinent and uses a condom drainage system. He requires medication and a careful diet to ensure regular bowel movements. At present Simon

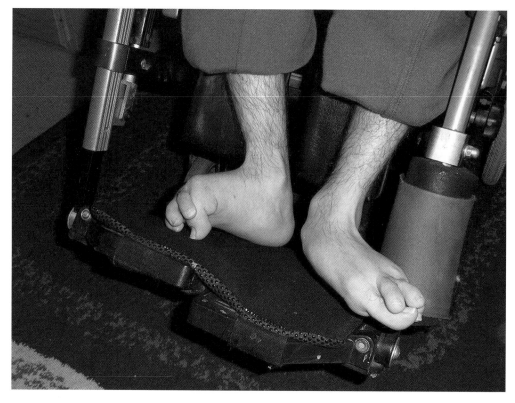

Figure 15.3. Simon's abnormal and painful foot and toe positions.

receives his medication via the PEG tube and takes all his nutritional needs orally. However, Vivien is reporting increasing concerns with eating, as Simon is coughing during and after meals, suggesting he might be aspirating, and she also reported that she feels he has been losing weight. Simon's support workers are also concerned about his eating and the company providing support workers has just banned staff from giving Simon oral feeds until he has been assessed by a speech pathologist.

Stage 5: contextual factors

Personal factors
Simon enjoys interacting with others and his daily programme reflects this. He particularly enjoys going to the football and tennis and watches a variety of sports on television. He vocalizes his enthusiasm when a point is scored. He has a very happy disposition and will try most new adventures. Recently he flew to spend a week at a leisure resort with his mother. Simon is very close to his mother and is much happier when she is around, although he has developed good rapport with a favourite support worker.

Environmental factors
Vivien does not work, and is supported by a carer support pension. Vivien and Simon live in a government funded home and in addition to the support workers that visit each weekday, Simon accesses respite six weekends per year and one annual weekly holiday. Vivien is pleased with the amount of respite she is allocated. However, they are often unable to find support workers to employ through the week. At the end of the financial year Simon may be left with funds allocated to this purpose. Sometimes these funds can be used to purchase equipment.

Recently Simon's support workers reported they were unhappy with the physical environment in the home and sent a list of issues that they wanted addressed. They included: uneven surface on the driveway; difficult access to the house as the front ramp is too narrow; the lip at the door entrance requires the wheelchair to be lifted over the raise; there is no second exit that can be used in case of an emergency; there are no paths in the back area for Simon to access the backyard; the shower recess is very small with an entrance that is difficult to turn into; the carpet is thick making it difficult to push Simon in his wheelchair.

Stage 6: negotiate the management plan
Vivien and the team identified a number of issues that required referral to various health professionals. The cost of supplying many of Simon's equipment needs can be met by a variety of sources most of which require an application supported by professional recommendations, and each of which takes time to process. Often there is a specified government supported funding source for equipment and home modifications, but short falls are made up by application to other sources or by the family's personal resources. Coaching Vivien through the process of identifying priorities and managing short-term solutions as well as long-term outcomes are an important component of therapy at this stage of Simon's life. Vivien prioritized the issues so that the most urgent were dealt with first and the team agreed that a review in 3 months would allow them to assess progress.

(1) Eating and swallowing needs: Vivien was most concerned about Simon's coughing and weight loss and thought that the referral to a speech pathologist and dietician for a swallowing and nutrition assessment were the most urgent needs.

(2) Equipment review: Simon requires a referral to occupational therapy and physiotherapy to review his wheelchair, bath chair and other equipment needs. Repairing the bath chair is the most urgent equipment requirement.

(3) Home modifications: the occupational therapists will need to urgently conduct a home visit to assess and advise on the environmental issues identified by the support workers, as Vivien was concerned that the workers would decide not to provide services until the issues were resolved.

(4) Skin and joint integrity and pain: Simon requires referrals to occupational therapy for a resting splint and a soft splint for his right hand, Simon's left hand is less flexed and the skin is not as compromised. He also requires a referral to

physiotherapy for a stretching/exercise programme for carers to carry out. Simon is sitting in his chair for around 8 hours every day and it is important to allow him time out of the chair to experience different positions and passively stretch his limbs and spine. A referral to an orthopaedic surgeon to review his abnormal and painful toe postures is also recommended.

(5) Dental care: Simon will be referred to the dental hospital for ongoing dental care.

(6) Long-term care: Vivian has requested a referral to a social worker to discuss long-term residential options.

Stage 7: implement plan

Urgent needs

DIET AND MEALTIME MANAGEMENT

The speech pathologist diagnosed oropharyngeal dysphagia. When fed, Simon expended a great deal of energy coordinating chewing and had a poorly controlled swallow resulting in frequent bouts of coughing. Videofluoroscopy assessment showed trace amounts of liquids falling into his trachea, although soft foods appeared to be swallowed safely. It was recommended that when fed orally Simon revert back to having a minced/soft/moist food diet and that he sit in an upright position with his head forward and chin tucked in midline. The food should be given on a spoon pushed lightly down on the mid to back portion of the tongue. The speech pathologist was also concerned by the amount of saliva that Simon needed to swallow and referred this back to the clinic for the physician to consider medication that might help.

The dietician assessed Simon's intake and found that although he only ate small amounts at any meal his diet was high in fat from chips, take away food and chocolates. A more suitable diet was discussed with Vivien. Simon and Vivien agreed that he would also start having some of his food through his PEG to ensure he was eating enough and to reduce the concern regarding aspiration.

REVIEW AND REPLACE EQUIPMENT

The occupational therapist coordinated a home visit with a shower chair supplier to review the damaged chair and obtain a quote for a more suitable reclining chair. A repair request was sent to the government funding body. At the same time Simon was assessed for an adult reclining chair.

The review of the wheelchair found that the heavy wood attachment with padding to protect his elbows was adding significant weight to the chair. Vivien agreed to remove the wood and padding and use gel sleeves to protect Simon's elbows. As Simon does not push his chair the push rings were also removed reducing the weight slightly. A power-assist unit, that provides additional motorized assistance, would help carers when taking Simon into the community therefore a funding application to retrofit this unit was made.

HOME ASSESSMENT

Vivien, the occupational therapist and an architect from the disability service within the local architectural centre, discussed the issues identified by the support workers. Along with providing advice regarding solutions and feasibility of the modifications, the architect drew up the plans the therapist used when applying for funding approval.

The following modifications were proposed:

- widen the front ramp access so it complies with the relevant architectural standards;
- widen the front door and install a small rubberized ramp to remove the small step;
- install a wall and door directly to the right inside the front door to give Simon his own private area where his bed and hoist are currently set up;
- change the windows that overlook the back patio into sliding doors and create a second access ramp at the rear of the house;
- modify the main bathroom by removing the bath and fitting a step-less shower base. Remove the separating wall between the bathroom and toilet to improve access;
- change the small bathroom at the rear of the house into an en-suite for Vivien. Install a second toilet.

Moderately urgent needs

PAINFUL TOES

Simon was referred to an orthopaedic surgeon for assessment of his toe deformities, which were causing pain.

HAND SPLINTS

An occupational therapist who understood hypertonicity associated with spastic cerebral palsy was located. The therapist fabricated a resting hand splint for Simon's right arm to be worn overnight and for at least 4 hours during the day. It is important that a long slow stretch be applied (Copley and Kuipers, 1999). Vivien requested that only one hand be splinted at this time. She agreed that soft splints for his right hand would reduce the moisture in Simon's palm during the day.

Less urgent needs

MAINTAINING JOINT RANGE

Vivien was given a referral to a physiotherapist who would develop a stretching and exercise programme for the support workers to use with Simon.

DENTAL CARE

Because of Simon's complex dental needs, a referral to the dental hospital was made where alternatives to manage him during dental examinations and treatment, such as sedation or general anaesthetic, can be provided.

The social worker discussed availability of permanent residential care as Vivien is a single mother and her health has deteriorated over the last year. Simon is also becoming more difficult to care for at home. Nevertheless Vivien is very reluctant to have Simon go into care full time as she feels his health may be compromised. There are financial implications for Vivien too as she is not of an age to receive an age pension (state pension) and without the carers' allowance she does not know how she could survive financially.

Stage 8: evaluate outcomes

At the 3-month review Vivien reported she was pleased with the number of issues that had been addressed already although waiting for funding was frustrating. Simon was now having 60% of his nutritional needs met via the PEG, which had taken the pressure off meal times. He was just eating those foods he enjoyed by mouth and there were fewer episodes of coughing. When Simon was weighed he had gained 2 kg and his BMI was 18.5.

The wheelchair was now a little lighter to push and the bath chair had been repaired but Vivien was still waiting to hear if she could use left-over support worker funds to pay for the retrofit power assist which would cost more than 2000 Australian dollars and a new bath chair. The recommendations for the home modifications had all been lodged with the appropriate government organization.

After 2 months of using the splints Vivien noticed a significant ease in flexing Simon's right wrist and extending his right metacarpophalangeal joints. Simon's right hand does not smell now and the palms are not sweaty. Vivien has not yet followed up on the referral to the physiotherapist. She has made an appointment with the orthopaedic surgeon and the dental hospital but both have long waiting times.

Overall Vivien is satisfied that progress is being made on the issues identified. Simon's support workers are happy that the requests they made have been responded to and his community programme continues to work well for him.

Box 15.2 Key clinical messages

- Adults with severe and complex disabilities require regular, ongoing management of a wide range of issues including posture, joint contractures, provision and maintenance of equipment and environmental adaptations, gastrointestinal and nutritional concerns, and dental and general health issues.
- Families of people with severe and complex disabilities require ongoing assistance with negotiating services and funding sources for the individual with disability, and support to prioritize and manage their own health.

References

Boldingh EJ, Jacobs-van der Bruggen MA, Lankhorst GJ & Bouter LM (2004) Assessing pain in patients with severe cerebral palsy: development, reliability, and validity of a pain assessment instrument for cerebral palsy. *Arch Phys Med Rehabil*, 85, 758–66.

Bourke-Taylor H, O'Shea R & Gaebler-Spira D (2007) Conductive education: a functional skills program for children with cerebral palsy. *Phys Occup Ther Pediatr*, 27, 45–62.

Brehaut JC, Kohen DE, Raina P, Walter SD, Russell DJ, Swinton M, O'Donnell M & Rosenbaum P (2004) The health of primary caregivers of children with cerebral palsy: how does it compare with that of other Canadian caregivers? *Pediatr*, 114, e182–91.

Canadian Association of Occupational Therapists (CAOT) (2002) *Enabling Occupation: An Occupational Therapy Perspective*. Ottawa: Canadian Association of Occupational Therapists.

Copley J & Kuipers K (1999) *Management of Upper Limb Hypertonicity*. San Antonio, TX: Therapy Skill Builders.

Donkervoort M, Roebroeck M, Wiegerink D, van der Heijden-Maessen H, Stam H & The Transition Research Group South West (2007) Determinants of functioning of adolescents and young adults with cerebral palsy. *Disabil Rehabil*, 29, 453–63.

Eliasson AC, Krumlinde-Sundholm L, Rösblad B, Beckung E, Arner M, Öhrvall A & Rosenbaum PL (2006) The Manual Ability Classification System (MACS) for children with cerebral palsy: scale development and evidence of validity and reliability. *Dev Med Child Neurol*, 48, 549–54.

Gething L, Papalia DE & Olds SW (1995) *Life Span Development*. Sydney: McGraw-Hill Companies.

Gough M (2009) Continuous postural management and the prevention of deformity in children with cerebral palsy: An appraisal. *Dev Med Child Neurol*, 51, 105–11.

Graham F, Rodger S & Ziviani J (2009) Coaching parents to enable children's participation: an approach for working with parents and their children. *Aust Occup Ther J*, 56, 16–23.

Graham HK (2004) Mechanisms of deformity. In: Scrutten D, Damiano D & Mayston MJ (eds) *Management of the Motor Disorders of Children with Cerebral Palsy*. London: Mac Keith Press.

Hallet KB, Lucas JO, Johnston T, Reddihough D & Hall RK (2007) Dental health of children with cerebral palsy following sialodochoplasty. *Spec Care Dentist*, 15, 234–8.

Hanna S, Rosenbaum PL, Bartlett DJ, Palisano RJ, Walter SD, Avery LM & Russell DJ (2008) Stability and decline in gross motor function among children and youth with cerebral palsy aged 2 to 21 years. *Dev Med Child Neurol*, 51, 295–302.

Houlihan CM, O'Donnell M, Conaway M & Stevenson RD (2004) Bodily pain and health-related quality of life in children with cerebral palsy. *Dev Med Child Neurology*, 46, 305–10.

Levitt, S. (1995) *Treatment of Cerebral Palsy and Motor Delay*. Oxford: Blackwell Scientific Publications.

Levitt S (2004) *Treatment of Cerebral Palsy and Motor Delay*. Malden, MA: Blackwell.

McCarthy JJ, D'Andrea LP, Betz RR & Clements DH (2006) Scoliosis in the child with cerebral palsy. *J Am Acad Orthop Surg*, 14, 367–75.

Palisano RJ, Rosenbaum PL, Bartlett D & Livingston MH (2008) Content validity of the expanded and revised gross motor function classification system. *Dev Med Child Neurol*, 50, 744–50.

Pountney TE, Mandy A, Green E & Gard PR (2009) Hip subluxation and dislocation in cerebral palsy: A prospective study on the effectivess of postural management programmes. *Physiother Res Int*, 14, 116–27.

Sullivan PB, Lambert B, Rose M, Ford-Adams M, Johnson A & Griffiths P (2000) Prevalence and severity of feeding and nutritional problems in children with neurological impairment: Oxford Feeding Study. *Dev Med Child Neurol*, 42, 674–80.

Theroux MC & Akins RE (2005) Surgery and anesthesia for children who have cerebral palsy. *Anesthesiol Clin North Am*, 23, 733–43.

Chapter 16

The adult years

Karen J Dodd, Nicholas F Taylor and Christine Imms

Case study: Teresa

A multidisciplinary team working in a small non-government organization that provided services and support for people with developmental disabilities of all ages received a request to work with Teresa. Teresa, a sociable and verbally articulate 45-year-old woman with spastic quadriplegic cerebral palsy, initiated the referral with her widowed mother, Jean. The steps involved in the clinical reasoning process used in this chapter are summarized in Figure 16.1 and described in Chapter 1.

Stage 1: initial data collection

Teresa and Jean attended the first appointment together. Teresa lived at home with her 69-year-old mother who was retired. Teresa worked full time as a receptionist at a local real estate agency and had done so for the past 10 years. Teresa's father had died 2 years earlier, and her older sister and brother, who were both married with families of their own, lived nearby.

Teresa's usual method of mobility was a self-propelled manual wheelchair (Gross Motor Function Classification System [GMFCS] level IV; Palisano et al, 2008; see Box 16.1 and Chapter 2). She could sit-to-stand with the physical assistance of one person. She could sit independently on a chair with a back support, but was insecure sitting on a stool. She could not independently transfer from the ground to a chair or to her wheelchair. She was able to roll independently and sit up on the edge of her bed. Teresa was classified at Manual Ability Classification System (MACS, Eliasson et al, 2006) level II (see Chapter 2). She could toilet, shower and dress her top half independently, but required light assistance dressing her bottom half. Teresa could drive an adapted car independently and felt confident driving herself around her local community. However, she did not like driving in unfamiliar places, in heavy traffic or at night.

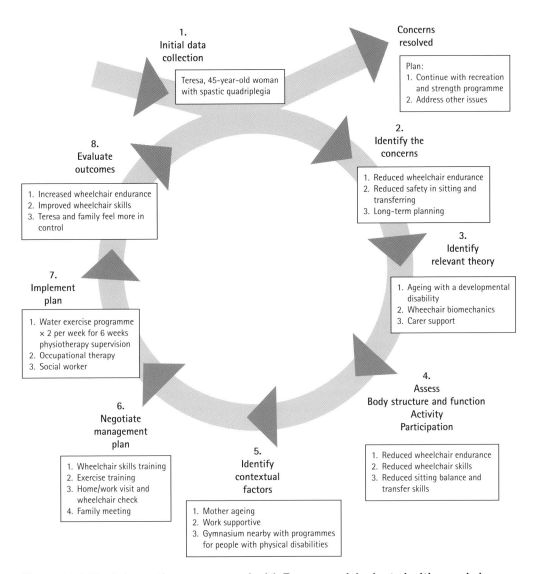

Figure 16.1 The intervention process used with Teresa: model adapted with permission from the Canadian Occupational Performance Process Model (CAOT, 2002).

Teresa had received physiotherapy and occupational therapy services as a child but she had not had direct therapy for the past 25 years. Teresa visited her local general practitioner for minor health concerns such as urinary tract infections, influenza and upper respiratory tract infections around five times a year. Teresa went through menopause about 3 years ago but had not received advice about the major changes that can occur in quality of life and health in the years around the menopause.

> **Box 16.1 GMFCS level IV snapshot**[1]
>
> Proportion of people with cerebral palsy classified as GMFCS IV: 9–15%
>
> Proportion of people classified as GMFCS level IV who:
>
> - have a severe intellectual disability (IQ <50) about 25%;
> - have a severe visual impairment 25–37%;
> - have epilepsy about 50%;
> - have behavioural problems less than 5%;
> - have hip displacement requiring surgery about 45%;
> - use a feeding tube 11%;
> - walk alone at home by age 4–12 years 0%;
> - walk with support at home by age 4–12 years 7%.

Stage 2: identify and prioritize concerns

Teresa and Jean were worried because Teresa's ability to sit-to-stand and step independently had deteriorated over the past 5 years. She had experienced four or five falls during transfers and dressing over the last year. Teresa had also noticed that she could not propel her wheelchair as far or as fast as she used to because she tired quickly. Teresa reported experiencing a long-standing moderate aching pain in her lower back, which did not stop her from doing things but was often worse at the end of a working day. The deep gnawing pain was getting her down.

Jean was finding it more difficult to provide the physical support that Teresa was increasingly requiring. Teresa and Jean had sought the referral after a recent fall when Jean needed help from the ambulance service to get Teresa off the floor because Jean did not have the strength to assist her.

Teresa and Jean clearly had a close relationship but apart from the physical and functional problems they mentioned, both appeared worried and, at times, almost agitated. Jean was becoming increasingly worried about what would happen to Teresa if she was no longer able to provide the amount of care and support that Teresa needed. Teresa was worried about being a burden on her mother, and wondered if her change of life was contributing to their problems. Teresa and Jean were very concerned that they could not maintain their current living arrangements.

---

1   See Chapter 2: p. 17 for details of the sources used to derive these data.

The most important concerns identified during the first interview were:

- increased risk of falls when transferring and dressing (Figure 16.2);
- reduced distance and speed of mobility in her manual wheelchair;
- moderate low back pain;
- support for Teresa's primary carer and the longer-term issues for ongoing care as Teresa's mother aged;
- support and advice for Teresa on managing the symptoms of her menopause.

Stage 3: identify relevant theory

Ageing with a developmental disability

The number of adults with cerebral palsy is increasing in most Western societies. This growth is due to the increased survival of low-birthweight infants and increased longevity of the adult population. Studies show that from 65 to 90% of children with cerebral palsy survive into adulthood (Rapp and Torres, 2000; Zaffuto-Sforza, 2005), which means there are large numbers of adults who need support and services from the health and human services sectors. Although there is an increasing need for

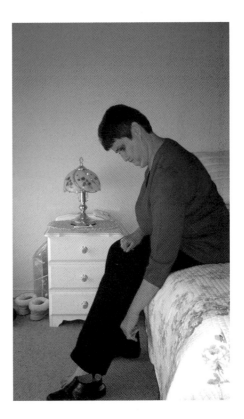

Figure 16.2 Teresa.

services, in most communities appropriate services are scarce and therefore more difficult to access for adults with cerebral palsy (Elrod and DeJong, 2008). This is particularly true for adults with cerebral palsy who have lived independently or with the support of their families in the general community. Because these adults and their families have coped successfully for many years they often have inadequate knowledge of what services are available. For these people it is often difficult to cope with the combined effects of the impairments associated with cerebral palsy and the effects of ageing. A gradual decline in functional ability is often not noticed, or not acted on, until a crisis arises.

As adults with cerebral palsy often have limited contact with physiotherapists and occupational therapists, therapists should assess the suitability of, and wear and tear on, adapted equipment and mobility devices. Advances in rehabilitation technology make it particularly important to conduct a home visit to assess the usefulness of equipment currently in the home, and the need for other equipment or adaptations that will optimize independence and safety. Teresa had purchased her wheelchair from a local independent living centre and it required some maintenance. The brakes were not functioning optimally on both sides and on questioning Teresa reported that on more than one occasion the wheelchair had slipped during transfers and this had contributed to her falling.

Chronic musculoskeletal pain is relatively common in adults with cerebral palsy, with around a third of the population experiencing chronic pain (Jahnsen et al, 2004). Back pain is the most common problem (Jahnsen et al, 2004). There is evidence that pain in adults with cerebral palsy is significantly associated with chronic fatigue, low life satisfaction and deteriorating physical function (Jahnsen et al, 2004). Physical fatigue is also common in adults with cerebral palsy (Jahnsen et al, 2003; Kemp and Mosqueda, 2004) and there is evidence that fatigue has an impact on the preservation of functional skills and life satisfaction (Jahnsen et al, 2003).

Teresa's reported difficulties with low back pain and increasing fatigue were consistent with the functional impairment syndrome identified as an important phenomenon in adults with disabilities. This syndrome includes pain, fatigue and weakness and occurs in increasing proportions of adults with disability as they age (Kemp and Mosqueda, 2004). Along with these physical symptoms, untreated depression is also a potential problem for adults with cerebral palsy (Kemp and Mosqueda 2004).

Little research has been completed on the issue of menopause and disability. Symptoms associated with menopause are variable, and whether or not a woman with a disability attributes her emotional and physical symptoms to menopause may depend on her self-definition (Morrow, 2003). However, increased musculoskeletal pain, and an increased risk of osteoporosis, can be associated with menopause and may be relevant for Teresa (Morrow, 2003). If Teresa has osteoporosis, her falls will markedly increase her fracture risk. Some of the symptoms of menopause may be alleviated by hormone therapy, which can also increase bone density (Royal Australian and New Zealand College of

Obstetricians and Gyaecologists [RANZCOG] 2006). However, long-term hormone therapy is not recommended because of the increased risk of breast cancer (RANZCOG, 2006). Providing emotional support and information about choices is very important in the management of menopause (Morrow, 2003).

Carer support
Approximately one third of adults with cerebral palsy live at home (Murphy et al, 2000). At the same time that the physical needs of the adults with cerebral palsy increase, many of their parents are becoming elderly. These carers start to lose the physical capacity to care for the day-to-day needs of an adult with cerebral palsy. In addition, they begin to lose their own support networks as other adult children leave home or, as occurred in Teresa's case, one parent becomes unwell or dies. Parents of adults with cerebral palsy often become increasingly distressed about what will happen to their grown-up child when they can no longer provide adequate support. Key elements to support transition to adult-centred health care have been identified as adequate preparation, flexible timing of the provision of services and support, the provision of care coordination and the introduction of interested adult-centred health care providers (Binks et al, 2007; see Chapter 14). The distress exhibited by Jean could be an example of parental grief associated with having a child with a disability. Many parents with a disabled child suffer sorrow, particularly during times of transition (Renzinbrinck and Bruce, 2008). Teresa and Jean's concern about how they were coping at home highlighted the need for the therapist to inquire about the capacities of the family and their plans for future care and support.

Biomechanical considerations
Wheelchair propulsion is highly inefficient with a gross mechanical efficiency of at most 10% (Veeger, 1989). Prolonged wheelchair use places high energy and mechanical demands on the user. It is possible that Teresa's musculoskeletal aches and pains were related to the high mechanical demands of prolonged wheelchair use.

Despite being a long-term user, if Teresa's wheelchair skills were deficient or inefficient, this might increase energy demands and contribute to reduced wheelchair endurance. Wheelchair skills include being able to move footrests and other accessories out of the way, manoeuvring skills such as being able to turn a chair 180° in place, transfer skills and obstacle negotiating skills, such as being able to go up an incline (Kirby et al, 2002).

Stage 4: assessment of body function, activity and participation
Table 16.1 describes the list of assessments that was developed based on the initial discussion with Teresa and Jean and with consideration of relevant theory.

Assessment of activity

WHEELCHAIR ENDURANCE
Wheelchair endurance was tested by measuring how far Teresa could propel her wheelchair in 6 minutes on a flat standardized course. The test was completed twice,

Table 16.1 Assessments for Teresa

Body function and structure	Activity	Participation
Muscle strength 1 repetition maximum for inclined waist press Grip strength	*Wheelchair endurance* 6-minute distance test	Qualitative report
Sitting balance Modified functional reach test	*Wheelchair skills* Wheelchair Skills Test	
	Sit-to-stand Timed sit-to-stand (3 times)	
	Low back function Oswestry Disability Questionnaire	
	Self-reported activitiy limitation Patient Specific Functional Scale	
	Activity limitation Functional Independence Measure (FIM)	

with the first trial regarded as practice. Medium distance wheelchair tests, assessing the distance travelled in 12 minutes, have been found to be responsive to change in young people with cerebral palsy, with improvements of 29% reported after an 8-week strength training programme (O'Connell and Barnhart, 1995). Improvements in medium distance wheelchair range were also highly associated with improvements in upper limb muscle strength (O'Connell et al, 1992).

WHEELCHAIR SKILLS
Teresa's wheelchair skills were assessed with the Wheelchair Skills Test (Kirby et al, 2002, MacPhee et al, 2004; see Appendix, p. 296). Twenty-five skills were assessed in four levels: basic skills, wheelchair manoeuvring and daily living skills, obstacle negotiating skills and advanced wheelchair skills. Each skill was scored on a 3-point ordinal scale: 0 if unable to complete the skill safely; 1 for partial completion; and 2 for successful and safe completion. The total score is recorded as a percentage of the total possible score of 50.

TIMED SIT-TO-STAND
Sit-to-stand was assessed by measuring the time it took for Teresa to move independently from sit-to-stand three times (see Appendix, p. 296).

LOW BACK PAIN AND FUNCTION

Activity limitation related to Teresa's low back pain was assessed with the Oswestry Disability Questionnaire (Fairbank et al, 1980). This widely used functional back scale asks how back pain has affected the person in ten areas such as personal care, lifting, sitting, social life and travelling (Fairbank et al, 1980). There are three categorical descriptors: 0–20% indicates minimal activity limitation due to low back pain; 20–40% moderate disability; 40–60% severe disability; and greater than 60% disability indicates that back pain impinges on all aspects of the person's life (Fairbank et al, 1980). A change of 10% in the Oswestry Disability Questionnaire indicates that the person being assessed has changed beyond measurement error (Davidson and Keating, 2002). For Teresa, the scale was adjusted to make it meaningful for her. For example, the section that asks about 'walking' was amended to ask about 'locomotion with your wheelchair'. The Oswestry Disability Questionnaire also includes one item that asks about pain intensity on an ordinal scale from zero (I have no pain at the moment) to five (the pain is the worst imaginable at the moment).

SELF-REPORTED ACTIVITY LIMITATION

The Patient Specific Functional Scale (Stratford et al, 1995) assessed difficulties with three activities that Teresa identified as important to her. Teresa identified

* standing from sitting;
* stepping; and
* getting from the car park to the office in her wheelchair.

She rated each task on a 0 (unable to perform activity) to 10 (able to perform activity) scale. The item scores of the three activities are averaged, with a lower score indicating greater activity limitation. A change of at least 2 units on the scale can be interpreted as being due to change beyond measurement error (Stratford et al, 1995). A possible limitation of the scale for Teresa is that most of the scale's development and testing has been on people with musculoskeletal impairment.

GENERALIZED ACTIVITY LIMITATION

The motor subscale of the Functional Independence Measure (FIM, see Appendix, p. 292) was used as a global measure of Teresa's activity limitation.

ASSESSMENT OF MOBILITY DEVICE

A thorough assessment of Teresa's manual wheelchair showed that neither of the brakes was functioning well. The right footplate was loose and did not clip back securely during transfers. It had swung back on several occasions and hit Teresa's ankle painfully. The tyres of the chair were badly worn, which made them slip on wet surfaces.

In an attempt to relieve the pain in her back, Teresa had placed several cushions in her wheelchair. However, the very soft seat cushion facilitated hip flexion (and posteriorly tilted pelvis) in sitting when Teresa was at her desk at work. This increased trunk flexion made it difficult for Teresa to alter her sitting posture during the day. In addition, the soft seat made it more difficult for Teresa to move from sit-to-stand because as she tried to rise she tended to sink into the cushion. Adding a seat cushion had also raised Teresa's sitting height, so her footplates were slightly too low for comfortable foot placement.

Table 16.2 summarizes the findings from the assessments of Teresa's activity performance.

Body function and structure

MUSCLE STRENGTH
Muscle strength was measured using a one-repetition maximum (1RM) inclined waist press (see Appendix, p. 288). The inclined waist press involved Teresa seated in her wheelchair facing away from a pulley-operated weight stack. She then pushed away from herself against resistance starting at waist level and inclined slightly towards the floor. The amount of weight that could be pushed on each side through full range to full elbow extension in the position of slight shoulder flexion was recorded. The inclined waist press was relevant to Teresa because it replicated the muscle actions required by her to propel her wheelchair.

Table 16.2 Assessment of activity

Activity		
Wheelchair endurance (6-min test)	174 metres	
Wheelchair Skills Test	62% (31/50)	
Sit-to-stand	8.3 seconds	
Back function (Oswestry Scale)	18% Pain intensity: minimal	
Self-reported activity limitation (Patient Specific Functional Scale) (Score range 0–10)	Sit-to-stand Stepping Wheelchair from car to work Average	4.0 2.0 6.0 4.0
Functional Independence Measure (Score range 13–91)	74/91	
Wheelchair assessment	Brakes, footplates and cushioning need attention	

SITTING BALANCE

Assessment of sitting balance was important as Teresa's interview had identified sitting balance and a lack of safety during transfers as problems. Adequate sitting balance in wheelchair users is a prerequisite to perform upper limb movements necessary for activities of daily living (Sprigle et al, 2007). The Pediatric Reach Test (Bartlett and Birmingham, 2003; see Appendix, p. 295) was used to assess Teresa's sitting balance.

Table 16.3 summarizes the assessment findings of the tests of body structure and functioning for Teresa.

Participation

Teresa's societal participation was assessed within the interview with her and her mother, Jean. Table 16.4 summarizes some of the key qualitative findings noted during the interview. The responses were organized according to domains considered important in the evaluation of societal participation: getting around, looking after self, work and leisure, getting on with people, awareness of surroundings and ability to afford things (Harwood and Ebrahim, 1995).

Stage 5: contextual factors: environmental and personal

Environmental factors

Teresa's mother Jean was her main carer but she was finding it increasingly difficult to provide adequate support for Teresa although they were both keen at this stage for Teresa to remain living in the family home. Teresa's older brother and sister and their families were supportive but they were very busy. They visited Teresa and her mother about once a fortnight.

Teresa had worked full time for 10 years at a small real estate agency located in her local shopping mall (Figure 16.3). She was a valued employee, who was good with customers

Table 16.3 Assessment findings for the tests of body structure and function

Body structure and function		
Muscle strength 1RM inclined waist press	Right Left	8 kg 12 kg
Sitting balance Pediatric Reach test	Total Forward Left Right	98 cm 38 cm 28 cm 32 cm
1RM, one-repetition maximum.		

Table 16.4 Societal participation (key findings from interview)

Participation	
Getting around	*Teresa*: 'I find I get tired now just getting from my car to my desk at work – it feels like I've done a day's work before I start.'
Looking after self	*Mother*: 'I think we are OK now, but I worry about what will happen in the next 10 years – I am not getting any younger. While my other grown-up children do visit us, I don't think they have the time to do much more. . .we have started talking more about where Teresa might go to live if I can't look after her any more.'
	Teresa: 'I have always needed my mother to help me a bit with little things like getting my shoes on, but I seem to need more help with these things recently. I do worry what I will do when mum can no longer support me. It's probably time for me to look around to see what's available – you know in terms of other places to live.'
	Teresa: 'I feel like I am ageing quickly. Things like realizing that I will now never have children and the problems I have been having at home bring it all to me.'
	Mother: 'I think it might be good to see if someone could look at the set up of our house. Perhaps we should get some rails for the bathroom and the toilet, and I have heard that there might be equipment that we could get that Teresa could use to help dress herself. . .'
Work and leisure	*Teresa*: 'I guess my focus has been so much on keeping my independence that I have never really developed many leisure activities – there just hasn't seemed to be enough time. I know though that I have to take more care of myself. I suppose I really should get fitter so that I can keep up.'
	Teresa: 'I really like my job. I have been there for 10 years now and the time has just flown.'
Getting on with people	*Teresa*: 'I love my job. I especially like my boss and the clients that come in – that's something I really value and I would hate to have to leave.'
	Note: no comments were made about 'being able to afford things' or 'awareness of surroundings'.

Figure 16.3 Teresa at work.

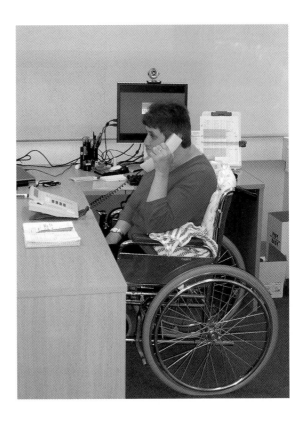

and dependable. The manager of the agency, Michael, was supportive of Teresa and happy to consider flexible working hours. There was a community gymnasium and aquatic centre located about 1 kilometre from the real estate agency that offered a range of group land and water exercise programmes and had convenient parking. A physiotherapist conducted classes each week in the gymnasium and aquatic centre for children and some adults with disabilities.

Personal factors
Teresa was coping well at work but she felt increasingly tired and she was also worried about her mother's health. Teresa was very sociable and had several close friends who she had met through her work and who she saw frequently. Teresa wondered if some of her problems were to do with her menopause. Teresa had no cognitive impairments.

Teresa wanted to make changes to her lifestyle to become fitter and to help arrest the physical decline she had noticed. She preferred to participate in a group activity, but didn't want to travel far. She was happy to participate in a programme designed for adults with chronic health conditions or disabilities because she had found that it was important for the group leader to have some knowledge of conditions that might impact on health or well-being. She was prepared to implement a regular day-time programme up to 3 times a week, because she didn't like to drive at night.

Stage 6: management plan

Summary of assessment findings

The assessment confirmed and documented the main problems prioritized by Teresa and her mother. She had limited wheelchair endurance and speed, and some difficulties manoeuvring the chair around her environment. Teresa's inclined waist press scores indicated that a relative lack of strength in the muscles that propel her wheelchair, especially on the right, could be contributing to her reduced wheelchair endurance. Her moderate scores in the Paediatric Reach Test, the sit-to-stand test and difficulty stepping confirmed Teresa's concerns about safety in sitting and her increased risk of falling when transferring. Her problems in this area were also identified by some items in the Wheelchair Skills Test.

Despite these specific problems, Teresa scored well on the FIM mobility subscale even if she was starting to require some assistance. Her score of 18% on the Oswestry Disability Questionnaire indicated that her long standing back problem was only minimally disabling.

Teresa's wheelchair brakes, footplates and tyres all needed attention and the cushions changed to provide more upright sitting posture especially as her wheelchair was used as her chair at work. Because Teresa's back pain was often more severe after a long day at work the occupational therapist and physiotherapist arranged to assess the ergonomics of her office furniture to make sure that this was not contributing to her back pain. In addition, Teresa and Jean had both indicated it would be helpful to have an assessment of their home to see if adaptations might help them, or if there was equipment available that would increase Teresa's independence in dressing.

Teresa's statement that she 'felt she was ageing quickly' and the keen awareness that she would not have children of her own, suggest that the link between her problems and her menopause should be fully explored. Both Teresa and Jean were concerned about long-term care. Teresa was socially integrated into her local community (with family, work and a few friends) even if she had not developed any community leisure activities.

Negotiated treatment plan

Based on the assessment findings and after further discussion with Teresa and her mother the following multidisciplinary management plan was developed.

PHYSIOTHERAPY

A series of weekly appointments with the physiotherapist over 6 weeks focused on problem-solving and skills training. The key elements of the physiotherapy programme were as follows:

- wheelchair skills training programme;
- exercise training:

- resistance training programme for the major muscles involved in wheelchair propulsion
- referral to a supervised water exercise class at the local gymnasium
- initial management of back pain;
- organization of repairs to wheelchair, and for optimal seating.

OCCUPATIONAL THERAPY

The occupational therapist negotiated a short-term plan to conduct equipment, home and workplace assessments to

- advise on strategies and organize for supply and installation of assistive devices to increase safety in transfers and independence with self-care, particularly dressing;
- advise and help organize optimal ergonomic adjustments to working environment;
- evaluate the home for her risk for falls and to provide recommendations about safe practices.

Teresa also indicated that there were other issues she would like assistance with, but that she would prefer to resolve them over a longer period. Therefore, the occupational therapist agreed that when Teresa's short-term goals had been met and she had completed her physiotherapy training programme the occupational therapist would:

- explore the potential need for a driving assessment and further driver training following Teresa's comment about not wanting to drive at night or in unfamiliar places;
- collaborate with the social worker to begin future planning with Teresa and her family for independent or assisted living arrangements;
- further explore Teresa's opportunities for and satisfaction with her social and recreational participation.

SOCIAL WORK

The social worker arranged to meet with Teresa and her mother to

- assess and then advise on how to obtain any financial, physical or other community supports that might be able to be provided to Teresa and her mother;
- help identify and negotiate for any family supports available to Teresa;
- investigate options for future housing needs;
- investigate options for ongoing care coordination for Teresa and her family.

Stage 7: implement plan

Wheelchair review

Teresa's wheelchair still fitted her, but it had not been regularly maintained since its purchase. Arrangements were made to have the chair serviced by the supplier and Teresa's brother, Dominic, offered to learn how to undertake basic care including the following:

- checking the rear wheel alignment to ensure the chair ran straight;
- looking for signs of wear including problems with the spokes, any sideways movements in the wheels, loose nuts or bolts, stability and fit of removable parts such as foot and arm rests and the ease with which the chair folded;
- the tyre pressure and wear of the tyres;
- the effectiveness of the brakes.

Once the chair was in good repair, the therapist reviewed Teresa's seating posture. Because Teresa can adjust her position frequently in her wheelchair she has not had any pressure ulcers in the past so the cushions in Teresa's wheelchair were replaced with a high-density foam seat, which was rounded at the front. This provided comfort but also provided a firm base from which Teresa could sit more erect and from which she could transfer into and out of the chair more easily. A firm lumbar roll was also provided to support her lumbar spine during sitting.

Raising the footplates of the wheelchair slightly ensured that Teresa's hip and knees were maintained in 90° of flexion, with the thighs approximately horizontal and her feet resting comfortably on the footplates. Teresa needed to use the armrests of her chair to support herself when she was transferring in and out of her chair. Therefore, they were placed at a height measured from under her elbow to the cushion surface when her shoulders were in neutral and elbows flexed to 90° (Dudgeon and Deitz, 2008).

Wheelchair skills training

Teresa started a training programme designed to improve her skills at using her wheelchair. Improvements of about 25% in wheelchair skills have been reported after implementing a training programme for adult wheelchair users with musculoskeletal and neurological disorders (MacPhee et al, 2004). The skills that Teresa had not been able to complete successfully during the Wheelchair Skills Test formed the basis of her training programme. For Teresa, these included skills such as completing transfers, adjusting her footplates, turning through pylons while propelling forward, turning in a narrow space, and being able to pick an object off the floor. The programme consisted of a 30-minute session during each visit to the physiotherapist and applied principles of motor skill learning, including practice and feedback on knowledge of performance (Carr and Shepherd, 2000). During each session, practice of skills took place in a block manner. In addition, at the last part of each session, there was practice of all skills completed successfully in random order.

Exercise training: strength training

Teresa also started an exercise programme to improve the muscle performance of the major muscles involved in wheelchair propulsion (Taylor et al, 2004; see Chapter 4). The choice of exercise aimed to mimic the major muscles involved in wheelchair propulsion (Keyser et al, 2003) meaning that there was greater specificity of training and improved likelihood that benefits would carry over into improved wheelchair use. There is evidence that increasing upper limb strength can improve wheelchair endurance (O'Connell and Barnhart, 1995).

Teresa was taught a single exercise, the seated inclined waist press, to be completed with elasticized bands at home three times per week (Table 16.5). Adults living in the community can increase muscle strength using elasticized bands at home and they provide an efficient and feasible method of strength training (Dodd et al, 2004). To help monitor progress Teresa completed an exercise log of each training session, recording band resistance (colour), number of sets and number of repetitions completed. Exercise dosage was consistent with guidelines of the American College of Sports Medicine (2002). The initial training intensity was set by Teresa's therapist as three sets of between 8 and 10 repetitions of the exercise, with a 2-minute rest period between each set.

Teresa's therapist started her training with a yellow elasticized band on each side. To make it easier hand pieces were attached to the elasticized bands. During the inclined waist press, Teresa was encouraged to maintain a neutral upright trunk posture to promote core stability and improved sitting balance. By the end of week one, Teresa was very pleased because she could complete three sets of 14 repetitions on the left and three sets of 9 repetitions on the right side. To meet one of the key principles of progressive resistance training (to progress load) Teresa progressed to the higher resistance red band for training her left side in week two. After 3 weeks Teresa could complete three sets of ten repetitions with the yellow band on her right side and progressed to the red band.

Table 16.5 Teresa's strength training programme

Exercise	Starting position	Description	Dosage
Inclined waist press	Seated in wheelchair, hips and knees flexed, feet placed flat on footplates; wrist by waist with shoulder extended and elbow flexed; trunk neutral posture not leaning back; facing away from table	With band just on tension, slowly extend band forward inclined toward the floor until elbow fully extended. Maintain trunk posture throughout. Do separately for each arm	3 sets of 8–10 repetitions 2-minute rest between sets Complete exercise 3 times per week

Exercise training: water exercises
Teresa and her therapist decided to refer her to a twice-weekly, 45-minute water exercise class at the local gymnasium. This appealed to Teresa because she had enjoyed water exercises as a child, but had not been in a pool for many years. The aims of the programme were:

- to increase Teresa's fitness and exercise capacity;
- to see if water exercise would help to ease and manage Teresa's mild but chronic back pain; and
- to provide a fitness and leisure option that Teresa could continue in the community.

A recent systematic review found some evidence of benefits from water exercise programmes for young people with cerebral palsy (Getz et al, 2006). Teresa's programme was with a small group of people with physical disabilities supervised by a physiotherapist. Adequate supervision and expert instruction is important in setting up water exercise programmes for people with disabilities (Kelly and Darrah, 2005). Teresa's class was in the middle of the afternoon and she organized to make up time lost from work.

Water exercises can include specific activities completed in water, the Halliwick method or adapted swimming lessons (Getz et al, 2006). Teresa's aims were to increase exercise capacity. Therefore her programme focused on adapted swimming lessons and included supervised swimming drills with kickboards, flippers and other flotation devices. It was hypothesized that facilitating trunk stability through swimming might help Teresa's core stability and sitting balance during activities out of the pool. The programme began at a moderate level of intensity (five or six on a ten-point effort scale where ten represents highest effort), and after a few weeks progress towards vigorous intensity (seven or eight on the ten-point effort scale). This intensity of training is approaching recommended levels of aerobic training for older adults (Nelson et al, 2007; see Fitness training, Chapter 4).

Initial management of back pain
Teresa's low back pain was addressed initially through the water exercise group. There is strong evidence that people with long-standing back pain can reduce pain and increase activity with exercise programmes (Hayden, 2005). There is little evidence that one type of exercise is more beneficial than another; rather the key component is intensity: people with back pain benefit from exercise particularly if it is moderately intensive (Hayden, 2005). To manage the postural component contributing to Teresa's back pain, the physiotherapist liaised with the occupational therapist to ensure that her chair provided adequate lumbar support and an appropriate cushion to make ensure Teresa was not sitting with excessive hip flexion, as this transfers greater loads to the lumbar spine.

Home and work visit

WORK

The occupational therapist and the physiotherapist completed two joint visits to Teresa's workplace to assess the ergonomics of her workstation. After discussion with Teresa, it was decided that she would continue to use her manual wheelchair as her office chair because she wanted to have maximum mobility around the office, and she wanted to minimize transfers from seat to seat. Teresa would require an adjustable height desk.

Adjustments made to Teresa's workstation used the following guidelines (Jacobs, 2008).

- The desk height was positioned so work was performed at Teresa's elbow height.
- Her thighs were cleared between the chair and the under surface of the desk.
- The computer screen was located an arm's length from Teresa when she was sitting at the desk and the top of the screen located about 10 centimetres below her eye height.
- The keyboard was aligned with the computer screen (or the document holder if it was being used as the major viewing surface) and directly in front of Teresa so that there was no need to twist or rotate to use it. Teresa was reminded that the keyboard set up needed to allow her wrists and hands to be in a neutral position for most of the typing time, and that the mouse should be placed close to the side of the keyboard.
- It became clear that one of the major problems was the amount of uninterrupted time Teresa spent sitting in one position while working at her desk. So after Teresa trialled a few different programs, a software program was installed onto Teresa's computer that prompted rest breaks and demonstrated simple sitting exercises. Suppliers of these ergonomic stretch break programs can be located on the world wide web.

HOME VISIT

The occupational therapist also completed two home visits to assess the equipment and adaptations in her home. The Westmead Home Safety Assessment (Clemson, 1997) was used to review both Teresa's and her mother's risk of falls and identify environmental hazards. As well as Teresa's identified difficulties with transfers and dressing, assessment of the home revealed that her risk of falls in the toilet and shower, and her mother's risk of a back injury while assisting her, were high. After the home visit, they made an appointment with the independent living centre therapist to review equipment options and make selections. Centres for independent living are available in many communities where they provide specialist advice regarding equipment prescription, a library of equipment for short-term loan or trial and show rooms for viewing and trialling alternate brands and styles of equipment prior to purchase.

The following home modifications were completed.

- *Shower*: the door to the shower was removed and the raised lip around this opening was removed to enable easier access by Teresa with her wheelchair, and for Jean to access the shower if Teresa required assistance. To enable more independence, the plastic chair she had been using was replaced with a sturdy shower seat with armrests and also grab rails were installed in the shower cubicle. The shower head was fitted with a hand-held system with flexible tubing and the position of the taps altered to allow access without having to reach through the water to turn them on or off. Repositioning of the soap and other shelves allowed Teresa to reach them easily when seated.

- *Toilet*: Teresa selected an over-toilet frame to provide a safer means of transfer and greater stability during toileting and arranged for the toilet roll holder to be repositioned for easier access.
- *Dressing*: Teresa's difficulty with dressing her lower body related to maintaining her safe balance while reaching to her feet or pulling up and fastening her trousers or skirts while standing. Provision of a long-handled shoehorn and sock/stocking donning devices reduced the amount of reaching. Together the therapist and Teresa discussed a plan for gradually upgrading her wardrobe to include items that were simple to don and fasten but fashionable and attractive.

Family meeting

The social worker facilitated a number of meetings with Teresa, Jean and the extended family to discuss their long-term concerns. Through these discussions, the family came to a better understanding of Teresa and Jean's fears about the future. Teresa's brother and sister wanted to be involved in supporting Teresa, but everyone agreed that it was not desirable for Teresa to live with anyone else in the family. The social worker then organized for Teresa and her mother to view some of the alternative housing and support options that were available. Alternative accommodation was not necessary immediately but Teresa placed her name on the residential list so that if she required either temporary accommodation and ultimately, permanent accommodation this could be organized quickly.

The social worker also determined that Teresa and her mother were eligible for low-cost council home help. This service provided a weekly visit from a person to carry out light house duties around the home. In addition, Teresa's mother was eligible for a carer's allowance which supplemented the costs associated with supporting Teresa in the home. After further discussion the family decided it would be beneficial for a care coordinator to be appointed so that Teresa and her mother had a person they could contact as other issues arose.

During a subsequent session the social worker also explored feelings of distress exhibited by Teresa and Jean. As a result, the social worker referred Teresa to the local women's' health clinic as a resource for support with her menopause and provided Jean with a resource where she could seek more information about being a parent of an adult with a disability.

Stage 8: evaluate outcomes

After 6 weeks each outcome measure was readministered to determine the programme's effectiveness. Teresa's Wheelchair Skills Test increased from 62 to 78% and the 6-minute distance from 174 to 196 metres. She also demonstrated approximately 10% improvement in muscle strength for the wheelchair propulsion arm muscles, and her self-reported activity limitation of getting from the car to work had improved from 6 to 7.5. These were positive but modest improvements and may not represent real improvement over and above measurement error. However, there is a plausible relationship between these variables, that is, maybe the improved strength, wheelchair skills and swimming had increased Teresa's exercise capacity as represented by wheelchair endurance. This gave the therapist confidence that they were on the right track. The programme had only been going for 6 weeks and a longer-term programme might be required to get more substantial improvements.

Other assessments remained relatively unchanged e.g. Oswestry Disability Questionnaire (14%), sit-to-stand test (8.2 seconds), sitting balance (103 centimetres). Teresa's low back pain remained mild. The lack of change in sitting balance and sit–to-stand probably reflected that there were no targeted interventions for these problems. Teresa had not had any falls in the last 6 weeks but this may not represent improvement because she had only fallen four or five times in the last year.

Qualitative outcomes

For Teresa, a key benefit was 'getting things sorted out with her wheelchair and at home'. She now felt more confident with transfers and with getting herself dressed. She said 'how it was great to be involved in the pool and it seemed to give her more energy to do other things'. The pool gave her some 'freedom of movement'. Both Teresa and her mother valued the meetings facilitated by the social worker. Teresa was seen by a very supportive doctor at the women's health clinic. They had decided not to proceed with hormone therapy but she had provided Teresa with a lot of information and support. As Teresa said, 'I feel more in control now'. Teresa's mother said that she now had 'some peace of mind'.

Teresa was happy with her progress, and it was agreed that she would continue going to her water exercise class twice a week and continue with her home exercise strengthening programme three times a week. Therefore, the physiotherapist made a time to meet Teresa again in 6 weeks and they planned a burst of treatment later in the year focusing more on transfer and balance skills training. Teresa and the occupational therapist planned to meet again in the break between the physiotherapy interventions.

> **Box 16.2 Key clinical messages**
>
> ● It is important for therapists not to overlook the needs of adults with cerebral palsy and their families as they age.
> ● Like the rest of the community, adults with cerebral palsy require regular health checks from a primary physician, preferably someone who has a professional interest in people living with a congenital disability.
> ● Therapy for adults with cerebral palsy is often focused on resolving specific functional problems and helping as a resource to address health issues rather than ongoing regular therapy sessions.

References

American College of Sports Medicine (2002) Progression models in resistance training for healthy adults. *Med Sci Sports Exerc*, 34, 364–80.

Binks JA, Barden WS, Burke TA & Young NL (2007) What do we really know about the transition to adult-centred health care? A focus on cerebral palsy and spina bifida. *Arch Phys Med Rehabil*, 88, 1064–73.

Bartlett D & Birmingham T (2003) Validity and reliability of a pediatric reach test. *Pediatr Phys Ther*, 15, 84–92.

Canadian Association of Occupational Therapists (CAOT) (2002) *Enabling Occupation: An Occupational Therapy Perspective*. Ottawa: Canadian Association of Occupational Therapists.

Carr JH & Shepherd RB (2000) A motor learning model for rehabilitation. In: Carr JH & Shepherd RB (eds) *Movement Sciences Foundations for Physical Therapy in Rehabilitation*: 33–110. Gaithersburg, MD: Aspen.

Clemson L (1997) *Westmead Home Safety Assessment (WeHSA)*. Melbourne: Coordinates Publications.

Davidson M & Keating JL (2002) A comparison of five low back disability questionnaires: reliability and responsiveness. *Phys Ther*, 82, 8–24.

Dodd KJ, Taylor NF & Bradley S (2004) Strength training for older people. In: Morris M & Schoo A (eds) *Optimizing Exercise and Physical Activity in Older People*: 125–8. Edinburgh: Butterworth-Heinemann.

Dudgeon BJ & Deitz JC (2008) Wheelchair selection. In: Radomski MV & TromblyLatham CA (eds) *Occupational Therapy for Physical Dysfunction*. Baltimore, MD: Wolters Kluwer/Lipppincott Williams & Wilkins.

Eliasson AC, Krumlinde-Sundholm L, Rösblad B, Beckung E, Arner M, Öhrvall A & Rosenbaum PL (2006) The Manual Ability Classification System (MACS) for children with cerebral palsy: scale development and evidence of validity and reliability. *Dev Med Child Neurol*, 48, 549–54.

Elrod CS & DeJong G (2008) Determinants of utilization of physical rehabilitation services for persons with chronic and disabling conditions: an exploratory study. *Arch Phys Med Rehabil*, 89, 114–20.

Fairbank JC, Couper J, Davies JB & O'Brien JP (1980) The Oswestry Low Back Pain Disability Questionnaire. *Physiother*, 66, 271–3.

Getz M, Hutzler Y &Vermeer A (2006) Effects of aquatic interventions in children with neuromotor impairments: a systematic review of the literature. *Clin Rehabil*, 20, 927–36.

Harwood RH & Ebrahim S (1995) *Manual of the London Handicap Scale*. Nottingham: Department of Health Care of the Elderly, University of Nottingham.

Hayden JA, Van Tulder MW, Malmivaara AV & Koes BW (2005) Exercise therapy for treatment of non-specific low back pain. *Cochrane Database of Systematic Reviews* 2004, Issue 4. Art. No.: CD000335. DOI: 10.1002/14651858.CD000335.pub2.

Jacobs K (2008) *Ergonomics for Therapists*, 3rd edn. St Louis, MO: Mosby Elsevier.

Jahnsen R, Villien L, Stranghelle JK & Holm I (2003) Fatigue in adults with cerebral palsy in Norway compared with the general population. *Dev Med Child Neurol*, 45, 296–303.

Jahnsen R, Villien L, Aamodt G, Stranghelle JK & Holm I (2004) Musculoskeletal pain in adults with cerebral palsy compared with the general population. *J Rehabil Med*, 36, 78–84.

Kelly M & Darrah J (2005) Aquatic exercise for children with cerebral palsy. *Dev Med Child Neurol* 47, 838–42.

Keyser RE, Rasch EK, Finley M & Rodgers MM (2003) Improved upper-body endurance following a 12-week home exercise program for manual wheelchair users. *J Rehabil Res Dev*, 40, 510.

Kemp B & Mosqueda L (2004) *Aging with a Disability: What the Clinician Needs to Know*. Baltimore, MD: The John Hopkins University Press.

Kirby RL, Swuste J, Dupuis DJ, MacLeod DA & Monroe R (2002) The wheelchair skills test: a pilot study of a new outcome measure. *Arch Phys Med Rehabil*, 83, 10–18.

MacPhee AH, Kirby L, Coolen AL, Smith C, MacLeod DA & Dupois DJ (2004) Wheelchair skills training program: a randomised clinical trial of wheelchair users undergoing initial rehabilitation. *Arch Phys Med Rehabil*, 85, 41–50.

Morrow M (2003) Challenges of change: midlife, menopause and disability. *Womens Health Newsl*, 58, 8–12.

Murphy KP, Molnar GE & Lankasky K (2000) Employment and social issues in adults with cerebral palsy. *Arch Phys Med Rehab*, 81, 807–11.

Nelson ME, Rejeski WJ, Blair SN, Duncan PW, Judge JO, King AC, Macera CA & Castaneda-Sceppa C (2007) Physcial activity and public health in older adults: recommendations from the American College of Sports Medicine and the American Heart Association. *Circulation* 116, 1094–105.

O'Connell DG & Barnhart R (1995) Improvement in wheelchair propulsion in pediatric wheelchair users through resistance training. *Arch Phys Med Rehabil*, 76, 368–72.

O'Connell DG, Barnhart R & Parks L (1992) Muscular endurance and wheelchair propulsion in children with cerebral palsy or myelomeningocele. *Arch Phys Med Rehabil*, 73, 709–11.

Palisano RJ, Rosenbaum PL, Bartlett D & Livingston MH (2008) Content validity of the expanded and revised gross motor function classification system. *Dev Med Child Neurol*, 50, 744–50.

Rapp CE & Torres MM (2000) The adult with cerebral palsy. *Arch Fam Med*, 9, 466–72.

Renzinbrinck I & Bruce E (2008) *Parental Grief and Adjustment to a Child with a Disability*. Victoria: Department of Human Services (http://www.education.vic.gov.au/ocecd/earlychildhood/library/publications/ecis/grief.html).

Royal Australian and New Zealand College of Obstetricians and Gynaecologists (2006) *College Statement: Management of Menopause*. East Melbourne: The Royal Australian and New Zealand College of Obstetricians and Gynaecologists.

Sprigle S, Maurer C & Holowka M (2007) Development of valid and reliable measures of postural stability. *J Spinal Cord Med*, 30, 40–9.

Stratford PW, Gill C, Westaway M & Binkley J (1995) Assessing disability and change on individual patients: a report of a patient specific measure. *Physiother Can*, 47, 258–63.

Taylor NF, Dodd KJ & Larkin H (2004) Adults with cerebral palsy benefit from participating in a strength training programme at a community gymnasium. *Disabil Rehabil*, 26, 1128–34.

Veeger HEJ (1999) Biomechanics of normal wheelchair propulsion In: van der Woude LHV (ed.) *Biomedical Aspects of Manual Wheelchair Propulsion: The State of the Art*. Amsterdam: IOS Press.

Zaffuto-Sforza CD (2005) Aging with cerebral palsy. *Phys Med Rehabil Clin N Am*, 16, 235–49.

Appendix

Assessment of the individual with cerebral palsy

This Appendix provides a brief introductory section on the measurement properties to consider when choosing an assessment tool. A description of some of the common assessment procedures used throughout the cases in Parts 2, 3 and 4 of the book (Chapters 5 to 16) is then provided, organized according to the International Classification of Functioning, Disability and Health (ICF) framework (World Health Organization, 2001).

Measurement properties

Determining which assessment to use involves knowledge of the properties of the assessment tools themselves. The important elements to understand include purpose, validity, reliability, responsiveness and clinical utility.

Purpose

Each assessment or test will have been designed for a specific purpose including description, prediction and/or evaluation. If you wish to evaluate the outcomes of intervention then choose assessments that were designed to be evaluative. If you need to predict future outcomes, you need to know the predictive ability of the assessment you choose. An important issue when deciding on the purpose of the assessment is whether you wish to assess capability (what a person can do, often in a clinical or laboratory setting) or performance (which reflects what a person usually does in their everyday life) (World Health Organization, 2001). An example of a scale that measures capability is the Gross Motor Function Measure (GMFM) (Russell et al, 2002) whereas the Functional Mobility Scale (FMS) (Harvey et al, 2007) measures performance.

Validity

There are many different types of validity but the bottom line is whether the assessment measures what it purports to measure: does it fulfil its intended purpose? Validity of a measure cannot be proven; rather the developers of a measure should provide evidence in support of the validity of their measure, about whether useful inferences can be based on the assessment findings (Streiner and Norman, 2003). Subsequent research then provides further evidence of validity. Assessments only have evidence of validity for the populations they were developed for, or with whom they were subsequently validated. For example, if a tool was designed for adults it cannot be assumed to be valid for children, if it was designed for individuals with spinal cord injury it cannot be assumed to be valid for those with cerebral palsy.

Responsiveness

If you wish to understand whether an intervention has been effective or if a natural change has occurred in a performance or condition, then the assessment tool you choose must be able to measure change: that is, be responsive. Responsiveness is a form of validity – longitudinal construct validity – that shows that the tool is valid for measuring clinically important change.

Reliability
Tests and assessments that have undergone rigorous development usually report varying types of reliability, for example, retest and inter-rater reliability. Reliability gives an indication of the degree of error or unpredictable variability in the measurement. Reliability matters because true differences or changes can be obscured by error if an assessment has low reliability. We require reliable assessments; however, it can be difficult for the clinician to decide how reliable an assessment should be. Some authors have reported that coefficients greater than 0.75 are considered to represent good reliability (Portney and Watkins, 2000). Others, however, have argued that reliability is more easily interpreted if reported in the units of measurement, rather than as a correlation coefficient. For example, reporting reliability in the units of measurement can allow the clinician to decide if a change (Keating and Matyas, 1998) in scores on reassessment (step 8 of the clinical intervention model) is due to real change or random variation in the measurement.

A test or assessment is only as reliable as the person who has administered it. Thus, regardless of the level of reliability reported in any research, if you are administering an assessment, *your* reliability counts. You will only be reliable if you

- read and understand the assessment manual or other protocol;
- undertake the training that is specified for each assessment;
- administer the assessment according to the instructions each time;
- score the assessment according to the criteria each time.

In addition, a useful professional development exercise involves periodic establishment of your own intra-rater reliability on any measure that you routinely use. This can be done simply by re-scoring a number of individuals (perhaps ten) and looking at the level of agreement between scores and investigating areas that appear to be less reliable.

Clinical utility
Utility includes consideration of elements such as time taken to administer and score, invasiveness to the individual, cost, availability and ease of administration, which must all be weighed against the usefulness (or otherwise) of the information gathered.

Some common assessment tools

The ICF (World Health Organization, 2001) provides a useful framework to organize assessments and to assist therapists in deciding which assessment is most appropriate. Figure A.1 provides an example of how the ICF can be used to prioritize the choice of assessments depending on which component of functioning is being targeted for improvement. As the ICF was published in 2001 and many of the assessments and tests used today are older, not all fit neatly into one category or another. Some assessments cross the levels of the ICF or could be administered in such a way as to target different domains. For example, the Canadian Occupational Performance Measure (COPM)

(Law et al, 1990) can be administered so that it elicits either participation or activity level issues.

Body function and structure

Body functions are the physiological functions of body systems, while body structures are anatomical parts of the body and their components. Impairments are significant deviations or loss in body function or structure (World Health Organization, 2001) (Figure A.2).

General Movements Assessment (GMA)

The GMA is a standardized video recorded assessment of the spontaneous movement repertoire of infants from preterm until approximately 20-weeks post-term age (Einspieler et al, 2004). In the initial phase from preterm up until 6 weeks, general

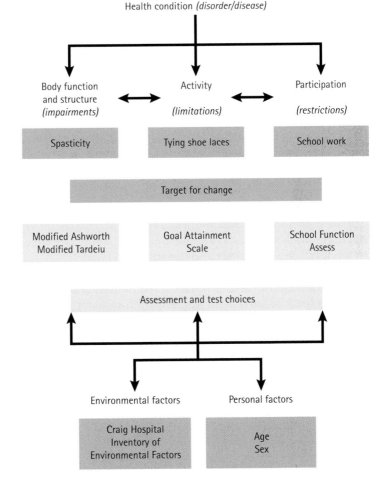

Figure A.1. Using the International Classification of Functioning, Disability and Health to help choose appropriate assessments. Adapted from WHO (2001) International Classification of Functioning, Disability and Health: Short Version: 26. Geneva: World Health Organization.

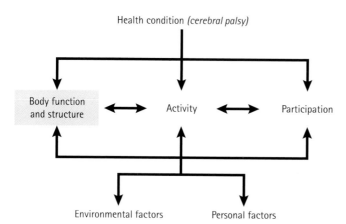

Figure A.2. The International Classification of Functioning, Disability and Health – Body function and structure. Figure used with permission from WHO (2001) International Classification of Functioning, Disability and Health: Short Version: 26. Geneva: World Health Organization. Copyright 2001 by the World Health Organization.

movements are classified as either normal or abnormal. Normal general movements are characterized by a large variability in speed, amplitude, force and intensity; whereby rotations of the arms, legs and trunk are superimposed with flexion and extension so that the overall picture of the sequence of these movements is fluent and elegant. There are three main types of abnormal general movements.

(1) Poor repertoire, where the sequence of movement components is monotonous rather than complex.

(2) Cramped synchronized, where the general movements appear rigid and stiff, with simultaneous contractions and relaxation of the trunk and limb muscles.

(3) Chaotic general movements where the movement amplitude is large and the movements disorganized (Bos et al, 2001).

During the second period, from 9 weeks until 20 weeks, 'fidgety' movements are classified as either present, abnormal or absent. Fidgety movements are movements of the neck, trunk and limbs of small amplitude, moderate speed and variable acceleration in all directions (Einspieler and Prechtl, 2005).

A basic training course of 3–4 days is required in order to be able to administer and score the General Movement Assessment. Inter-rater (κ=0.84–0.92) and intra-rater reliability (κ=1.0) has been found to be excellent (Spittle et al, 2008). General movements also have been shown to have good predictive validity for cerebral palsy (Prechtl et al, 1997; Guzetta et al, 2003; see Chapters 5 and 6).
(Sue Greaves)

The Melbourne Assessment of Unilateral Upper Limb Function
The Melbourne Assessment has demonstrated evidence of validity for measurement of unilateral quality of upper limb movement in children with cerebral palsy aged 2.5 to 15 years (Randall et al, 2001, 2008). It provides reliable measurement of the components of movement that are required in functional tasks, including range of

movement, fluency, target accuracy and dexterity of grasp and release. The child is videotaped performing 16 upper limb tasks from which the varying movement components are scored according to specified criteria. Raw scores are converted to a percentage score, with scores of 100% indicating unimpaired quality of upper limb movement. The Melbourne Assessment has been used as an outcome measure in a number of trials that have evaluated the effectiveness of upper limb interventions for children with cerebral palsy (e.g. Wallen et al, 2007; Jannink et al, 2008; Motta et al, 2008; van Meeteren et al, 2008; see Chapters 11 and 12).
(Christine Imms)

Mirror movement assessment
Presence of mirror movements can be evaluated using the protocol developed by Woods and Teuber (1978). With elbows resting on a table and forearms facing up, the child is videotaped performing the following tasks with both left and right upper limbs:

- rapid tapping of the index finger on the distal joint of the thumb of the same hand;
- rotation of the fist by alternating supination and pronation of the forearm;
- repetitive touching of each fingertip to the tip of the thumb of the same hand, in the order thumb to second, third, fourth, fifth, second, third, fourth, fifth and so on.

Using video footage, the child is rated during each task on the following five-point ordinal scale for mirror movements appearing in the opposite hand to the one intentionally moved. The possible score for each hand ranges from 0 to 12.

(0) No clearly imitative movement.
(1) Barely discernible repetitive movement.
(2) Either slight but unsustained repetitive movement, or stronger, but briefer, repetitive movement.
(3) Strong and sustained repetitive movement.
(4) Movement equal to that expected for the intended hand.

Although Woods and Teuber provide a standard protocol for assessing the presence and extent of mirror movements, no published evidence on the measurement properties of the scale has been located (see Chapter 8).
(Brian Hoare)

Muscle endurance
Muscle endurance can be measured by counting the number of repetitions completed using a weight equal to 50% of one-repetition maximum (1RM). One study has demonstrated evidence of construct validity of measuring muscle endurance this way in people with neurological conditions, finding large and clinically significant increases after a strength training programme (Taylor et al 2006; see Chapter 13).
(Karen Dodd and Nicholas Taylor)

Muscle strength
Dynamic muscle strength can be measured using a one-repetition maximum (1RM). The test involves recording how much weight an individual can move, just once with control, through the full range of available motion and then back to the starting position. One-repetition maximum can be measured with high levels of retest reliability ($r=0.89$) and responsiveness in people with cerebral palsy (Taylor et al, 2004b). Measurement of dynamic muscle strength requires the use of a weights machine (with the weights on a stack), or the use of free weights such as dumb bells. However, for those not familiar with lifting weights it is safer to assess 1RM on a weights machine. In measuring 1RM, the therapist is required to identify the person's best effort within three or four goes, and to make sure that the person rests sufficiently (usually 90 seconds to 2 minutes) between efforts, so that muscle fatigue does not affect the amount of weight that can be lifted.

If the therapist does not have access to a weights machine, an alternative is to use a lightweight hand held dynamometer to assess isometric muscle strength. The therapist uses the device to resist muscle contraction with force gradually built up over 1 to 3 seconds (Damiano and Abel, 1998). It has been found that the most reliable method is to take three measures, with the first regarded as familiarization and the final score obtained by averaging the second and third measures (Taylor et al, 2004a). There is evidence of high retest reliability using this method with young people with cerebral palsy (intra-class correlation coefficient (ICC) >0.80), however, it can be difficult to document change in an individual (Taylor et al, 2004a; see Chapters 13 and 16).
(Karen Dodd and Nicholas Taylor)

Pain Assessment Instrument for Cerebral Palsy (PAICP)
The PAICP was developed as a measure of pain for people with cerebral palsy whose mental age is 4 years or older (Boldingh et al, 2004). For testing, individuals do not need to be verbal, but do need to have adequate vision to see the images (which can be enlarged if needed) and able to indicate their choice using any method. The authors report that establishing the mental age of the individual can usually be reliably reported by caregivers who know the individual well. Alternately, the Columbia Mental Maturity Scale which is also a non-verbal measure, can be used (Burgemeister et al, 1954 as cited in Boldingh et al, 2004). The PAICP uses a series of seven faces to indicate level of pain, from neutral (face one) to very painful (face seven). The tool was validated with 164 adults with severe cerebral palsy using a series of pictures of situations that were either likely to be painful or not. Test developers indicated that additional drawings can be added to assess specific situations. Test–retest stability for each item was adequate with modified kappa values all above 0.48 and most above 0.69. Correlations between the individual with cerebral palsy and proxy respondents (either a physiotherapist or caregiver) were generally low suggesting that it is important to obtain reports of pain directly from the individual (all but three items Spearman's *rho* ≤0.28; see Chapter 15).
(Christine Imms)

Pick-up Test
The Pick-up Test reported by Krumlinde-Sundholm and colleagues involves a timed task of how quickly an individual picks up 10 wooden blocks measuring 10 mm per side out of a box measuring 120 × 120 × 40 mm (Krumlinde-Sundholm et al, 1998; Krumlinde-Sundholm and Eliasson, 2002). The length of time taken, in seconds, is recorded for the impaired hand in two trials, one with vision and one with vision occluded. The individual's 'functional sensibility' (Krumlinde-Sundholm and Eliasson, 2002) is determined by the difference in time taken between the two performances. No impairment in functional sensibility (score 1) is determined when the time taken with vision occluded is <2.5 times the time taken with vision. Deficits in functional sensibility are scored at 2, when the time taken is >2.5 times that with vision, or scored 3 when the task could not be performed without vision. Validity of the Pick-up Test is supported with evidence from a trial that included 25 children with hemiplegia and 19 children without impairments, and compared outcomes using differing tests of sensation (Krumlinde-Sundholm and Eliasson, 2002). Krumlinde-Sundholm and Eliasson's study also provided support for the clinical usefulness of the results of the Pick-up Test as the results provided a clear indication of the amount the children relied on vision to support their motor performance (see Chapter 8).
(Christine Imms)

Spinal Alignment and Range of Motion Measure (SAROMM)
The SAROMM (Bartlett and Purdie, 2005) has been developed to provide an overall estimate of flexibility and posture for children with cerebral palsy with the aim of identifying areas that might benefit from therapy to either prevent the development of secondary impairments associated with contractures, or minimize the progression of existing limitations. The SAROMM comprises two subsections: spinal alignment (4 items); and range of motion and muscle extensibility (11 items, tested bilaterally making a total of 22 items for the subsection). Each item is scored on a five-point ordinal scale, from zero (representing ability to align normally with no passive limitations) to four (severe deviations in spinal alignment or limitations in joint range of motion or muscle extensibility).

Construct validity of the SAROMM has been evaluated in children with cerebral palsy aged 3–18 years, with results showing that the age and the Gross Motor Function Classification System (GMFCS) level of participants were significantly associated with the SAROMM score contributing to almost half of variance in the score (Eliasson et al, 2006). High levels of inter-rater and retest reliability have been reported for subscales and total scores (ICC >0.80) (Bartlett and Purdie, 2005; see Chapter 2).
(Karen Dodd)

Tardieu scale
To measure spasticity using the modified Tardieu scale (Boyd and Graham, 1999), passive muscle stretch is performed at two specified velocities: 'as slow as possible' (signified as V1) and 'as fast as possible' (signified as V3). It is important to assess the child in the same position on each occasion and the neck must remain in a constant position throughout the assessment and from one test to another.

Two dimensions of spasticity are measured. First, the intensity and duration of the muscle reaction to stretch is rated on the following six-point ordinal scale.

Quality of muscle reaction (signified as X):

(0) No resistance throughout the course of the passive movement.
(1) Slight resistance throughout the course of the passive movement with no clear catch at a precise angle.
(2) Clear catch at a precise angle, interrupting the passive movement, followed by release.
(3) Fatigable clonus (less than 10 seconds when maintaining the pressure) appearing at a precise angle.
(4) Infatigable clonus (more than 10 seconds when maintaining the pressure) at a precise angle.
(5) Joint immovable.

Second, the joint angle at which this muscle reaction is first felt is measured. The joint angle (in degrees) when passively stretching the muscle as slow as possible (signified as R2) and as fast as possible (signified as R1) is measured relative to the position of minimal stretch of the muscle (corresponding to angle zero) for all joints except at the hip where it is relative to the resting anatomical position. If the difference in joint angle between the fast and slow passive stretch (i.e. R2–R1) is low this is interpreted as evidence of minimal spasticity.

To evaluate change in spasticity, the quality and the intensity of the muscle reaction (i.e. X) can be compared before and after treatment. In addition, the joint angle of the muscle reaction at a very slow passive stretch (R2) before and after treatment, and the joint angle of the catch at a fast velocity passive stretch (R1) before and after treatment can be compared.

Recent findings found the modified Tardieu scale had poor reliability as a measure of upper limb spasticity due to large inter-session variation and difficulty in applying standardized velocities (Mackey et al, 2004). Despite these limitations for research purposes, the modified Tardieu scale is a very useful clinical tool when used to identify spasticity in larger muscles (Patrick and Ada, 2006). A recent systematic review identified the scale as the only clinically valid measure of spasticity currently available (Scholtes et al, 2006; see Chapters 7–10, 12, 13).
(Brian Hoare and Karen Dodd)

Activity level assessment
Activities are the execution of a task or an action by an individual, and activity limitations are difficulties an individual may have in performing activities (World Health Organization, 2001) (Figure A.3).

Figure A.3 The International Classification of Functioning, Disability and Health – Activity. Figure used with permission from WHO (2001) International Classification of Functioning, Disability and Health: Short Version: 26. Geneva: World Health Organization. Copyright 2001 by the World Health Organization.

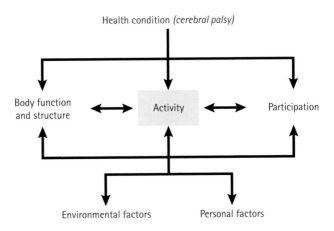

Assisting Hand Assessment (AHA)
The AHA assesses a child's ability to use the assisting hand in bilateral activity. Toys, selected by the test developers to elicit bimanual activity, are presented to children in a semi-structured play session. The play session is video recorded and then scored according to how effectively the child uses the affected (assisting) hand on 22 criteria such as, stabilizing objects by weight, grasp and coordination of both hands together, release and manipulation of objects within the hand. There is good evidence in support of its inter- and intra-rater reliability in children with cerebral palsy (Krumlinde-Sundholm and Eliasson, 2003; Krumlinde-Sundholm et al, 2007), and responsiveness has been demonstrated in at least one trial (Eliasson et al, 2005; see Chapter 6).
(Margaret Wallen and Christine Imms)

Canadian Occupational Performance Measure (COPM)
The COPM (Law et al, 2005) is a client-centred tool, which guides individuals and/or families to identify areas of performance that the client needs or wants to learn in relation to self-care, leisure and productive activities. In the child, productive occupations include learning through movement and play or attending school. The client and/or family prioritize the identified issues and rate the top five issues on two scales: perception of current 'performance' and 'satisfaction' with current performance. Scores closer to ten (on the ten-point rating scales) indicate better performance and increased satisfaction. The COPM was originally validated for people 8 years and older, but it has become convention for parents to be proxy-respondents for younger children (Wallen et al, 2008). Cusick et al (2007) have provided evidence of the validity of an adapted version for children aged 2–8 years. The COPM is responsive to clinical change (Carswell et al, 2004), with a two-point difference in scores interpreted as clinically meaningful. Responsiveness in trials with children with cerebral palsy has also been demonstrated (e.g. Healy and Rigby, 1999; Reid, 2002; Greaves, 2004; Lowe et al, 2006; Wallen et al, 2007; see Chapters 7, 11, 14).
(Margaret Wallen and Christine Imms)

Functional Independence Measure (FIM)
The FIM is a widely used scale designed to document disability in motor and cognitive functions of rehabilitation patients (Keith et al, 1987). The motor subscale of the Functional Independence Measure (FIM) can be used as a global measure of activity limitation in adults. The motor subscale of the FIM measures 13 items scored on a scale from 1 (total assist) to 7 (complete independence). The 13 items include 6 items about self-care (e.g. bathing, dressing – upper and lower body), 2 items on sphincter control, 3 items on transfers and 2 items on locomotion. The motor subscale score is obtained by adding the scores of the 13 items, resulting in a score between 13 and 91, with 91 indicating complete independence. The FIM has demonstrated evidence of high inter-rater and retest reliability across a wide variety of settings and raters (Ottenbacher et al, 1996a). The FIM has also been applied to adults with cerebral palsy to document levels of activity limitation (Andren and Grimby, 2004a, 2004b; Donkervoort et al, 2007; see Chapter 16).

In addition to the FIM, the WeeFIM is a valid and reliable measure of independence for children aged 6 months to 7 years (Ottenbacher et al, 1996b). The WeeFIM has been shown to be responsive to change over 12 months in a population of children with chronic disabilities including cerebral palsy (Ottenbacher et al, 2000). The WeeFIM measures functional independence on a seven-point rating scale ranging from complete independence to complete dependence across six subscales. In particular, the test measures how much assistance the child requires to complete the tasks. The subscales can be collapsed into motor (self-care, sphincter control, transfers and locomotion) or cognitive (communication and social cognition) scales.
(Karen Dodd, Nicholas Taylor and Christine Imms)

Functional Mobility Scale (FMS)
The FMS is a six-level categorical scale that quantifies the amount of assistance required for mobility in the different environmental settings of the home, school and community (Graham et al, 2004). It is based on clinician interpretation of child or parent report (Figure A.4). The FMS can detect change in mobility status (both deterioration and improvement) in children with spastic diplegia following single event multilevel surgery (Harvey et al, 2007; see Chapters 9 and 10).
(Adrienne Harvey)

Goal Attainment Scaling (GAS)
The GAS (Kiresuk and Sherman, 1968) is an individualized measure of goal achievement. The therapist works with the client and family to identify meaningful goals for intervention. The client's baseline performance of the goal is observed and described. The scaling then requires that the client and therapist identify the anticipated level of achievement following intervention, along with a less than expected and more than expected level of achievement. This results in a five-point ordinal scale ranging from minus two (baseline performance); minus one (less than expected achievement); 0 (expected outcome following intervention); plus one (more than expected achievement); and plus two (much more than expected achievement). Each step of the scale is written in behavioural and measurable terms.

Rating 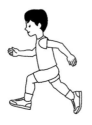 **6**

Independent on all surfaces:

Does not use any walking aids or need any help from another person when walking over all surfaces including uneven ground, curbs etc. and in a crowded environment.

Rating 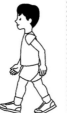 **5**

Independent on level surfaces:

Does not use walking aids or need help from another person.* Requires a rail for stairs.

*If uses furniture, walls, fences, shop fronts for support, please use 4 as the appropriate description.

Rating 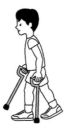 **4**

Uses sticks (one or two):

Without help from another person.

Rating 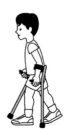 **3**

Uses crutches:

Without help from another person.

Rating 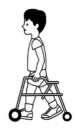 **2**

Uses a walker or frame:

Without help from another person.

Rating 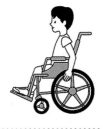 **1**

Uses wheelchair:

May stand for transfers, may do some stepping supported by another person or using a walker/frame.

Walking distance	Rating: select the number (from 1–6) which best describes current function
5 metres (yards)	
50 metres (yards)	
500 metres (yards)	

Rating **C**   **Crawling:**
Child crawls for mobility at home (5m).

Rating **N**   **N = does not apply:**
For example child does not complete the distance (500 m).

Figure A.4 The Functional Mobility Scale (FMS). Figure used with permission of Adrienne Harvey.

Validity, including responsiveness of the GAS for children with cerebral palsy has been reported (Cusick et al, 2006). The GAS's collaborative approach has the flexibility required for family directed service, allowing individualized assessment that is specific and sensitive (King et al, 1999). Although setting goals that are the appropriate 'fit' to the child's abilities has been recognized as a difficulty inherent in goal construction (Cusick et al, 2006), incorporating a SMART approach – setting Specific, Measurable, Acceptable, Relevant and Time-related goals can assist this process. Additionally, extensive training in goal selection, scale development and rating may improve reliability of this measure (King et al, 1999; Steenbeek et al, 2007).

Following intervention, the scores achieved for each goal may be converted to produce one-overall score called a T-score (Kiresuk et al, 1994). However, the most appropriate way for clinicians to determine the impact of intervention for individuals in clinical practice is to describe the level of achievement on individual goals (see Chapter 5).
(Margaret Wallen and Christine Imms)

Gross Motor Function Measure (GMFM–88 and GMFM–66)
The GMFM is a criterion referenced measure used to evaluate change in gross motor function over time, or following intervention, in children with cerebral palsy (Russell et al, 1989). It measures gross motor items through five dimensions based on typical development up to five years of age. There are 88- and 66-item versions, both with five dimensions: lying and rolling; sitting; crawling and kneeling; standing; and walking, running and jumping. Each item is evaluated on a four-point scale (Russell et al, 2002). The GMFM was designed and validated for children with cerebral palsy aged from 5 months to 16 years. The GMFM–66 was developed after application of Rasch analysis to the original scale, which eliminated 22 items and resulted in a unidimensional scale with interval level data and good psychometric properties (Russell et al 2002; Avery et al, 2003). The GMFM has been used widely in clinical practice and research to evaluate the effects of interventions (see Chapters 5, 6, 9, 10, 12 and 13).
(Nicholas Taylor and Karen Dodd)

The Peabody Developmental Motor Scale–2 (PDMS–2)
The PDMS–2 is a standardized norm-referenced test designed to measure fine and gross motor skills of children from birth to 6 years (Folio and Fewell, 2000). The scales consist of six subtests that assess reflexes, body control and equilibrium, locomotion, object manipulation, grasping and visual–motor integration. A total of 249 items, which take 45 to 60 minutes to administer, are scored on a three-point scale (zero, one and two, with two assigned when the child achieves the specified item criterion) and summed to give gross motor, fine motor and total composite scores. Some recent reports have questioned the measurement properties of the PDMS–2 in typically developing infants; with a lack of concurrent validity between PDMS–2 and the Bayley Scales of Infant Development Motor Scale (Connolly et al, 2006), and ceiling effect and mis-fitting of items in a Rasch analysis of the fine motor scale (Chien and Bond, 2009). However, when evaluated on a sample of 32 children with cerebral palsy the PDMS–2 demonstrated high levels of retest reliability over 1 week (ICC=0.99–1.00) and high

levels of responsiveness over 3 months (responsiveness coefficients >1.6) (Wang et al, 2006; see Chapter 6).
(Sarah Foley, Susan Greaves and Christine Imms)

Pediatric Evaluation of Disability Inventory (PEDI)

The PEDI is a discriminative and evaluative assessment designed to measure functional capabilities for children with disabilities aged 6 months to 7.5 years (Haley et al, 1992). It comprises three scales that measure different aspects of a child's ability to perform, or be assisted with, various daily living activities. The Functional Skills scale comprises three content domains: self-care, mobility and social function. Two additional scales, Caregiver Assistance and Environmental Modifications, clarify how much assistance is needed and whether environmental modifications are required to support performance. Together the three scales provide different but strongly related aspects of functioning (Ostensjo et al, 2003). Several studies support the PEDI as a valid and reliable assessment of daily living skills in children with disabilities (Feldman et al, 1990; Haley et al, 1991; Nichols and Case-Smith, 1996) and there is evidence that it is responsive to change, especially in younger children (Vos-Vromans et al, 2005; see Chapters 5 and 6).
(Sarah Foley, Susan Greaves and Christine Imms)

Pediatric Reach Test

The Pediatric Reach Test (Bartlett and Birmingham, 2003) assesses standing and sitting balance. The test is a version of the Functional Reach Test (Duncan et al, 1990), incorporating side reaching as well as forward reaching during sitting. The starting position is seated on a surface without back or side support and with feet flat on floor. The distance reached forward, and to each side is measured with a tape measure. For standing balance, the test measures the distance a person can reach forward and to each side without losing balance or taking a step. The difference between starting position and reach position is recorded, and the sum of the differences for the three positions (forward, left and right) give a composite measure of balance. The Pediatric Reach Test has high retest reliability (ICC=0.84) in children with cerebral palsy (Bartlett and Birmingham, 2003). Retest reliability of the standing section was also high (r >0.85) in a group of young people with cerebral palsy, and evidence of validity was found with moderate to high correlations with laboratory tests of stability using a force platform (see Chapters 13 and 16).
(Karen Dodd and Nicholas Taylor)

The Sitting Assessment for Children with Neuromotor Dysfunction (SACND)

The SACND was designed to provide a clinical assessment of the quality of sitting at rest and during upper-extremity reaching movement of children with neuromotor disability aged from 2 to 10 years (Reid, 1997). The instrument contains two 5-minute modules. In the rest module the child sits independently on a bench while listening to a story or watching a video, whereas in the reach module the child sits on a bench and reaches towards objects on a board with the preferred hand centrally, up and down, and to each side. Each module assesses postural tone, proximal stability, postural alignment and balance. Each of the four items in the two modules is given a score of

one (for the most mature or normal response) to four (for the most immature or an abnormal response). The total score in the rest and reach modules are the sum of each of the four item scores. Complete instructions for scoring and administration are contained in the SACND manual (Reid, 1997). Preliminary research on two therapists rating 20 children with a range of neuromotor disabilities including cerebral palsy reported excellent inter-rater reliability (κ ranged from 0.91 to 1.0) (Reid et al, 1995), and there is evidence of construct validity in that the scale detected hypothesized improvements in sitting with provision of a saddle seat in six children with spastic diplegia (Reid, 1996). An example of the clinical application of the SACND to evaluate the effect of therapy on the sitting ability of a child with cerebral palsy is described by Knox (2002) (see Chapter 6).
(Susan Greaves, Karen Dodd and Nicholas Taylor)

Six-minute Walk Test
Walking endurance can be assessed by measuring how far a person can walk in 6 minutes on a flat standardized course. The test is completed twice, with the first trial regarded as practice. The 6-minute Walk Test showed high retest reliability (ICC=0.94–0.97) in young people with cerebral palsy (Andersson et al, 2006), and the test was responsive when used with young adults with cerebral palsy who improved by 86 m (31%) after a 10-week strength training programme (Andersson et al, 2003; see Chapters 13 and 14).
(Karen Dodd and Nicholas Taylor)

Timed sit-to-stand test
The timed sit-to-stand test is administered by measuring the time it takes to independently move from sit-to-stand three times. Timed sit-to-stand was a reliable measure of performance over time in older people and people with physical disabilities (Bohannon, 1995). In adults with cerebral palsy the timed sit-to-stand test showed high levels of retest reliability ($r=0.87$), and evidence of construct validity in that it was able to detect an improved performance in sit-to-stand after a 10-week training programme (Taylor et al, 2004b; see Chapter 16).
(Karen Dodd and Nicholas Taylor)

Timed stairs test
The timed stairs test is based on two items of the Gross Motor Function Measure (Russell et al, 2002). The test requires participants to walk up and down three steps of standard size (17.5 cm) as quickly as possible, using rails if required. The time taken to complete the task is measured using a stopwatch. A trend to reduced time to complete this test was observed after 6 weeks of strength training in young people with spastic diplegic cerebral palsy (Dodd et al, 2003; see Chapter 13).
(Karen Dodd and Nicholas Taylor)

Wheelchair Skills Test
The Wheelchair Skills Test assesses 25 skills in four areas: basic skills; wheelchair manoeuvring and daily living skills; obstacle negotiating skills; and advanced wheelchair skills (Kirby et al, 2002; MacPhee et al, 2004). Each skill is scored on a

three-point ordinal scale: zero if unable to complete the skill safely, one for partial completion and two for successful and safe completion. The total score is a percentage of the total possible score of 50. The test developers reported that the Wheelchair Skills Test had good to excellent reliability (inter-rater reliability r=0.95), and demonstrated evidence of construct validity in that it was able to detect hypothesized changes in a mixed group of adult wheelchair users receiving rehabilitation (MacPhee et al, 2004; see Chapter 16).
(Karen Dodd and Nicholas Taylor)

Participation
Participation is involvement in a life situation and participation restrictions are problems an individual may experience in a life situation (World Health Organization, 2001) (Figure A.5).

The Children's Assessment of Participation and Enjoyment (CAPE)
The CAPE is a 55-item questionnaire that measures how many activities a child or youth participates in, as well as the intensity of that participation (King et al, 2004). In addition, scores for who the child participates with (alone, with family or friends) and where (at home or in the broader community), and how much they enjoy their participation are obtained. It is appropriate for young people aged 6 to 21 years with and without disabilities. The CAPE provides three levels of score: overall participation, as well as domain scores for formal and informal activities, and scores in five activities types: recreational, active-physical, social, skill-based, and self-improvement (King et al, 2004).

A recent systematic review concluded that the CAPE was one of the measures of participation suitable for use in young people with cerebral palsy (Sakzewski et al, 2007). The CAPE has been used in studies in at least three different countries providing some evidence of cross-cultural validity (Law et al, 2004; Engel-Yeger et al, 2007; Imms et al, 2008). As the CAPE is a relatively new tool there are no studies

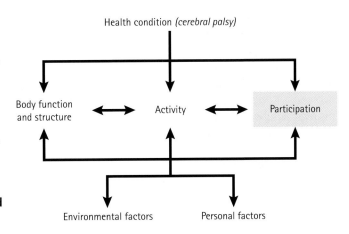

Figure A.5 The International Classification of Functioning, Disability and Health – Participation. Figure used with permission from WHO (2001) International Classification of Functioning, Disability and Health: Short Version: 26. Geneva: World Health Organization. Copyright 2001 by the World Health Organization.

providing evidence of the tool's responsiveness. The Preferences for Activity of Children (PAC) is a companion measure to the CAPE and provides a measurement of whether children and youth prefer particular types of activities (King et al, 2004; see Chapters 12 and 13).
(*Christine Imms*)

Life–H

The LIFE–H was developed based on the disability creation model and includes 77 items in 12 domains of social participation (Fougeyrollas et al, 1998). The 12 domains include nutrition, fitness, personal care, communication, housing, mobility, responsibilities, interpersonal relationships, community life, education, employment and recreation. Test–retest reliability of the LIFE–H for children is 0.73 (Fougeyrollas et al, 1998) and the measure has evidence of good content and construct validity (Noreau et al, 2007). The LIFE–H has two scores for each item – level of difficulty in performing the item and the type of assistance required in order to do each item. Scores on the LIFE–H range from zero (not able to do an item) to nine (able to participate in an item with no restrictions). Scores are calculated for each domain using a transformed score range of 0–10 (see Chapter 14).
(*Mary Law and Debra Stewart*)

School Function Assessment (SFA)

The SFA (Coster et al, 1998) was designed to evaluate the ability of a child in primary (elementary) school to complete the academic and social activities required within a school environment. The scale has three parts: I participation; II task supports; and III activity performance. The participation section evaluates the child's ability to take part in six domains of the school environment: classroom (special or regular), playground/recess, transport to and from school, bathroom/toilet, transitions to and from class and snack/meal time. Task supports examines the type of assistance usually required by the child (either adult help or adaptations). Activity performance evaluates the ability of the child to complete school-related activities (Coster et al, 1998). A professional who knows the child's school-based performance and participation well, completes the SFA. It has demonstrated validity for assessment of the child's function within the school environment (Sakzewski et al, 2007), and has been used within population-based studies of participation of children with cerebral palsy (Schenker et al, 2005, 2006), but was not found to be as responsive as other paediatric measures in one study (Wright et al, 2005; see Chapter 12).
(*Christine Imms*)

Contextual factors

Contextual factors comprise environmental and personal factors. Environmental factors make up the physical, social and attitudinal environment in which people conduct their lives, and personal factors are the particular background of an individual's life, and comprise features of the individual that are not part of the health condition, such as age and sex (World Health Organization, 2001) (Figure A.6).

Figure A.6 The International Classification of Functioning, Disability and Health – Contextual factors. Figure used with permission from WHO (2001) International Classification of Functioning, Disability and Health: Short Version: 26. Geneva: World Health Organization. Copyright 2001 by the World Health Organization.

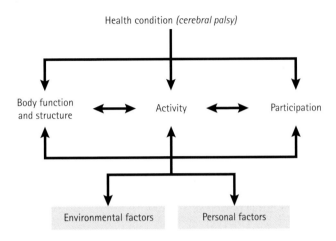

Environmental factors

CRAIG HOSPITAL INVENTORY OF ENVIRONMENTAL FACTORS (CHIEF)
The CHIEF (Whiteneck et al, 2004) has been used to assess environmental factors influencing the participation of children and youth with physical disabilities, including cerebral palsy (Law et al, 2007). Respondents rate the frequency with which they encounter barriers (daily, weekly, monthly, less than monthly, or never) on the 25 items of the CHIEF. The CHIEF was developed and tested with individuals with disabilities aged 16 to 95 years but is valid for individuals with and without disabilities. The CHIEF has demonstrated high levels of reliability (ICC=0.93) and evidence of construct validity by showing that compared with non-disabled people, people with disabilities encounter more environmental barriers (Harrison-Felix, 2001; see Chapter 14).
(Mary Law and Debra Stewart)

Personal factors

THE SELF-PERCEPTION PROFILE FOR ADOLESCENTS
This scale was designed to assess young persons' perceptions of themselves across the domains of scholastic competence, social acceptance, athletic competence, physical appearance, job competence, close friendship, romantic appeal and behavioural conduct. In addition, the individual provides a global perception of their worth or esteem as a person (Harter, 1988). The scale is suitable for adolescents for whom the subscales of job competence, romantic appeal and close friendship may be appropriate, and builds on the Self-Perception Profile for Children (Harter, 1985). The children's scale has demonstrated moderate to high retest reliability ($r=0.56–0.80$) for young people with cerebral palsy (Dodd et al, 2004). If required, there is also a version suitable for children under 8 years of age (Harter and Pike, 1984).

The 45-item adolescent questionnaire uses a structured alternative format in which the respondent is asked to select which of the two alternative statements for the 45 items

they were most like and whether the selected statement was 'sort of true' or 'really true'. Scores for questions in each domain are added and averaged to obtain separate domain scores for self-concept. A score of at least 2.5 out of 4 in a domain indicates a positive self-concept for that domain (see Chapter 13).
(Karen Dodd and Nicholas Taylor)

References

Andersson C, Grooten W, Hellsten M, Kaping K & Mattsson E (2003) Adults with cerebral palsy: walking ability after progressive strength training. *Dev Med Child Neurol*, 45, 220–8.

Andersson C, Asztalos L & Mattson E (2006) Six-minute walk test in adults with cerebral palsy: a study of reliability. *Clin Rehabil*, 20, 488–95.

Andren E & Grimby G (2004a) Activity limitations in personal, domestic and vocational tasks: a study of adults with inborn and early acquired mobility disorders. *Disabil Rehabil*, 26, 262–71.

Andren E & Grimby G (2004b) Dependence in daily activities and life satisfaction in adult subjects with cerebral palsy or spina bifida: a follow up study. *Disabil Rehabil*, 26, 528–36.

Avery LM, Russell DJ, Raina PS, Walter SD & Rosenbaum PL (2003) Rasch analysis of the Gross Motor Function Measure: validating the assumptions of the Rasch model to create an interval-level measure. *Arch Phys Med Rehabil*, 84, 697–705.

Bartlett D & Birmingham T (2003) Validity and reliability of the pediatric reach test. *Pediatric Physical Therapy*, 15, 84–92.

Bartlett D & Purdie B (2005) Testing of the spinal alignment and range of movement: a discriminative measure of posture and flexibility for children with cerebral palsy. *Dev Med Child Neurol*, 47, 739–43.

Bohannon RW (1995) Sit-to-stand test for measuring performance of lower extremity muscles. *Perceptual Motor Skills*, 80, 163–6.

Boldingh EJ, Jacobs-van der Bruggen MA, Lankhorst GJ & Bouter LM (2004) Assessing pain in patients with severe cerebral palsy: development, reliability, and validity of a pain assessment instrument for cerebral palsy. *Arch Phys Med Rehabil*, 85, 758–66.

Bos AF, Einspieler C & Prechtl HF (2001) Intrauterine growth retardation, general movements, and neurodevelopmental outcome: a review. *Dev Med Child Neurol*, 43, 61–8.

Boyd RN & Graham HK (1999) Objective measurement of clinical findings in the use of botulinum toxin type A for the management of children with cerebral palsy. *Eur J Neurol*, 6, S23–35.

Carswell A, McColl MA, Baptiste S, Law M, Polatajko H & Pollock N (2004) The Canadian Occupational Performance Measure: a research and clinical literature review. *Can J Occup Ther*, 71, 210–22.

Chien CW & Bond TG (2009) Measurement properties of the Fine Motor Scale of the Peabody Developmental Motor Scales – second edition : a rasch analysis. *Am J Phys Med Rehabil*, 85, 376–86.

Connolly BH, Dalton L, Smith JB, Lamberth NG, McCay B & Murphy W (2006) Concurrent validity of the Bayley Scales of Infant Development II (BSID-II) Motor Scale and the Peabody Developmental Motor Scale – II (PDMS-2) in 12-month old infants. *Pediatr Phys Ther*, 18, 190–6.

Coster W, Deeney TA, Haltiwanger JT & Haley SM (1998) *School Function Assessment*. San Antonio, TX: The Psychological Corporation.

Cusick A, Lannin NA & Lowe K (2007) Adapting the Canadian Occupational Performance Measure for use in a paediatric clinical trial. *Disabil Rehabil*, 29, 761–6.

Cusick A, McIntyre S, Novak I, Lannin NA & Lowe K (2006) A comparison of goal attainment scaling and the Canadian Occupational Performance Measure for paediatric rehabilitation research. *Pediatr Rehabil*, 9, 149–57.

Damiano DL & Abel MF (1998) Functional outcomes of strength training in spastic cerebral palsy. *Arch Phys Med Rehabil*, 79, 119–25.

Dodd KJ, Taylor NF & Graham HK (2003) A randomized clinical trial of strength training in young people with cerebral palsy. *Dev Med Child Neurol*, 45, 652–7.

Dodd KJ, Taylor NF & Graham HK (2004) Strength training can have unexpected effects on the self-concept of children with cerebral palsy. *Pediatr Phys Ther*, 16, 99–105.

Donkervoort M, Roebroeck M, Wiegerink D, van der Heijden-Maessen H, Stam H & The Transition Research Group South West Netherlands (2007) Determinants of functioning of adolescents and young adults with cerebral palsy. *Disabil Rehabil*, 29, 453–63.

Duncan PW, Weiner DK, Chandler J & Studenski S (1990) Functional reach: a new clinical measure of balance. *J Gerontol*, 45, M192–7.

Einspieler C & Prechtl HF (2005) Prechtl's assessment of general movements: a diagnostic tool for the functional assessment of the young nervous system. *Ment Retard Dev Disabil Res Rev*, 11, 61–7.

Einspieler C, Prechtl HF, Bos AF, Ferrari F & Cioni G (2004) *Prechtl's Method on the Qualitative Assessment of General Movements in Preterm, Term and Young Infants.* London: Mac Keith Press.

Eliasson AC, Krumlinde-Sundholm L, Shaw K & Wang C (2005) Effects of constraint induced movement therapy in young children with hemiplegic cerebral palsy: an adapted model. *Dev Med Child Neurol*, 47, 266–75.

Eliasson AC, Krumlinde-Sundholm L, Rösblad B, Beckung E, Arner M, Öhrvall A & Rosenbaum PL (2006) The Manual Ability Classification System (MACS) for children with cerebral palsy: Scale development and evidence of validity and reliability. *Dev Med Child Neurol*, 48, 549–54.

Engel-Yeger B, Jarus T & Law M (2007) Impact of culture on children's community participation in Israel. *Am J Occup Ther*, 61, 421–8.

Feldman AB, Haley SM & Coryell J (1990) Concurrent and construct validity of the Pediatric Evaluation of Disability Inventory. *Phys Ther*, 70, 602–10.

Folio MR & Fewell RR (2000) *Peabody Developmental Motor Scales: Examiners Manual.* Austin, TX: Pro-Ed.

Fougeyrollas P, Noreau L, Bergeron H, Cloutier R, Dion S-A & St Michel G (1998) Social consequences of long term impairments and disabilities: conceptual approach and assessment of handicap. *Int J Rehabil Res*, 21, 127–41.

Graham HK, Harvey A, Rodda J, Nattrass GR & Pirpiris M (2004) The Functional Mobility Scale (FMS). *J Pediatr Orthop*, 24, 514–20.

Greaves SM (2004) *The Effect of Botulinum Toxin A Injections on Occupational Therapy Outcomes for Children with Spastic Hemiplegia.* Bundoora, School of Occupational Therapy, La Trobe University.

Guzetta A, Mercuri E, Rapisardi G, Ferrari F, Roversi MF, Cowan F, Rutherford M, Paolicelli PB, Einspieler C, Boldrin A, Dubowitz L, Prechtl HF & Cioni G (2003) General movements detect early signs of hemiplegia in term infants with neonatal cerebral infarction. *Neuropediatr*, 34, 61–6.

Haley S, Coster W, Ludlow L, Haltiwanger J & Andrellos P (1992) *Pediatric Evaluation of Disability Inventory (PEDI). Version 1. Development, Standardization and Administration Manual.* Boston MA, New England Medical Centre Hospitals.

Haley SM, Coster W & Faas RM (1991) A content validity study of the Pediatric Evaluation of Disability Inventory. *Pediatr Phys Ther*, 3, 177–84.

Harrison-Felix CL (2001) *The Craig Hospital Inventory of Environmental Factors.* San Jose: The Center for Outcome Measurement in Brain Injury (http://tbims.org/combi/chief/).

Harter S (1985) *The Manual for the Self-perception Profile for Children.* Colorado: University of Denver.

Harter S (1988) *The Manual for the Self-perception Profile for Adolescents.* Colorado: University of Denver.

Harter S & Pike R (1984) The pictorial scale of perceived competence and social acceptance for young children. *Child Devel*, 55, 1969–82.

Harvey A, Graham HK, Morris ME, Baker R & Wolfe R (2007) The Functional Mobility Scale: ability to detect change following single event multilevel surgery. *Dev Med Child Neurol*, 49, 603–7.

Healy H & Rigby P (1999) Promoting independence for teens and young adults with physical disabilities. *Can J Occup Ther*, 66, 240–49.

Appendix

Imms C, Reilly S, Carlin J & Dodd K (2008) Diversity of participation in children with cerebral palsy. *Dev Med Child Neurol*, 50, 363–9.

Jannink MJ, van der Wilden GJ, Navis DW, Visser G, Gussinklo J & Ijzerman M (2008) A low-cost video game applied for training of upper extremity function in children with cerebral palsy: a pilot study. *Cyberpsychol Behav*, 11, 27–32.

Keating J & Matyas T (1998) Unreliable inferences from reliable measurements. *Aust J Physiother*, 44, 5–10.

Keith RA, Granger CV, Hamilton BB & Sherwin FS (1987) The Functional Independence Measure: a new tool for rehabilitation. *Advances in Clinical Rehabilitation*, 1, 6–18.

King GA, Law M, King S, Hurley P, Rosenbaum PL, Hanna S, Kertoy MK & Young N (2004) *Children's Assessment of Participation and Enjoyment and Preferences for Activities of Kids*. San Antonio, TX: PsychCorp.

King GA, McDougall J, Palisano RJ, Gritzan J & Tucker MA (1999) Goal attainment scaling: Its use in evaluating pediatric therapy programs. *Phys Occup Ther Pediatr*, 19, 31–52.

Kirby RL, Swuste J, Dupuis DJ, MacLeod DA & Monroe R (2002) The wheelchair Skills Test: a pilot study of a new outcome measure. *Arch Phys Med Rehabil*, 83, 10–18.

Kiresuk TJ & Sherman RE (1968) Goal Attainment Scaling: a general method for evaluating comprehensive community mental health programs. *Community Ment Health J*, 4, 443–53.

Kiresuk TJ, Smith A & Cardillo JE (1994) *Goal Attainment Scaling: Applications, Theory and Measurement*. Hillsdale, NJ: L Erlbaum Associates.

Knox V (2002) Evaluation of the Sitting Assessment for Children with Neuromotor Dysfunction as a measurement tool on cerebral palsy. *Physiother*, 88, 534–41.

Krumlinde-Sundholm L & Eliasson AC (2002) Comparing tests of tactile sensibility: aspects relevant to testing children with spastic hemiplegia. *Dev Med Child Neurol*, 44, 604–12.

Krumlinde-Sundholm L & Eliasson AC (2003) Development of the Assisting Hand Assessment: a Rasch-built measure intended for children with unilateral upper limb impairments. *Scand J Occup Ther*, 10, 16–26.

Krumlinde-Sundholm L, Eliasson AC & Forssberg H (1998) Obstetric brachial plexus injuries: Assessment protocol and functional outcome at the age 5 years. *Dev Med Child Neurol*, 40, 4–11.

Krumlinde-Sundholm L, Holmefur M, Kottorp A & Eliasson AC (2007) The Assisting Hand Assessment: current evidence of validity, reliability and responsiveness to change. *Dev Med Child Neurol Suppl*, 49, 259–64.

Law M, Baptiste S, Carswell A, McColl M, Polatajko H & Pollock N (2005) *Canadian Occupational Performance Measure*. Ottawa, ON, CAOT Publications ACE.

Law M, Baptiste S, McColl M, Opzoomer A, Polatajko H & Pollock N (1990) The Canadian Occupational Performance Measure: an outcome measure for occupational therapy. *Can J Occup Ther*, 57, 82–7.

Law M, Finkelman S, Hurley P, Rosenbaum PL, King S, King G & Hanna S (2004) Participation of children with physical disabilities: Relationships with diagnosis, physical function and demographic variables. *Scand J Occup Ther*, 11, 156–62.

Law M, Petrenchik T, King G & Hurley P (2007) Perceived environmental barriers to recreational, community, and school participation for children and youth with physical disabilities. *Arch Phys Med Rehabil*, 88, 1636–42.

Lowe K, Novak I & Cusick A (2006) Low-dose/high concentration localised botulinum toxin A improves upper limb movement and function in children with hemiplegic cerebral palsy. *Dev Med Child Neurol*, 48, 170–5.

Mackey AH, Walt SE, Lobb G & Stott NS (2004) Intraobserver reliability of the modified Tardieu scale in the upper limb of children with hemiplegia. *Dev Med Child Neurol*, 46, 267–72.

MacPhee AH, Kirby L, Coolen AL, Smith C, MacLeod DA & Dupois DJ (2004) Wheelchair skills training program: a randomised clinical trial of wheelchair users undergoing initial rehabilitation. *Arch Phys Med Rehabil*, 85, 41–50.

Motta F, Stignani C, Antonello CE, Motta F, Stignani C & Antonello CE (2008) Upper limb function after intrathecal baclofen treatment in children with cerebral palsy. *J Pediatr Orthop*, 28, 91–6.

Nichols DS & Case-Smith J (1996) Reliability and validity of the Pediatric Evaluation of Disability Inventory. *Pediatr Phys Ther,* 8, 15–24.

Noreau L, Lepage C, Boissiere L, Picard R, Fougeyrollas P, Mathieu J, Desmarais G & Nadeau L (2007) Measuring participation in children with disabilities using the Assessment of Life Habits. *Dev Med Child Neurol,* 49, 666–71.

Ostensjo S, Carlberg EB & Vollestad NK (2003) Everyday functioning in young children with cerebral palsy: Functional skills, caregiver assistance, and modifications of the environment. *Dev Med Child Neurol,* 45, 603–12.

Ottenbacher KJ, Hsu Y, Granger CV & Fiedler RC (1996a) The reliability of the functional independence measure: a quantitative review. *Arch Phys Med Rehabil,* 77, 1226–32.

Ottenbacher KJ, Taylor ET, Msall ME, Braun S, Lane SJ, Granger CV, Lyons N, Duffy LC (1996b) The stability and equivalence reliability of the Functional Independence Measure for children (WeeFIM). *Dev Med Child Neurol,* 38, 907–16.

Ottenbacher KJ, Msall ME, Lyon N, Duffy LC, Ziviani J, Granger CV, Braun S & Feidler RC (2000) The WeeFIM instrument: its utility in detecting change in children with developmental disabilities. *Arch Phys Med Rehabil,* 81, 1317–26.

Patrick E & Ada L (2006) The Tardieu Scale differentiates contracture from spasticity whereas the Ashworth Scale is confounded by it. *Clin Rehabil,* 20, 173–82.

Portney LG & Watkins MP (2000) *Foundations of Clinical Research: Applications to Practice.* Upper Saddle River, NJ: Prentice Hall Health.

Prechtl HF, Einspieler C, Cioni G, Bos AF, Ferrari F & Sontheimer D (1997) An early marker for neurological deficits after perinatal brain lesions. *Lancet,* 349, 1361–3.

Randall M, Carlin J, Chondros P & Reddihough D (2001) Reliability of the Melbourne Assessment of Unilateral Upper Limb Function. *Dev Med Child Neurol,* 43, 761–7.

Randall M, Imms C & Carey L (2008) Establishing validity of a modified Melbourne assessment for children aged 2–4 years. *Am J Occup Ther,* 62, 373–84.

Reid D (1996) The effects of the saddle seat on seated postural control and upper extremity movement in children with cerebral palsy. *Dev Med Child Neurol,* 38, 805–15.

Reid D (1997) *The SACND: A Standardised Protocol for Describing Postural Contol.* San Antonio, TX: Psychological Corporation.

Reid D, Schuller R & Billson N (1995) Reliability of the SACND. *Phys Occup Ther Pediatr,* 16, 23–32.

Reid DT (2002) Benefits of a virtual play rehabilitation environment for children with cerebral palsy on perceptions of self-efficacy: a pilot study. *Pediatr Rehabil,* 5, 141–8.

Russell D, Rosenbaum PL, Avery LM & Lane M (2002) *Gross Motor Function Measure (GMFM-66 & GMFM-88) User's Manual.* London: Mac Keith Press.

Russell DJ, Rosenbaum PL, Cadman DT, Gowland C, Hardy S & Jarvis S (1989) The gross motor function measure: a means to evaluate the effects of physical therapy. *Dev Med Child Neurol,* 31, 341–52.

Sakzewski L, Boyd R & Ziviani J (2007) Clinimetric properties of participation measures for 5- to 13-year-old children with cerebral palsy: a systematic review. *Dev Med Child Neurol,* 49, 232–40.

Schenker R, Coster W & Parush S (2005) Participation and activity performance of students with cerebral palsy within the school environment. *Disabil Rehabil,* 27, 539–52.

Schenker R, Coster W & Parush S (2006) Personal assistance, adaptations and participation in students with cerebral palsy mainstreamed in elementary schools. *Disabil Rehabil,* 28, 1061–9.

Scholtes VA, Becher JG, Beelen A & Lankhorst GJ (2006) Clinical assessment of spasticity in children with cerebral palsy: A critical review of available instruments. *Dev Med Child Neurol,* 48, 64–73.

Spittle AJ, Doyle LW & Boyd RN (2008) A systematic review of the clinimetric properties of neuromotor assessments for preterm infants during the first year of life. *Dev Med Child Neurol,* 50, 254–66.

Steenbeek D, Ketelaar M, Galama K & Görter JW (2007) Goal attainment scaling in paediatric rehabilitation: a critical review of the literature. *Dev Med Child Neurol,* 49, 550–6.

Appendix

Streiner DL & Norman GR (2003) *Health Measurement Scales: A Practical Guide to their Development and Use.* Oxford: Oxford University Press.

Taylor NF, Dodd K & Graham HK (2004a) Test-retest reliability of hand-held dynamometric strength testing in young people with cerebral palsy. *Arch Phys Med Rehabil,* 85, 77–80.

Taylor NF, Dodd KJ & Larkin H (2004b) Adults with cerebral palsy benefit from participating in a strength training programme at a community gymnasium. *Disabil Rehabil,* 26, 1128–34.

Taylor NF, Dodd KJ, Prasad D & Denisenko S (2006) Progressive resistance exercise for people with multiple sclerosis. *Disabil Rehabil,* 28, 1119–26.

van Meeteren J, Roebroeck ME, Celen E, Donkervoort M & Stam HJ (2008) Functional activities of the upper extremity of young adults with cerebral palsy: A limiting factor for participation? *Disabil Rehabil,* 30, 387–95.

Vos-Vromans DCWM, Ketelaar M & Görter JW (2005) Responsiveness of evaluative measures for children with cerebral palsy: The Gross Motor Function Measure and the Pediatric Evaluation of Disability Inventory. *Disabil Rehabil,* 27, 1245–52.

Wallen M, O'Flaherty SJ & Waugh MA (2007) Functional outcomes of intramuscular Botulinum Toxin type A and occupational therapy in the upper limbs of children with cerebral palsy: a randomised controlled trial. *Arch Phys Med Rehabil,* 88, 1–10.

Wallen M, Ziviani JM, Herbert RD, Evans R & Novak I (2008) Modified constraint-induced therapy for children with hemiplegic cerebral palsy: a feasibility study. *Dev Neurorehabil,* 11, 124–33.

Wang HH, Liao HF & Hsieh CL (2006) Reliability, sensitivity to change, and responsiveness of the Peabody Developmental Motor Scales – second edition for children with cerebral palsy. *Phys Ther,* 86, 1351–9.

Whiteneck GG, Harrison-Felix CL, Mellick DC, Brooks CA, Charlifue SB & Gerhart KA (2004) Quantifying environmental factors: a measure of physical, attitudinal, service, productivity and policy barriers. *Arch Phys Med Rehabil,* 85, 1324–35.

Woods BT & Teuber HL (1978) Mirror movements after childhood hemiparesis. *Neurol,* 28, 1152–7.

World Health Organization (2001) *International Classification of Functioning, Disability and Health. Short Version.* Geneva: WHO.

Wright FV, Boschen K & Jutai J (2005) Exploring the comparative responsiveness of a core set of outcome measures in a school-based conductive education programme. *Child Care, Health Dev,* 31, 291–302.

Index

Other titles from Mac Keith Press

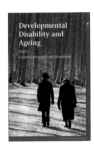

Developmental Disability and Ageing

A practical guide from Mac Keith Press

Edited by Gregory O'Brien and Lewis Rosenbloom

2009 • £20.00 • €23.00 • $34.95 • Paperback • 144 pp

ISBN 978–1–898683–61–2

This book is for clinicians and others who care for ageing adults with developmental disabilities. It is intended to inform understanding, promote assessment, assist in care planning, and especially to improve everyday living for this needy but often neglected group of vulnerable individuals. The authors base their guidance on evidence, focusing on important insights that will be valuable in the care of the individuals on whose behalf the book has been prepared.

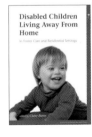

Disabled Children Living Away from Home in Foster Care and Residential Settings

A practical guide from Mac Keith Press

Edited by Clare Burn

2009 • £20.00 • €23.00 • $34.95 • Paperback • 144 pp

ISBN 978–1–898683–58–2

This book considers the key issues that must be addressed when disabled children move from the family home to new accommodation. It provides insights into the difficulties that these children face and looks at how the standards of care that they receive might be improved. It also makes suggestions about how professionals might work more effectively with each other and with the children's care-givers.

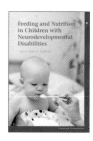

Feeding and Nutrition in Children
with Neurodevelopmental Disability

A practical guide from Mac Keith Press

Edited by Peter B. Sullivan

2009 • £20.00 • €23.00 • $40.00 • Paperback • 196 pp

ISBN 978–1–898683–60–5

This book is for all those who have responsibility for the nutritional and gastrointestinal care of children with neurodisability, providing an up-to-date account of the practicalities of assessment and management of feeding problems in these children. The emphasis throughout is on the importance of team-based care: it is written from a multidisciplinary perspective by a group of authors with considerable clinical and research experience in this area.

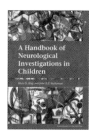

A Handbook of Neurological
Investigations in Children

A practical guide from Mac Keith Press

Mary D. King and John B.P. Stephenson

2009 • £39.95 • €46.00 • $69.95 • Paperback • 399 pp

ISBN 978–1–898683–69–8

The number of possible neurological investigations is now very large indeed, and uncritical investigations may be seriously misleading and often costly. The authors set out the investigations that are really needed to establish the cause of neurological disorders in children. Their problem-oriented approach starts with the patient's presentation, not the diagnosis. More than 60 case vignettes of real children illustrate clinical scenarios.

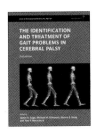

The Identification and Treatment of
Gait Problems in Cerebral Palsy (2nd edn)

Edited by James R. Gage, Michael H. Schwartz,
Steven E. Koop and Tom F. Novacheck

Clinics in Developmental Medicine 180–181

2009 • £125.00 • €143.80 • $199.00 • Hardback • 644 pp

ISBN 978–1–898683–65–0

The only book to deal specifically with the topic, this comprehensive, multi-disciplinary volume is essential for all those working in the field of cerebral palsy and gait. It is accompanied by two discs: the first presents a teaching video on normal gait and the second contains the videos and motion analysis data of the case examples in the book, as well as demonstrations of many of the surgical procedures referred to in the book.

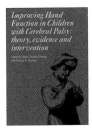

Improving Hand Function in
Children with Cerebral Palsy

Theory, evidence and intervention

Edited by Ann-Christin Eliasson and Patricia A. Burtner

Clinics in Developmental Medicine 178

2008 • £75.00 • €86.30 • $150.00 • Hardback • 442 pp

ISBN 978–1–898683–53–7

This book presents the fundamental theory behind the development of hand function in children with cerebral palsy. It then demonstrates how this theory can be translated into practice by those who provide assessment and intervention services to improve hand use in this population. Linking different fields of knowledge, this book highlights new perspectives and provides the best evidence for different types of intervention.

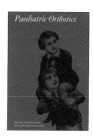

Paediatric Orthotics

Edited by Christopher Morris and Luciano Dias

Clinics in Developmental Medicine 175

2007 • £60.00 • €69.00 • $110.00 • Hardback • 248 pp

ISBN 978–1–898683–51–3

This is one of very few books on the subject of orthotics and the only book focusing solely on the orthotic management of children. It sets out the principles that are fundamental to orthotic management and then considers the appropriate orthotic management of the more common conditions in childhood in the context of multidisciplinary care. It thus provides both a basic grounding in the subject and practical guidance to help clinical practice.

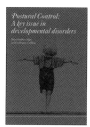

Postural Control

A Key Issue in Developmental Disorders

Edited by Mijna Hadders-Algra and Eva Brogren Carlberg

Clinics in Developmental Medicine 179

2007 • £45.00 • €51.80 • $79.99 • Paperback • 352 pp

ISBN 978–1–898683–57–5

Until now, knowledge about the nature of postural problems in children has been scattered, and this has hampered the development of appropriate therapeutic management strategies. This book is a breakthrough in that it introduces the reader to the complexity of typical and atypical postural development and provides suggestions for the day-to-day management of postural problems in children with developmental disorders such as cerebral palsy, developmental coordination disorder, muscle disorder and myelomeningocoele.